PRAISE FOR DR. RICHA
THE VITAMIN PRESCR

"Dosage charts indicating amounts, and an alphabetical list of ailments and recommended compounds make this a handy reference for those interested in a more natural approach to healing."

-Publishers Weekly

"An excellent introduction to some of the most exciting therapies for achieving optimal health. Dr. Firshein writes with the authority of experience."

-Julian Whitaker, M.D.,
author of Shed 10 Years in 10 Weeks

"The single most valuable medical sourcebook of the past three decades. It should be a fixture on bookshelves of everyone interested in achieving maximum health."

-Joseph T. Martorano, M.D.,
author of Unmasking P.M.S. and
Beyond Negative Thinking

"A good book for consumers seeking information on commonly prescribed nutrients."

-Library Journal

"Scientifically formulated and based on peer-reviewed clinical research, this book addresses the nutrients, herbs and vitamin supplements most often prescribed to combat disease, boost emotional and physical well-being, and improve overall health."

-Idea Health and Fitness Source

"Firshein has designed a life program, complete with the latest information on vitamins"

-Newsday

"The Vitamin Prescription For Life is a comprehensive, must have book on the subject of vitamins, nutraceuticals and natural therapies. This book is the best in it's class and it is essential for those that want to experience a healthier life, through natural therapies."

-Jordan S. Josephson, MD, FACS author of Sinus Relief Now

Books by Dr. Richard Firshein:

Reversing Asthma
7 steps to an asthma free child
The Nutraceutical Revolution*

The Vitamin Prescription
(for life)

The Vitamin Prescription (for life)

How Vitamins Can Be Your Natural Medicine

Dr. Richard N. Firshein

Library of Congress Control Number: 2008904963
ISBN: Hardcover 978-1-4363-4775-4
Softcover 978-1-4363-4774-7

This book was printed in the United States of America.

This book has been revised and updated and was originally published under the title "The Nutraceutical Revolution"
Cover photo by Roberto Ligresti
Back photo by Isabella Ginanneschi

To order additional copies of this book, contact:
Xlibris Corporation
1-888-795-4274
www.Xlibris.com
Orders@Xlibris.com
36672

In loving memory of
my mother and father

Acknowledgments

I have been fortunate to have so many talented people play such a crucial role in the writing and editing of this book. There are many people to thank.

My gratitude goes to Julie Grau, who understood my vision and believed in this book from the beginning.

Kris Dahl my agent at ICM, who has consistently exceeded my expectations.

Camille Chatterjee, my assistant during the writing of this book; and to Mary Angela Lauricella, for her extensive work in researching and proofreading. I would like to thank Jasmine Hedocil for all of her efforts in making sure that this book came to a successful completion.

Special appreciation goes to my office staff over the years. In particular I would like to thank Amy, Susan, Hazel, Vadim, Parikh, Therese, and Debra for their dedication and hard work. To Jill Neimark for the many hours spent during the preparation and writing of this book.

I would also like to thank the following people who have made, at one time or another an important contribution to this book or my life: Dr. Alan Lambert, Dr. Albert Knapp, Adam Zeliger, Dr. Ahron Friedberg, Aida Turturro, Ann Acheson, Ann Clairmont, Dr. Arthur Kennish, Beth Minardi, Bettina Witteveen, Carmine Minardi, Chris Blackwell, Csaba Lucas, Dr. Dan Firshein, Dana Goldstein, Daria Zeliger, David Beal, Donna Azarian, Duncan Kirk, Elie Tahari, Ellen Newhouse, Gail Firshein, Dr. Gary Ostrow, George Clairmont, Helene Levy, Dr. Holly Phillips, Vartan and Houri Geudelekian, Isabella Ginanneschi, Ira Levy, Dr. James Aisenberg, Dr. Jed Kaminetsky, Jim Gayneau, Joanne Sasso-Gayneau, Dr. Jonathan Charney,

John Azarian,, Dr. Jonathon Glashow, Dr. Jordan Josephson, Dr. Jordana Gilman, Joy Firshein, Dr. Karlene Chinquee, Larry Mullen Jr., Dr. Lewis Kohl, Lori Wasserman, Martin Elthrich, Mary Ching, Marilynn Hawkridge, Meg Friedman, Dr. Melissa Kohl, Michael Goldstein, Mistie Elthrich, Dr. Oz Garcia, Pankaj Shah, Paul Levy, Paul Sorvino, Dr. Phillip Bruder, Raoul Witteveen, Rhonda Levy, Richard Faherty, Dr. Ron Grelsamer, Dr. Ronald Hoffman, Rory Tahari, Rosella Galli, Sam Newhouse, Shari Dunaif, Sian Edwards Beal, Steve Dunaif, Dr. Steven Firshein, Susann Lucas, Sy Ethan , Dr. Stuart Young.

Special thanks to Dawn Perry for sharing her wonderful recipes in this book.

Finally, I want to thank my family and most importantly my wife Marcia for her love, and for making the world a more beautiful place to live in.

Contents

Index by Ailments and Corresponding Chapters

Arteriosclerosis *(Hardening of the Arteries). See also* Heart Disease
Magnesium CH 3
B vitamins CH 11
(Homocysteine)
Vitamin E CH 12

Arthritis
B vitamins CH 11
(Homocysteine)
Fish oil CH 4
Probiotics CH 6
SAMe CH 23
MSM CH 4
Glucosamine sulphate CH 4
Pycnogenol CH 23

Asthma
Ginkgo CH 13
Magnesium CH 3
Fish oil CH 4
NAC CH 14
Quercetin CH 17
Pycnogenol CH 23
Alkylglycerols CH 23

Atherosclerosis. *See also* Heart Disease
Resveratrol CH 23
Tocotrienols CH 12

Bladder Infection *(Urethritis). See also* Urinary Tract Infection
Cranberry CH 8
Probiotics CH 8

BPH
Saw palmetto CH 22
Nettles CH 22
Zinc CH 22
Pygeum africanum CH 22

Cancer
- Coenzyme Q_{10} CH 6
- Fish oil CH 4
- Isoflavones CH 5
- Vitamin E CH 12
- Tocotrienols CH 12
- Lutein CH 16
- Alkylglycerols CH 23
- Flaxseed CH 10
- B vitamins CH 11 (Homocysteine)
- Resveratrol CH 23
- Milk thistle CH 7

Candida
- Probiotics CH 8
- Flaxseed CH 10

Cardiomyopathy. *See* Heart Disease

Cataracts
- Lutein CH 16
- Vitamin E CH 12

Celiac Disease *(Gluten Enteropathy)*
- Glutamine CH 9
- Zinc CH 9

Cholesterol. *See also* Heart Disease
- Coenzyme Q_{10} CH 6
- Vitamin E CH 12
- Milk thistle CH 7

Chronic Fatigue. *See* Fatigue

Circulation
- Ginkgo CH 13
- Fish oil CH 4
- Vitamin E CH 12

Cirrhosis. *See* Liver Disease

Claudication
- Ginkgo CH 13
- Vitamin E CH 12
- Fish oil CH 4

Colitis
- Glutamine CH 9
- Zinc CH 9
- Probiotics CH 8
- Fish oil CH 3

Constipation
- Flaxseed CH 10
- Probiotics CH 8
- Magnesium CH 3

COPD *(Chronic Obstructive Pulmonary Diease)*
- NAC CH 14
- Vitamin E CH 12
- Magnesium CH 3

Crohn's Disease
- Glutamine CH 9
- Zinc CH 9
- Probiotics CH 8
- Fish oil CH 4

Depression
- Ginkgo CH 13
- St. John's wort CH 18
- SAMe CH 23

Diabetes
- B vitamins CH 11 (Homocysteine)
- Coenzyme Q_{10} CH 6
- Vitamin E CH 12

Magnesium CH 3
Lipoic acid CH 23
Pycnogenol CH 23
Milk thistle CH 7
Phosphatidyl serine CH 19

Diarrhea
Probiotics CH 8
FOS CH 8

Diverticulitis
Flaxseed CH 10

Dysbiosis
Probiotics CH 8
FOS CH 8

Emphysema
NAC CH 14
Magnesium CH 3
Selenium CH 12
Zinc CH 12

Exercise
BCAA CH 20
Whey protein CH 20

Fatigue
Tyrosine CH 15
Coenzyme Q_{10} CH 6
Ginseng
Ginkgo CH 13
Licorice CH 23

Flatulence
Probiotics CH 8

Food Allergies
Probiotics CH 8
Quercetin CH 17

Hypotension
- Tyrosine CH 15
- Ginseng CH 15
- Licorice CH 15

Hypothyroidism
- Tyrosine CH 15

Immune Disorders
- Glutamine CH 9
- Maitake mushroom CH 23
- Alkylglycerols CH 23
- Licorice CH 23

Impotence
- Ginkgo CH 13
- Arginine CH 23

Insomnia
- BCAA CH 20
- Valerian CH 18
- Passion flower CH 18

Irritable Bowel Syndrome
- Glutamine CH 9
- Flaxseed powder CH 10
- Probiotics CH 8

Liver Toxicity
- Milk thistle CH 7
- NAC CH 14
- Calcium-D-glucarate CH 23

Macular Degeneration
- Lutein CH 16
- Zeaxanthin CH 16
- Vitamin E CH 12

Memory
- Ginkgo CH 13
- Phosphatidyl serine CH 19

Obesity
- Chromium CH 23
- Green tea Extract 23

Menopause
- Black cohosh CH 21
- Dong quai CH 21
- Licorice CH 2

Menstrual Cramps
- Black cohosh CH 21
- Magnesium CH 3

Osteoporosis
- Magnesium CH 3
- Calcium CH 3
- Boron CH 3
- Isoflavones CH 5

Peptic Ulcers. *See* Heartburn

Periodontal Disease
- Co Q_{10} CH 6
- Aloe Vera CH 6

Peripheral Neuropathy
- Acetyl-L-carnitine CH 19
- Phosphatidyl serine CH 19
- Lipoic acid CH 23

Pregnancy
- Folic acid CH 11
- Calcium CH 3
- Magnesium CH 3

PMS
- Black cohosh CH 21
- Fish oil CH 6
- Dong quai CH 2

Author's Note

Patients with particular medical conditions should consult their physicians before beginning any nutritional program. This book is not intended to be a substitute for medical care or advice. Since nutraceuticals are used for specific medical conditions, they should be used under the guidance of a qualified medical practitioner. Anyone with a known medical condition, on medication, or with specific health concerns should consult their physician before beginning any treatment in this book.

Dosages are meant to be used as guidelines only and may vary according to the specific needs of each individual. Supplements should be incorporated into a comprehensive health program. Individuals seeking a healthier lifestyle should incorporate foods which contain the appropriate nutraceuticals or vitamins whenever possible. Good sources are highlighted within each chapter and at the end of this book.

1

Everyday Miracles

Today you can change your life, stay healthy and reverse aging with a specific roster of essential vitamins, minerals and nutraceuticals. "The Vitamin Prescription for Life" teaches you how a specific list of super-nutrients can do the work of natural medicines. The real miracle-nature's power to heal-has always been available to us. But now science has given us the tools to understand the mystery of healing foods and nutrients. We can study and isolate the chemical composition of plants, fruits and vegetables, fish, flowers, berries, and herbs. We can explain just why they powerfully impact our cells and our lives. These days, we know what a nutrient is doing to our blood, our cell membranes, even our DNA, and how it protects us from cancer or heart disease or thinning bones. And we can often measure the effects in our body within hours of ingestion. We can watch the miracle in action through the powerful lens of modern science.

And then we can change our lives. Today, front-page news about medical triumphs not only covers heart transplants or even the marvelous and sophisticated science that maps the human gene. It's about the power of nutrition. This kind of power:

- Tomatoes may cut the risk of deadly prostate cancer by nearly half.

- A modest dose of a single B vitamin, folic acid, can prevent tragic and common birth defects.

- Within weeks of eating fish or supplementing your diet with fish oils, your body's estrogen levels shift dramatically in favor of the most protective anticancer form of estrogen.

- Daily portions of broccoli can cause similar strong shifts in estrogen balance and prevent cancer.

- Taking fish oil capsules for a mere twelve weeks significantly slows the growth of colon tumors.

- Olive oil lowers the risk of breast cancer and heart disease.

- Green tea can reduce the risk of heart attacks.

Nudged between today's headlines is one of the great stories of our time: that nutrition can literally save lives. I don't claim to offer a cure-all for every person, nor can I magically pull anybody I treat back from the brink of death. What I do promise is that in many cases of ill health, from mild malaise to life-threatening disorders, nutritional medicine can make an astounding and life-altering impact. Moreover, we can do more than correct illness. We can prevent it when we understand how nutrients can help maintain our vitality and good health. You will find this book full of stories of healing that may surprise and inspire you.

The Common Thread

I've been practicing medicine for over twenty years, and although the field is deepening and refining itself every week, I've found that I often rely on a versatile, hardy, and relatively small army of researched nutrients to do much of the healing work. Some of these are "supernutrients" that seem to work to prevent disease across many categories. Soy, for instance, can help boost and balance hormones and can help prevent cancer. Fish oils seem to work wonders in chronic inflammatory diseases, from asthma to colitis, yet they are also useful for thinning the blood and thereby protecting the heart. Ginkgo, an ancient and powerful herb, also thins the blood, fights allergies, and improves circulation throughout the body, so that it is useful in everything from heart disease to Alzheimer's disease.

Many of these nutrients work synergistically. I have assembled nutritional programs that heal chronic illness, fight fatigue, boost the immune system, and help balance hormones. My programs combine both common and relatively unknown nutraceuticals: amino acids like glutamine and newer compounds like lutein and modified citrus pectin. You may be stumbling over these words now, but by the book's end, I hope they will be familiar friends to you.

What I try to offer you in this book is a healthy way of eating and living, along with the most powerful nutrients known to medicine. I call them super supplements, and I've studied both how they work and why they work.

These nutrients are part of an overall program that I offer my patients, including healthy lifestyle changes, exercise, and stress-reducing activities like meditation and yoga. I don't believe that nutrients are magic bullets all by themselves. They rarely heal illness if you go on eating an unhealthy diet laden with saturated fats, processed foods, and sugar. I do believe that if you eat well, live well, and *then* add one or more of the necessary "super" supplements, 80 percent of chronic illnesses can be reversed or prevented entirely.

Humanity's healthiest diets have evolved over tens of thousands of years, in far-flung and radically different climates, from the heart-protecting diet of the Eskimos, which is largely made up of fish, to the cancer-fighting rice-and-vegetable-based cuisines of the Chinese. Yet today all these far-flung foods are available to us, right here at home. Using everything from North Alaskan salmon to umeboshi plums, wild game to passion fruit, bok choy to spelt, we can create a biologically optimum diet that incorporates the latest findings on nutrition and healing. We now know what broccoli does inside the cells to help prevent cancer, how fish oil gets absorbed into the cell membrane and prevents inflammation, and just what chemical magic soybeans trigger to help prevent cancer.

Call it ancient wisdom transformed by science.

Nutrition in Action

John, a thirty-seven-year-old executive, was rushed to the hospital after collapsing. When he regained consciousness, his doctors told him he suffered from a severe case of adult-onset diabetes. His blood sugar reading was 830, nearly 700 points above normal. For the rest of his life, he was told, he would have to inject himself twice a day with insulin, or he would die.

John walked into my office emotionally shattered. He was clean-shaven and fit, with brown hair and blue eyes. He admitted that for months he'd been feeling thirsty and parched and had urinated frequently and that foods had begun tasting odd to him. But he'd had no idea he was suffering from adult-onset diabetes.

"Now I'm injecting myself with insulin twice a day just like they told me to. But I don't feel well. I'm fatigued. I still crave sweets like crazy. And I'm scared. I don't want to stay on a drug the rest of my life."

The tip-off, however, was when he told me he craved sweets. It turned out that John's diet consisted of meat, daily pasta, and lots of sugary sodas and fruits. It was a diet extremely high in simple sugars. I put him on exactly the opposite diet:

one that emphasized fish, vegetables, and beans and cut out all refined starches and most fruits.

But I didn't stop there. I knew John's body was depleted in certain nutrients and needed extra help. I also put him on special supplements, some of which included the following:

- Chromium picolinate, which stabilizes blood sugar and lowers insulin resistance
- Magnesium, which is often deficient in diabetics, perhaps because insulin surges deplete it
- Fish oils, which allow the body to utilize insulin more effectively
- *Garcinia cambogia*, another herb that helps the body metabolize fats and sugars more effectively

After only six weeks of nutritional healing, John was weaned off all his insulin, and his blood sugar was normal. Elated, he returned to his doctor for a checkup. His stunned physician didn't know what to say. John's diabetes stayed in remission for over two years.

Another patient, Alicia, an outgoing forty-eight-year-old kindergarten teacher with curly brown hair and a big smile, was told that she had breast cancer and must undergo surgery and radiation immediately. She was also told she might be left with disfiguring scars. She agreed to the treatment but came to see me as well, hoping to boost her immune system and heal as rapidly as possible. I have a very specific anticancer protocol that systematically starves the tumor while feeding the individual. We flooded her system with anticancer and immune-boosting nutrients and foods, as well as my anticancer diet, and added topical treatments such as aloe vera to minimize any scars from surgery and radiation. The nutrients I prescribed included the following:

- Large doses of antioxidants, especially vitamin C
- Omega-3 essential fatty acids, which are protective against cancer
- Topical aloe vera to be applied to her surgical wound

A few months later, Alicia's surgeon called to tell me she had recovered better than any patient he'd treated. He told me, "When Alicia went for a follow-up mammogram, they could not find the surgical scar. It had completely healed. What did you give her?"

The speed and power of nutritional healing are sometimes astonishing. Blood test results can change in a matter of weeks with the proper diet and supplements. In fact, many nutrients cause changes in the blood within hours—changes that can be measured. In other cases, the healing is slow but can reverse stubborn and persistent problems. For eighteen months, I worked with a man deformed by psoriasis. He was covered with red and scaly patches from head to toe. He reminded me of a raw, peeling fish. The cortisone his doctors had prescribed in ever-increasing doses no longer helped.

I tested him for food allergies and eliminated all possible allergenic foods from his diet. In addition, I prescribed these nutrients:

- Essential fatty acids, including those found in fish oil and primrose oil, which help stop inflammation

- Milk thistle and dandelion, herbs that help the liver detoxify harmful substances (Whenever a person suffers from skin problems like psoriasis, it's a reasonable bet that their liver is having trouble detoxifying.)

After eighteen months, not a single scaly patch was left. "I thought I would have to live the rest of my life with this disfiguring illness," he told me. "I thought I'd never go on a date or go to the gym. I'm in a state of shock."

Nutrients as Edible Vaccines

Vaccines can protect you from lethal illness. So can foods. Can we refer to our foods, then, as edible vaccines? As potent and protective agents that help prevent disease?

I like to think so. Consider this:

- Certain vitamins (such as vitamins C and A) can reduce the recurrence of bladder cancer by 50 percent.

- Flaxseed can slow tumor growth.

- Milk thistle can reverse liver enzyme elevation.

- Green tea, an ancient staple of Chinese society, has a powerfully protective effect against lung cancer, and in one study from the *Journal of the National Cancer Institute*, green tea drinkers had a 60 percent lower risk of cancer.

- Foods high in magnesium and potassium can lower high blood pressure in weeks.

- The nutrient coenzyme Q_{10} has heart-healing properties—in clinical studies, it has sometimes eliminated the need for blood pressure medication, and in one small study helped prevent breast cancer.

A little over half a century ago, vitamin C was first discovered. In 1958, free radicals were discovered. In the past two decades alone, an incredible amount of research on nutrients has spilled out of laboratories and universities. When we think of disease-fighting nutrients today, we don't just worry about vitamins A or E or C. We study the hormones and chemicals in plants and herbs. We study substances with long scientific-sounding names, like sulforaphanes (in broccoli). These compounds have now been found to be essential elements for our health. For instance, we know that a cell has to jump through many biochemical hoops before it becomes malignant. But at almost every hoop on the way to cancer, there are compounds in vegetables and fruits that can slow or even stop the process. Within hours after eating broccoli, sulforaphane is coursing through the bloodstream, activating enzymes that literally whisk carcinogens out of the cell so that the body can discard them. And within weeks of eating large amounts of broccoli, a compound called indole-3-carbinol dramatically lowers the form of estrogen that promotes cancer. These are dramatic and rapid shifts, and it turns out that most natural foods—from cumin to cauliflower, garlic to strawberries—provide potent health factors.

Where's the Catch?

No matter what your health history, you can start to change it within days just by changing your diet and adding the right supplements, because at the cellular level, your body responds almost immediately.

What's the catch? There is no catch—if you don't mind getting a Ph.D. in nutrition and studying all day every day.

I say that because there is now so much information available it can be dizzying. I did an Internet search recently on "phytochemicals and health" and found over eighty thousand references. As I began to leaf through the first few hundred of those studies I had printed out from my search, the results were tremendously exciting to read about.

Mass media regularly report nutritional discoveries fresh from the trenches of science, making all of us lay scientists. For instance, a drug company in Spain—Pharma Mar—was working with the National Cancer Institute to scour the earth's oceans in search of new medicines, medicines they might find in a frog's venom or an algae's protein. From a library of more than twenty thousand samples of marine organisms, nearly 350 compounds have already been isolated, and some have shown strong anticancer potential. William Shurtleff of the Soyfoods Center, a bookstore in Lafayette, California, even maintains a nutritional database on soy. It contains 45,000 articles. Add that to the fact that at the turn of the century, there were only two tofu suppliers in the entire country, and now we have two hundred suppliers producing 65 million pounds a year, and you begin to understand that this is not a revolution that can be overlooked.

This book is your guide into a new world, one rich with possibilities, where nutrition becomes high-tech medicine—where you can offer your body precisely what it needs at a cellular level to protect and heal itself. In this book, I offer you the twenty top nutrients that I use in my practice, and fifteen *new* nutraceuticals that are still so new they aren't widely known, but hold great promise. These are nutrients that I think of as magic molecules, smart nutrients with their own kind of intelligence. I feel myself to be a kind of fascinated outsider, peering into the intelligence of another world.

If you come along on the journey of this book, you will discover just how smart these magic molecules are. In the era of the gene, when we have mapped the genetic code, and when we regularly read reports about genes for cancer or other hereditary illnesses such as Alzheimer's, we are sometimes too impressed with science's technical prowess. Discovering a gene does not mean we understand how the symphony of genes works or just how potent a single gene might be. Sometimes we give away too much personal power. We believe that genes and tests and drugs have all the answers—when, instead, we should be asking questions. Not long ago, the *New York Times* headline stated: "A Single Gene Linked to 95% of All Breast Cancers." This is not true, as we have since discovered. That gene does not necessarily lead to breast cancer. It seems to be one flute playing in a whole orchestra—and we don't yet know how big a part that flute has. Genes rarely act alone. They usually act as a symphony, playing off each other. And they can be activated or calmed down—and that process depends in large part on environment, particularly diet.

Consider another important study by Erich V. Kliewer of the Australian National University and Ken R. Smith of the University of Utah. They studied women who had emigrated to Australia or Canada as adults. Nearly sixty groups of immigrants from all parts of the world were studied, and the breast cancer rate of their homelands was compared to that of their new environment. It inevitably adjusted itself to the new environment. Within a mere thirty years, the rate of breast cancer in these émigrés was indistinguishable from that of local residents. Noel Weiss, professor of epidemiology at the University of Washington School of Public Health in Seattle, remarked, "The importance of this study is that it reinforces our notion that your risk of breast cancer isn't something you're born with." We don't have to passively accept the "dictatorship" of the genes.

At the renowned Strang Medical Clinic, the impact of diet on the genes that regulate estrogen in our body was studied. One type of estrogen is associated with a low risk of cancer. Another type is associated with a high risk. Researchers found that merely by adding omega-3 fatty acids, from fish and fish oil, to the diet, the gene's activity changed within a mere matter of weeks. That means we can regulate our genes simply by altering the foods and supplements we take.

If that's not enough evidence, consider the widely reported research on birth defects and folic acid. A study in the *Lancet* reported that some mothers pass on a gene to their babies that causes birth defects like spina bifida. But this only happens if those mothers do not consume enough folic acid, a common B vitamin. That's because the "bad" gene cannot function properly unless it has extra folic acid. When it gets what it needs, it's fine. That same gene may be involved in heart disease as well, since it increases the risk of coronary illness by two to three times.

So come explore the same super-nutrients that I use every day to help my patients achieve optimal health. They can be your bridge to a better life where food and nutrition offer not just pleasure but optimal health. "The Vitamin Prescription for Life" gives you a detailed tour through the nutrients that address and often help heal the most common modern conditions, from allergies and asthma to eye problems, heart disease, cancer, reproductive difficulties, arthritis, poor digestion, fatigue, depression, anxiety, and more. In this book I will explain how and why these nutrients work, and I will offer the stories of many of my patients whose lives have changed through nutritional and integrative medicine.

2

My Own Odyssey

In this chapter, I will tell you a bit about my own personal experience with healing nutrients, as well as suggest a basic way of eating that is an absolutely necessary foundation for health. As I've said before, nutritional supplements are amazingly potent, but they are not a substitute for a good diet.

I have been asthmatic since I was a child. In my late twenties, however, I nearly died after an asthma attack spiraled out of control. I had been unable to sleep, after an interminable night of wheezing, and toward morning I took a few puffs from my bronchial inhaler. It was supposed to open up my lungs, but instead my throat began to close. I felt as if I'd been locked in an airless trunk. Every cell in my body seemed to be sounding an alarm. I kept trying to breathe, but even the deepest, most ragged breath left me dizzy and breathless.

My condition began spiraling dangerously out of control. My friends both physicians, rushed me to the Emergency room , where I was quickly triaged to the Intensive Care Unit, While I lay in the ICU unable to breathe or speak, starring at a machine that could forcibly pump air into my lung I was transformed. By evening I was simply unresponsive but I could hear the doctors discuss how difficult my situation was and even question whether or not I would "make it". That night, for a time , I was literally outside of myself, and seeing myself gasp for air became determined to do whatever was necessary to turn my health around. I struggled , with every breathe to survive that sleepless night and as morning came I was more determined than ever to begin this revolution. I began examining every detail of my life, a process that would change the way I lived and practiced medicine forever.

That attack was my wakeup call. For years my health had been deteriorating, but I didn't want to admit it. In 1981, I'd fallen ill with mononucleosis, which is caused by a virus. In 1982, I began to suffer from chronic fatigue syndrome, as well as muscle pain (fibromyalgia) in my legs. At one point, I was so ill I had to take all my courses and exams at home.

Yet by 1986, I'd become a practicing doctor, teaching and seeing patients in the clinic of the medical school where I'd graduated. I was living every day with battle fatigue, but I'd gotten used to it. After my hospitalization, I sought out expertise from a center specializing in the treatment of the most serious cases of asthma and have pioneered allergy tests for a wide range of foods, airborne toxins, food dyes, and additives.

Doctors at the center gave me capsules containing food extracts without telling me what was in each capsule. During one food challenge, my sinuses became congested, and I correctly guessed that the capsule contained tomato extract. It was easy to guess, since this particular congestion occurred whenever I ate tomatoes.

Foods can have profound effects on health. In my case, severe allergies made eating a difficult and even life-threatening experience. My body had been telling me the truth for years, but until that moment, I did not listen. Often it's hard for us to listen, even when the evidence is brutally obvious. In my case, each sensitivity expressed itself differently. Wheat might trigger an asthma attack; sesame might make my lips sting and swell.

Why did different foods affect me in such different ways? Because they contain distinctly different proteins. Over the next few years, I eliminated every single food to which I was sensitive. I stopped eating processed and junk foods. I purified my diet by sweeping it clean of unhealthy, fatty, and refined foods. I relied heavily on fish, fresh vegetables and fruit, whole grains, and free-range chicken. And I studied nutritional medicine closely so that I could flood my own body with healing nutrients in the form of supplements. I knew that after so many years of poor eating and ill health, my body needed as much help as possible.

I remember taking a trip down to Chinatown, in New York City, where I live. It was as if I'd been transported to another country: there in a small shop was a wizened old man behind a counter, measuring out what looked like barks and dried plants of mysterious origin. I told him my problem and was given several herbs, including ginkgo leaf and ginseng root, and ordered to cook them in soup for eight hours!

I started to shop for food in an entirely new way. I slowed down and started to notice the colors of fruits and vegetables, from purple potatoes to the gleam of fresh raspberries to the lemony yellow of summer squash. I learned that the vibrancy of color reflects a food's content of bioflavonoids and important antioxidants that help prevent disease. I began to understand the importance of freshness, ripeness, and flavor—all markers of important nutrients needed to maximize our health. I learned to hold and feel produce, to weigh it in my hands when I was testing for ripeness. I'd grown up eating iceberg lettuce: now I was discovering a whole new world of greens, from arugula to watercress, romaine, bibb, and Boston lettuce, dandelion greens, raw parsley, and spinach. And I was learning to combine them all into delicious creative salads, with fresh dressings made of lemon juice, honey, mustard, and spices.

I experimented with vegetables native to Asia, including bok choy, lotus root, bamboo shoots, and Chinese squash. I felt, in a way, like I'd traveled back centuries and come across some beautiful plant or root and foraged and picked it out myself, choosing the freshest and most unblemished specimen I could find. Suddenly I wasn't looking just at food but at a medicine chest filled with powerful nutrients that could detoxify my liver and recharge my own immune system. I was becoming connected to my health by understanding what I was putting into my body. I thought about the Chinese herbalist and the centuries of experience his culture had provided, the knowledge of foods that can enhance health and treat disease. I began to investigate herbal knowledge in other cultures.

I eventually bought a small rosemary tree and set up window boxes with herbs. Fresh herbs serve as a reminder to me that I am connected daily with nature and healing.

I began to look at my meals as medical miracles, as healing treasures. For the most part, I didn't miss chocolate, cakes, and hamburgers, though occasionally I craved them. And occasionally I ate them too. Nobody's perfect! But this began to change over time. The better I ate, the better I felt, and soon my desire for these foods diminished.

It worked. Now, years later, from the safe perch of recovered health and a nutritional practice that is both gratifying and inspiring, I can look back and see that period of my life as a healing crisis. I was burned and almost destroyed in the crucible of that crisis, but it was in the end a gift. I would not be the kind of doctor I am today if I had not almost died trying to be a different kind of doctor. I would not be out in the trenches, working with my patients to help them change their lives through nutrition. And, I'm glad to say, I'm only one of a growing number of physicians around the country who are as excited as I am about the healing potential of nutritional medicine.

The compounds in foods can harm or heal us. As Paul Lachance, professor of nutrition and food science at Rutgers University, says, the healing nutrients in foods, or nutraceuticals, "represent an alternative to high-tech rescue medicine. By using natural therapies, we could save several billion health care dollars and prevent 70 percent of our current diseases." Just by eating the right foods! We've come a long way.

The Key to Pleasure: Healthy Substitution

Why is it so hard for some of us to give up foods like ice cream, juicy steaks, and french fried potatoes, especially if we know that eating those foods regularly is actually making us ill and shortening our lives?

When I ask my patients why they continue to eat these foods, they say, "Because they taste good, and they make me feel good." For many of us, life's stresses and chronic illnesses are so difficult to handle that the quick, easy reward of food is the first thing we reach for. Food that is sweet or creamy or crispy or fatty. Rich, fried instantly gratifying food. Food that has good "mouth feel," as cooks are wont to say. Another reason is the unavailability of good food. Unfortunately, junk food is much more readily available than good foods, particularly in the winter months. But science has been at work rectifying this situation, so that many of the important nutrients found in food are also available in supplement form.

Most of the time, however, when I ask people to think about how they really feel within an hour or two of eating junk foods, they reply, "Well, actually, I felt tired. I had a headache. I had indigestion and gas."

The truth is that healthy foods can taste delicious too. And in the long run, health itself is the ultimate "feel good" reward. So the only answer is to replace our feel-good treats with healthy food.

My Healing Diet

Here's how I did it.

First, I changed what I drank. I used to drink processed iced tea with sugar. Now I put a whole pint of organic strawberries into a pitcher of green tea while it's still hot and then pour it over ice. Green tea and strawberries are loaded with plant chemicals that fight chronic illness. Ellagic acid in strawberries may help prevent cancer, and proanthocyanidins in green tea help prevent colon cancer and improve digestion. I recommend this tea to anyone who suffers from intestinal problems or is at risk of colon cancer.

In winter, I make a soup base out of pure vegetable stock made from onions (cancer fighter), parsley (blood purifier), carrots (loaded with carotene), and root vegetables like turnips and potatoes. I add cayenn (helps asthma and circulation) and ginger (good for digestion) and an assortment of vegetables, puree that stock, and freeze it. When I want my own homemade soup, it's ready to go. And it's truly healing. The same can be done with healthy juicing.

No more orange juice in a carton or apple juice from a jar. Instead, I make my own fresh juices. I've found that a combination of ginger and carrot juice in the morning is really energizing. And it's actually a lot more delicious!

From time to time, I test my own boundaries. For example, recently I was ordering organic pizza from a nearby gourmet shop for lunch every day. The pizza had a thin crispy whole-wheat crust and organic vegetables like yellow and red peppers, zucchini, onions, mushrooms, and tomatoes. Perfectly healthy, right? And delicious. Except after a few weeks, I noticed I was feeling fatigued after lunch. It turns out that although these days I can tolerate wheat, I can't eat it every day. I will start to develop my food sensitivities again.

So I stopped ordering my healthy pizza for a while and returned to the lunch that makes me feel the best: fish and whole grains, along with a fresh salad.

Why Food Is Not Enough

Even so, I learned that as powerfully healing as food can be, most of us need more than food in order to return to optimal health. The damage caused to tissue by illness and inflammation is tremendous, especially if the illness is chronic, and it needs to be corrected by flooding the body with nutrients targeted to that specific illness. Even for healthy people, supplements can be invaluable, because almost all of us have inherited genetic weaknesses that cause us to be more vulnerable to specific illnesses. We can correct many of those weaknesses by giving our body extra nutrients when needed.

My healing program focuses on supplements that I call nutraceuticals, nutrients that are pharmacologically active, almost like medicines. Yet they have very few harmful side effects.

To heal myself, I took high doses of vitamin C, vitamin E, zinc, antioxidants, and magnesium every day. I took fish oil capsules, which are known to fight asthma by reducing inflammation. They made a tremendous difference. Years later, I find that if I slack off in taking my daily nutrients, I begin to lose energy and become more susceptible to asthma.

But here's a good example of how powerful nutrients are. I recently stained the doors in my office, and the toxic odor of the chemicals in the stain filled every room. That led to an asthma attack. The first night of the attack, I had trouble sleeping, and I was weak. "Oh no," I thought. "It's come back, after all this time. Am I going to get sick again? I can't afford to!" The next day, I took extra healing nutrients, especially magnesium and vitamin C, ate only fresh fish and vegetables, and drank lots of green tea. It was a detoxifying and healing diet. My asthma symptoms completely vanished in a few days. Now I understand the anti-inflammatory benefits of magnesium and the antioxidant benefits of vitamin C.

That is the enormous and marvelous difference between my life then and now. Where once I was forced to take drugs and was chronically ill, now an occasional setback lasts only a day or two and can be healed with an extra boost from diet and nutrients.

"This is a very exciting time to be in nutrition and disease research," says Dr. Barbara Levine, coordinator of clinical nutrition research at the Memorial Sloan-Kettering Cancer Center. "While we used to look at nutritional deficiencies, now we are looking at the vitamins, minerals and phytochemicals in foods that may prevent and treat disease."

And the rest of America is just as excited. One out of four Americans take a vitamin supplement daily. Herbal products soared to $1.6 billion in sales.

Yet how can you decide which supernutrients you should take? Do some nutrients enhance others? What's safe? How much is safe? Since most herbs are not standardized, and each batch or bottle actually contains different amounts of potent chemicals, what should you do? Even if nutrients heal, how can you find your way through the incredible avalanche of information out there? Where can you turn to ask these questions? If you can't eat all the right foods, which nutrients can help you? And if you're eating well, which nutrients can enhance your health or longevity even further?

That's why you've come to this book—your personal user's manual to nutritional healing—to find out.

Stop Right Here

A lot of the answers to these questions are in this book. Though there may be literally thousands of studies out there on all the different chemicals found in nature that may heal us, there are certain basic building blocks that are essential and can help treat most common conditions. In fact, the more I study and use these nutrients, the more they amaze me, often because one nutrient seems to heal such a wide range of seemingly unrelated conditions. Consider magnesium, the first in my star parade: it can help prevent heart attacks, lessen the frequency and severity of asthma attacks, ease menstrual migraines, lessen postoperative pain, and dramatically lessen the complications of diabetes. How can one nutrient have so many functions?

The answer, it seems, is that these all-important basic nutrients work at the cellular level. They heal cells, and they help cells function normally. They get to the root cause of disease. A supplement such as fish oil that renders the cell membrane more stable will improve health throughout the body, whether it's brain function or liver function. A mineral such as magnesium that renders the cell membrane more fluid and flexible will allow it to receive needed nutrients more easily. You can see, then, how nutraceuticals are the essence of health and why the ones I describe in this book are truly a parade of stars. The Vitamin Prescription For Life will help you design a nutritional program based on the principles that I use in my practice, starting with building blocks such as fish oil and magnesium that will help you live a healthier more productive life.

3

Magnesium: Nature's Great Relaxer and Bone's Best Friend

It might be hard to believe, but a substance that could help prevent America's number one killer, heart disease, is right on the shelf of your local health food store. This natural mineral is found everywhere in life, from fish to barley to spinach. Magnesium. You've probably heard of it before but never really considered its importance. I believe magnesium is the most significant healing mineral we have.

Magnesium is one of the most essential nutrients in maintaining optimal health. It's a mineral that bathes the cell and seems to stabilize it, calming your body at a metabolic level, a microscopic level. If there is a tendency—whether in the cells of your heart or lungs, your muscles, or your blood vessels—to overreact, magnesium soothes and relaxes the body.

Research on magnesium's benefits dates back to the early 1930s, and recently we've seen a renaissance in our study of this mineral. It turns out that at the beginning of the century, most Americans got about 1,200 milligrams of magnesium a day in their diet, while today the minimum RDA is about 400 milligrams. And not all of us get even that. We don't eat enough whole grains, fruits, and vegetables to fulfill our needs for this crucial mineral. A recent Gallup survey revealed that 72 percent of adult Americans are falling short of the recommended dietary allowance for magnesium. It also found that an astounding 55 percent of adults consume 75 percent or less of the recommended daily allowance, while 30 percent are eating less than half the required amount.

Modern chemical farming and food processing are partly to blame for our magnesium deficiency. Worse yet, we lose almost 40 percent of the magnesium content in our food when it is cooked. And our bodies need magnesium more than ever, since our polluted air and water can interfere with its function in the body.

The elderly are even more at risk than the young. The Gallup survey showed that magnesium consumption decreases with age. Seventy-nine percent of adults fifty-five and over eat well below the RDA for magnesium, and 66 percent receive less than three-quarters of their allowance from food.

A dietary deficiency of magnesium can be a major factor in the development of life-threatening illnesses like heart disease and diabetes, as well as in chronic fatigue syndrome, asthma, muscle cramps, and migraine headaches, and is even implicated in osteoporosis. Study after study clearly shows that magnesium is the missing link between these ailments and good health. In fact, I take it every day myself to prevent asthma attacks.

How can such a common mineral be so significant—and overlooked?

The Secret of Magnesium

Magnesium might be called life's lubricant. It's like an hour of intercellular meditation that relaxes and expands blood vessels, stops muscles from cramping, prevents inflammation, and allows energy to be used more efficiently. How does it do this? One simple way is this: magnesium blocks the influx of calcium into the cells.

Magnesium and calcium compete and cooperate, one flowing into the cell while the other flows out, and it is the balance of both that is supremely important. They allow the cell to excrete what it does not need or want and to absorb necessary nutrients. Calcium both elevates your blood pressure when necessary (say, during exercise) and contracts your muscles. However, while calcium is essential for contraction, excess availability of calcium can lead to serious problems—a state of sustained contraction that can show up in many different illnesses. Even in rigor mortis, a stiffening of the body that occurs after we die, calcium remains in the cell, while magnesium drains out.

When magnesium levels are low, the body releases stress hormones and substances that constrict blood vessels and cause the blood to clot more easily. In turn, stress of any kind, whether physical or emotional, increases the need for magnesium. Take the stress of marathon running: magnesium supplements improve endurance and reduce cramps and fatigue in athletes. And in these runners, magnesium is commonly depleted. In fact, one study of five marathon runners found that the four runners who did not receive any magnesium supplements experienced a steady fall in blood levels of magnesium during the race (monitored by blood samples drawn at six different times).

Stop Heart Attacks and Strokes

Despite the incredible advances modern medicine has made in the last twenty years, heart attacks are still the nation's single leading cause of death. Even though we understand the importance of a diet low in saturated fats, and the preventive impact of exercise, most of us know little about magnesium, the one mineral that can do the most to help us.

Many researchers now believe that magnesium deficiency can be linked to hardening of the arteries and hypertension. They've discovered that many heart attack victims have low magnesium levels in their blood and heart muscles. Researchers even consider magnesium deficiency a contributing factor in atherosclerosis, the accumulation of fats within the arterial walls.

Research into magnesium and heart disease is so encouraging that I don't know why every cardiologist doesn't prescribe this mineral as a matter of course. This mineral can treat mild to moderate hypertension as well as some drugs. For instance, a recent study in the *British Medical Journal* of one hundred middle-aged and elderly men and women found that magnesium supplements lowered blood pressure by almost eight points. Another study of thirty thousand male health professionals found that the combination of dietary fiber, potassium, and magnesium lowered the risk of high blood pressure. A study of German men found that magnesium was beneficial in treating heart attacks, helping to minimize damage. And a study of early deaths resulting from strokes found that magnesium supplementation was a significant protector.

I've seen this repeatedly in my own practice. George Lloyd, a thirty-one-year-old interior designer with a bright future (and a hot temper), was literally saved by magnesium. His job was extremely deadline driven and required fantastic precision as well as an ability to understand global trends. The first time he walked into my office, he told me that he'd already been in the hospital twice for an inflammation of the pancreas and for diabetic complications, and now he had elevated blood pressure as well. He was on medication for his diabetes and blood pressure. I knew I had my work cut out for me—and for him.

Blood tests showed elevated liver enzymes and elevated triglycerides. His blood sugar was also elevated, despite his medication.

There was no question that these were a lot of problems for someone so young, and he showed no signs of lessening the intense pace of his career. "I've worked ten years to get to this place!" he practically shouted. "I've given up a social life, friendships, and a chance at an early family. I'm not about to give up now!"

I agreed with him: he should not give up the life he wanted, but I would have to introduce a lifestyle that would make that possible. The first thing we changed was his diet, taking him off junk food and sodas and putting him on healthy fiber-rich foods such as brown rice, barley, healthy vegetables, and lots of fresh fish. I also started him on daily green leafy vegetables, which are high in magnesium, as well as an exercise program.

Magnesium is a hidden star in the treatment of diabetes *and* the care of hypertension. His elevated triglycerides were a marker for insulin resistance, a condition that affects up to 20 percent of the population and is an independent risk factor for heart disease. It is often found in families with a history of diabetes. I knew that magnesium helped the body handle insulin more efficiently and reduced its damaging effects on blood vessels. Magnesium, then, was an answer to both his hypertension and his diabetes.

Indeed, within weeks, magnesium lowered his blood pressure. I then started him on a biofeedback relaxation program, along with specific aerobic exercises and yoga to build muscle tone and resistance. It's taken time, over a year now, but his blood pressure, which was once unrestrained, is now under control. He says that his last year has been his most successful to date.

How Does It Work?

How does magnesium heal the heart and blood vessels? Like a symphony conductor, magnesium orchestrates the complex process that keeps the heart beating with regularity and precision. In its function as a cellular lubricator, magnesium is critical to the continued health of our hearts. A severe lack of magnesium can cause muscle spasms, and without enough magnesium present in the blood to play the role of the body's great relaxer, a coronary artery supplying the heart muscle with oxygen can suddenly clamp shut without warning.

Amazingly enough, 25 percent of all heart attacks occur in people with clean coronary arteries that are otherwise free of the junk-food-created garbage usually associated with heart disease. So what's killing these healthy people? Numerous studies suggest that people who die suddenly from ischemic heart disease, an oxygen-starved heart, often have tissues severely depleted of magnesium.

In a recent study at Johns Hopkins, eighteen subjects admitted for cardiac surgery were discovered to have extremely low levels of intracellular magnesium, and intravenous magnesium corrected these levels.

I recently treated a thirty-six-year-old woman who suffered from mitralvalve prolapse, a common heart ailment in which a valve in the heart does not close firmly, causing blood to leak backward. Although this is usually not dangerous, it can sometimes cause complex and debilitating symptoms, including chest pain, fatigue, rapid heartbeat, and frequent heart palpitations. Doctors sometimes prescribe drugs known as beta-blockers to steady the rhythm of the heart. Yet this condition is often remarkably responsive to magnesium, which studies show can eliminate symptoms in 50 percent of cases over a six-month period. I prescribed daily magnesium. Her symptoms steadily improved, and she was able to continue on oral magnesium alone, without symptoms returning.

When we lack magnesium, calcium deposits can accumulate in our soft tissues. The risk of a spasm in the muscular tissue surrounding a coronary artery—the source of all blood and oxygen for the heart—is greater. Since most women taking calcium to prevent bone loss are postmenopausal (and at greater risk for heart disease), magnesium should be a staple of their diet as well.

Many individuals with coronary artery disease are usually placed on drugs called calcium channel blockers, which function to increase magnesium in the cell; their side effects include dizziness, fatigue, and disorientation.

The *American Heart Journal*, in an editorial written by leading heart disease researchers, described magnesium as "nature's channel blocker." Magnesium is critical in maintaining the natural balance of calcium both inside and outside cells. Without it, the calcium scale tips too far in one direction, leading to a variety of conditions that can affect the heart and blood vessels. These include problems such as hypertension and heart disease.

WHAT'S HIDING IN YOUR RED BLOOD CELLS?

I use a special test to measure how well your red blood cells are able to carry magnesium. Often, a regular blood panel will show adequate levels of magnesium, which can mask a true underlying deficiency. Magnesium may be floating in the blood itself, but cells may not absorb it. If magnesium cannot actually get into the cell, it cannot work. Since magnesium is carried to cells all over the body through the blood, and the proper functioning of red blood cells is greatly dependent on magnesium, a test for red blood cell (RBC) magnesium levels is important. Many patients with asthma, heart disease, and diabetes have low levels.

This Mineral May Banish Fatigue for Good

"I'm so tired." I hear that statement from many of my patients. No matter what the illness—whether it's as serious as diabetes or heart disease or as mild as allergies and malaise—fatigue is often a cardinal symptom. Clearly, it's an immensely important signal that something has gone awry. Patients who are fatigued are frightened as well—they wonder if they're ever going to feel energetic again. And because it is so commonplace, even among those of us who are healthy, I am addressing it first.

Sometimes I think that, just as the Eskimos have dozens of words for "snow"—words that describe whether the snow is soft, fresh, days old, turning to ice—we ought to have different words for different kinds of fatigue. The fatigue that hits when you've just gone for an hour's bike ride or a mile-long swim. The fatigue that fells you when you get a bad flu, and every bit of your body seems to hurt. The fatigue that follows a sleepless night.

I've had patients tell me that their fatigue is so persistent it seems to have penetrated to the very core of their being. Those suffering from fibromyalgia, an increasingly common muscle disorder, experience deep, painful muscle fatigue.

What, then, is fatigue?

It's a good question and a hard one to answer. Fatigue is both the most common and the most elusive condition I see. It's the problem few doctors take seriously, yet it's the symptom of a wide range of illnesses. How do you actually describe fatigue? You can't measure it in the blood or urine. There is no test to prove that somebody is exhausted. Fatigue is unlike other conditions. You can see the changes in an arthritic joint, you can measure blood sugar elevation in diabetes, you can perform pulmonary function tests in asthma, and you can run an EKG in heart disease. You can even measure high levels of viral antibodies in the blood of patients suffering from chronic fatigue syndrome (CFS)—an immune disorder in which fatigue is a major symptom—but this is not diagnostic.

But if you are simply tired—just plain old exhausted—the only proof is that you say so. How is a doctor going to treat that?

As noted before, magnesium allows our muscles to relax. If our bodies become calcium deficient, we can borrow from the large reserves contained in our bones, but when our bodies become magnesium deficient, we must borrow from the already low supply in our muscles. But as our muscles lose magnesium, calcium charges in to replace it, and, as a result, our muscles grow tense and cramped. This can result in debilitating problems, especially the exacerbation of chronic fatigue symptoms.

Magnesium has had a profound impact in the treatment of this disease.

Chronic fatigue syndrome, according to the Centers for Disease Control, is a diagnosis of exclusion, meaning that certain conditions must be ruled out before a true diagnosis can be made. There are specific major and minor criteria that must be fulfilled for at least a six-month period. Some of the conditions that are ruled out include hypothyroidism, Lyme disease, and other chronic illnesses such as diabetes, hypoglycemia, or multiple allergies.

A recent article in *Health Watch*, a publication of the CFS Research Foundation, showed magnesium to be the single most critical supplement for patients with

CFS. It is known that intracellular magnesium deficiencies exist in patients with this disorder.

A lack of magnesium in the cells would disrupt the flow of energy that causes muscle relaxation and a regular heartbeat. Some pioneering doctors have started treating CFS patients with magnesium injections and found them helpful. One patient of mine, a fifty-year-old industrial engineer, suffered with chronic fibromyalgia, a painful muscle condition, as well as severe fatigue. When I tested his magnesium levels, I found them to be very low. Weekly injections were able to bring him back to a normal level of energy, and his muscle pain diminished dramatically.

Another patient of mine improved with magnesium, along with other supplements and dietary changes. Joan was a forty-five-year-old psychiatrist with an easy smile and genuine warmth who came to me in desperation. She had suffered from symptoms of chronic fatigue for over ten years. Her condition began as an acute viral illness, with sore throat, muscle and joint pains, fever, and flulike symptoms. Yet instead of getting better, she just got worse and worse, until she was barely able to continue working. Like many patients with this ailment, she'd never had a significant previous medical condition. She was a hard worker and dedicated to her patients. She worked long hours. Before she came to me, she had tried innumerable treatments, from consulting a psychiatrist herself to trying antidepressants, acupuncture, homeopathy, natural remedies in health food stores, and regular "mainstream physicians." Since she had just begun a separation from her husband, she was usually told her condition was related to stress and depression. In other words, a psychiatrist—a medical doctor—was told her own condition was psychosomatic, or "all in your head."

When I saw her, ten years after her initial symptoms had begun, she was indeed depressed and demoralized from the lack of understanding she'd received.

"I know something is wrong," she insisted, "but no one believes me." A series of blood tests suggested she was right. She had high levels of antibodies to Epstein-Barr virus, *Cytomegalovirus*, and HHV-6, a herpes virus. Antibodies to three different viruses is unusual; although many people are exposed to viruses like Epstein-Barr, for some as yet unknown reason, certain people become quite ill as a result, often chronically. Joan's natural killer cells were at a very low level of 10 (normal ranges from 20 to 250). Her red blood cell magnesium, one of the markers I use to diagnose this condition, was also low. We were beginning to understand Joan's problem. Now we had to solve it.

As part of the treatment for CFS, I take a comprehensive look at the patient's condition and check for any allergies the patient might have, since 80 percent of chronic fatigue patients suffer from them. I also check for nutritional and hormonal deficiencies. Fortunately for Joan, with the exception of several key foods to which she was allergic, these tests came back normal.

I treated Joan with a variety of supplements, and magnesium was first on the list. I find 500 milligrams of magnesium aspartate per day is an optimal oral dose.

Magnesium alone, of course, can only do part of the job in a severe and chronic illness. Joan's complete program included antioxidants such as vitamin C, energy-boosting amino acids such as tyrosine, the herb ginkgo to improve cerebral circulation, coenzyme Q_{10} to energize the cellular mitochondria, and Siberian ginseng, an excellent herb that helps patients cope with stress more effectively.

Within a few weeks of beginning this supplement program, Joan felt her energy increase. Today, Joan is once more an active, vibrant member of her community. She regularly takes her magnesium supplements and is determined never to let her system deteriorate again. Other nutraceuticals which are helpful include NADH, Tyrosine and D-Ribose.

A Mineral Meant for Women?

Women might be pleased to learn that by adjusting their diet slightly and adding daily magnesium supplements, they could banish the more unpleasant symptoms of PMS. It's been discovered that women suffering from headaches, intense muscle cramps, and fatigue had extremely low levels of RBC magnesium, leading many researchers to conclude that such painful problems, usually treated with aspirin or Tylenol, could be caused by magnesium deficiency.

In a recent study reported in *Family Practice News*, women were given doses of oral magnesium three times a day for two weeks prior to the onset of menstruation. This managed to reduce the severity of PMS and the duration and intensity of PMS-related migraines. A study, in the journal *Headache*, found that women suffering from migraines triggered by their menstrual cycle had lower levels of magnesium.

There is also a tremendous need for magnesium in the early stages of pregnancy, and researchers estimate that pregnant women only get 50 to 60 percent of the RDA of magnesium in their diet. Studies have shown that magnesium helps prevent migraine headaches, especially in pregnant women.

I've been impressed by magnesium's ability to alleviate PMS symptoms. One patient, Victoria Hanover, was a forty-seven-year-old executive at one of the largest banks in the world, and the mother of three. Yet she'd suffered all her life from PMS, monthly migraines linked to her menstrual cycle, and mitral valve prolapse.

When she described her symptoms, we realized that they all occurred at the same time, toward the end of the month before her period. Her symptoms worsened after drinking wine and eating bread. That was a clear sign that she had underlying food allergies, and indeed, tests showed she was allergic to yeast-enriched foods, such as (as her allergic reactions indicated) wine and bread.

I took her off these foods and treated her with multivitamins and high doses of magnesium. In the case of the heart, magnesium (240 milligrams a day in divided doses) is essential for the normal contraction and relaxation phases of the heart. I knew we'd have to wait a month to see how she'd improve, and, to my delight, her headaches decreased significantly. They lasted for only two days, rather than a week, before her period, and were less intense. She noticed no skipped heartbeats, either—a previously troubling symptom of her mitral valve prolapse.

Symptoms during subsequent menstrual cycles continued to improve, and over the past three years, there's been a dramatic overall improvement in her health. About a year ago, Victoria decided to stop taking her magnesium supplements. She thought maybe she'd grown out of her phase of poor health. But her symptoms returned in the first cycle, and, by the second, they were as bad as they'd been when I first saw her. Now she's back on those supplements and never skips them. Other patients have been able to get off them.

Even when migraines are not premenstrual, magnesium can help. A 1996 study in a journal devoted to studying only headaches evaluated eighty-one patients between the ages of eighteen and sixty-five. One group was given 600 milligrams of magnesium daily, while the other group took a placebo. After twelve weeks, there were 41 percent fewer headaches in the magnesium group and only 15 percent fewer headaches in the placebo group.

BRITTLE BONES: DON'T RELY ON CALCIUM ALONE

Calcium builds healthy bones, right? Yes and no. Though calcium has been hailed as an osteoporosis preventive, it is not the only answer. Magnesium is just as important. In fact, calcium may increase the risk of blockages in your heart if taken in doses that are too high.

Milk mustaches on celebrities, bottles of calcium stacked on shelves in pharmacies, drugstores, supermarkets, and health food stores, and countless articles on calcium's benefits have obscured the importance of its sister mineral, magnesium. Magnesium can combat osteoporosis too. Magnesium can help prevent fractures and increase bone density. It appears to have a direct effect on the parathyroid hormone, which is associated with low calcium levels. Many elderly patients have problems with malabsorption of minerals, and they may be using diuretics for blood pressure problems. In both cases, magnesium is excreted, and low levels of the mineral contribute to porous, brittle bones.

I advise supplementation with both calcium and magnesium as a preventive measure for all my patients who are going through menopause or have passed through menopause already.

Breathe Easy at Last

Asthma is epidemic in our time. Fifteen million Americans now suffer from this devastating condition, and it is the primary cause of hospitalization in children. We spend $6 billion a year on asthma treatment, and our solution so far has been the use of potent and sometimes harmful drugs, along with minimal exposure to allergens when possible.

Many studies show that magnesium is a key mineral in treating asthma. A European study found that magnesium diminishes the "bursting" of inflammatory white blood cells that often occurs in asthma and begins a cascade of reactions that result in wheezing and rawness. A study of asthmatic children treated with IV magnesium showed that this mineral alone improved lung function, and another study of IV magnesium in adults found that the mineral dramatically reduced hospitalizations.

Is it really possible that something as simple and abundant as magnesium might arrest devastating asthma symptoms? I take it myself for my own asthma, and it has helped tremendously. I've also seen it work in my practice again and again. Magnesium, along with fish oils and other herbs and nutrients, is a mainstay of my natural approach to reversing asthma. Every asthmatic patient of mine takes oral magnesium.

How does it work? Magnesium relaxes the bronchial muscles and prevents them from overreacting to allergic stimuli. It also seems to quench or calm the allergic response. In a sense, magnesium's effect is not that different than bronchodilators and steroids, but instead of causing side effects like dry mouth and nervousness, magnesium leaves the patient in a calm state of well-being.

Andrew Jenkins was an irrepressibly buoyant six-year-old boy when he first came to see me. He had been to the emergency room four times in the past year because of his asthma. Like most kids, his favorite foods were pizza, hamburgers, and ice cream. He was a very finicky eater who wouldn't go near a vegetable. Andrew was a smart young boy, however, and his condition was causing him great misery. Medications made him shaky; days came when he couldn't play with his friends, and, worse yet, there were the constant visits to the emergency room with the dreaded injections, poking, and prodding that both parents and child hated.

Although it's true that children who don't like vegetables usually have a higher aversion to pills than normal, we were able to start him on 90 milligrams of magnesium, 200 milligrams of vitamin C (a natural antihistamine and free radical quencher), 1 teaspoon of flaxseed oil (to provide important fatty acids that most asthmatics lack), and 50 micrograms of selenium (a building block for glutathione reductase, the body's premier detoxifying enzyme)—all to be taken twice a day. You may be surprised that a young boy may need help in detoxifying, but any chronic disease creates free radical damage and inflammation that stress the body's detoxification system.

I gave Andrew a pulmonary function test, which was critical to see if his airways were obstructed. Another common way for testing breathing capacity is for patients to blow into a tube called a peak flow meter, which registers how forcefully the air is blown out of their lungs. Good lung function should register at least 80 percent on a pulmonary function test, but Andrew's numbers were astonishingly low. One test registered below 50 percent of normal function. He began his nutritional and medical treatments, and when he returned, we redid the tests. The percentages had doubled. His symptoms improved, but on questioning his mother, I learned she had only been able to keep him on the magnesium (180 milligrams a day) and the diet. It took some extra coaxing to get him to comply with the entire program.

In the three years that I've treated him, he's had only one visit to the emergency room, compared with the four hospitalizations the year before he came to see me. Today, he's a healthy young boy coping with his asthma. Although his improvement may seem hard to believe, research studies confirm my experience with children. In a study conducted at the University of Florida in Gainesville, six severely asthmatic children who were given an infusion of magnesium sulfate all showed sustained clinical improvement afterward. These children had not responded to steroids, bronchodilator therapy, or other drugs.

Whether magnesium is given to children or adults suffering from asthma, it is one of the most effective and natural aids available.

Can Magnesium Keep Diabetes Under Control?

A Gallup survey of five hundred adults with diabetes reported that 83 percent consumed insufficient magnesium from foods. Both type I and type II diabetics are susceptible to magnesium depletion, but type II patients are at a greater risk. Magnesium depletion is a common but sometimes unnoticed problem in diabetic patients, damaging their heart function and glucose control.

Magnesium deficiency is the most common disturbance in mineral metabolism observed in insulin-dependent diabetics. The body needs magnesium to create insulin naturally, and studies have shown that insulin resistance is definitely connected with magnesium depletion. A Viennese study found that low magnesium actually contributes to insulin resistance, and there was a marked improvement in the control of diabetes when magnesium was added to the diet.

Research indicates that raising the low magnesium levels in diabetic patients improves cardiovascular function and glucose control. As you may recall, the health of my patient George, who suffered from hypertension and diabetes, improved markedly with the addition of magnesium. Although magnesium cannot eliminate diabetes, it can help enhance insulin function, thereby preventing or warding off many of the serious complications associated with this illness, such as blood vessel damage.

Magnesium and You

Magnesium is one of the most important and healing minerals in the body. It can help prevent some of the most serious ailments we face: heart disease, asthma, and diabetes. It can also treat less serious but nonetheless frustrating chronic conditions such as fatigue, mitral valve prolapse, and muscle aches and spasms.

Now that you know that magnesium is just as important as vitamin C or vitamin E, you can add it to your diet, through foods and supplements.

Magnesium-rich foods are available at your local health food store and even at the corner grocery. Rich food sources of magnesium include wheat germ, wheat bran, nuts, soybeans, whole grain oats and barley, corn, fish, and various green leafy vegetables. Bottled mineral waters also contain magnesium. And for those of us who need extra magnesium in addition to our diet—perhaps because of an inherited risk for heart disease or diabetes—magnesium supplements are easily available at your health food store. I recommend magnesium aspartate, which is easily absorbed, or citrate, which is the least expensive type of magnesium available. For the average individual, I would recommend between 300 to 500 milligrams daily. For serious conditions like heart disease or diabetes, higher doses may be recommended; however, magnesium can trigger diarrhea. Higher doses should be monitored by a knowledgeable physician.

Even after all my experience with magnesium's healing powers and the many patients I've seen it help, I sometimes find myself amazed to think that such a simple mineral could help in such a wide range of health problems. Sometimes the simplest cures are the best.

HOW MUCH SHOULD I TAKE?

For General Health

100-250 milligrams a day
Divide dosage. Take after meals.

Special Conditions

Leg cramps	300-400 mg/day
Fatigue	400-600 mg/day
Heart attack	400-600 mg/day
Hypertension	400-700 mg/day
Palpitations	300-500 mg/day
Asthma	200-600 mg/day
Fibromyalgia	400-600 mg/day
PMS	400-600 mg/day
Migraines	400-600 mg/day
Osteoporosis	400-600mg/day

4

Fish Oil: Firefighter of the High Seas

Keith Preston was a twenty-eight-year-old banker who had married his high school sweetheart. Soon afterward, she got pregnant, and they bought a new house. Then Keith was diagnosed with a painful form of arthritis.

Keith's future seemed hostage to his illness. His doctors had told him he would probably suffer with this disease the rest of his life. They placed him on daily doses of Naprosyn, a potent anti-inflammatory drug; but the joints in his knees, hands, and feet continued to swell. After three years like this, Keith's marriage began to suffer. He was embarrassed to go out in public and socialize. He began to withdraw emotionally from his wife and baby daughter. His doctors then recommended a drug called methotrexate, a powerful chemotherapy agent with side effects that include liver and kidney damage.

Keith came to me believing there was no hope yet, paradoxically, pleading with me to help him. He couldn't imagine a life on these powerful prescription drugs, especially since they weren't even keeping his illness in remission.

Not surprisingly, none of his doctors had asked him what he ate. It turned out that Keith's diet was just the opposite of what he needed—it was high in the kind of foods that trigger inflammation in individuals who are vulnerable to autoimmune conditions. He regularly ate red meat and fried foods, which tend to promote inflammation. On top of that, he was fond of refined starches and sugars, and he almost never ate fish, which contains essential oils that help quench inflammation.

Keith's diet was stimulating inflammation in the body, unchecked by needed essential fatty acids. I helped Keith change his diet to one that included daily fish, vegetables, fruits, and whole grains.

Keith was given a complete evaluation, laboratory tests including tests for his omega-3 fatty acid levels, a history, and a physical, along with dietary analysis. He was found to be lacking in vitamin B_{12} and folic acid. Most people with a chronic illness tend to deplete their body's stores of nutrients faster than normal, and Keith was no exception. I started him on a treatment program that included extra doses of B vitamins and a good multivitamin.

The most crucial element in Keith's treatment program, however, was fish oil. Fish oil is the nutritional star in any anti-inflammation program. Most Americans, like Keith, get almost none of the essential oils they truly need. His blood tests confirmed what I thought: he had extremely low levels of DHA and EPA. I prescribed Keith six 500-milligram capsules a day.

Most patients who suffer from an inflammatory-related ailment, when asked about their diet, usually reply with some variation on this theme:

"Oh, I grab a bagel with cream cheese for breakfast. Then maybe a cheeseburger for lunch, some potato chips for a snack, and then, because I'm watching my weight, some pasta for dinner."

The health food version of this is: "Oh, I like crunchy granola with skim milk for breakfast. Then a tuna salad sandwich for lunch, some oil-free baked potato chips for a snack, and then, because I'm watching my weight, some pasta with low-fat tomato sauce and fruit for dessert."

"So, any salad or greens?" I ask.

"Sure, sure," they say.

"And what type of salad dressing do you use?"

"Oh, whatever they give me." (The healthy version: "Olive oil and balsamic vinegar.")

"How about fish?"

"Oh, sometimes. But I like steak better." (Or: "I eat chicken without the skin, and I guess I eat fish once a week or so.")

Most of these patients have no idea that, healthy diet or not, they are almost entirely deficient in the necessary oils to fight inflammation. Only 10 percent of vegetarians truly eat healthy diets, according to a recent study; most still eat a lot of junk food.

Once I put Keith's diet back on track, we began to see some astounding results. Within a couple of months, his joint swelling vanished, as did his pain. He stopped taking his drugs and remained well. At that point, he even stopped taking his supplements, thinking he perhaps had experienced some kind of spontaneous cure. Within weeks, his symptoms began to reappear. Once he started back on his supplements, the disease vanished again. His joints were mobile. He was able to play basketball on the weekends. He was just like any other guy. He started to enjoy life again.

Keith's experience with this disease, and his body's ability to control it completely with a proper diet and supplements, was staggering to him. He actually went into therapy for six months in an effort to cope with the emotional seesaw he'd been through—imagining, at twenty-eight, that he'd be deformed for life, watching his marriage almost disintegrate, being told by his doctors that the only option was ever more powerful drugs, and then finding himself restored to health in a matter of months simply by observing dietary changes and taking a few potent supplements.

Putting Out Fires

Because fish oils quench inflammation, I like to call them nature's firefighters. Fish oils have shown dramatic benefits in an astounding range of conditions—many of which are triggered by some form of chronic inflammation. Here are some examples:

Arthritis: I have seen fish oil turn around many cases of arthritis. A study in the *Annals of Rheumatology* found that patients treated with fish oil or primrose oil showed a significant improvement in their symptoms, and by the end of a year, they had dramatically reduced the level of their medications.

Asthma: A recent study in the *International Archives of Allergy and Applied Immunology* examined the effect of fish oil on asthmatics over a one-year period. After nine months, the lung function of the subjects taking fish oil increased by 23 percent, while those given placebos saw no discernible improvement.

Inflammatory Bowel Disease: Fish oils are beneficial in ulcerative colitis and Crohn's disease (when the patients are not too ill to absorb fats). A recent Italian study showed that coated fish oil capsules, which pass through the stomach without being dissolved and reach the gut fully preserved, produced significant improvement in symptoms of inflammatory bowel disease. There were also improvements in the cells of the colon. Bleeding diminished, as did abdominal distention and pain, and bowel movements were more fully formed.

Heart Disease: Fish oil has a profoundly beneficial effect on heart disease. A recent study showed that when men who otherwise ate a standard American diet ate fish twice a week, their death rates plummeted by 50 percent. A study in the *Archives of Internal Medicine* showed that fish oils in moderate amounts reduced triglycerides and harmful cholesterol, both shown to be risk factors for heart disease.

Blood Pressure: Fish oil can lower high blood pressure. A 1990 study in the *American Journal of Hypertension* showed that in patients with hypertension, fish oil supplements reduced blood pressure, lowered triglyceride levels, and increased the amount of time the body takes to form a blood clot.

Cancer: I consider fish oils an absolutely essential supplement for my patients with a history of cancer. Cancer cells can grow and spread by creating inflammation. Research suggests that essential fatty acids slow down cancer growth, impairing the malignant cells' ability to function efficiently. In one study, increasing the proportion of red blood cell omega-6 fatty acids significantly reduced the risk of prostate cancer. Another study showed that fish oil may protect against colon cancer, and a study reported in the *Journal of the National Cancer Institute* suggests that a diet rich in omega-3 fatty acids can suppress breast cancer cell growth.

Diabetes: Fish oils can help prevent the damage to blood vessels that is so common in diabetes and is actually the underlying cause for many of the devastating complications of the disease—from kidney failure to gangrene to heart disease. A 1980 study published in Germany found that essential fatty acids improved the action of insulin and reduced the development of blood clots.

PMS: I often prescribe fish oils, among other nutrients, to treat symptoms of PMS. A study in the *European Journal of Clinical Nutrition* looked at 181 healthy Danish women between the ages of twenty and forty-five. Menstrual pain was significantly higher in those who did not include omega-3s in their diet or whose bloodwork showed unfavorable ratios of omega-3 and omega-6. The study concluded that marine fatty acids are linked to reduced symptoms of PMS.

An Inflammatory Issue

How can something as simple as an essential fatty acid change someone's life as profoundly as Keith's was changed? What is occurring in the body?

The answers will teach you about more than fish oils, or their plant counterpart, flaxseed oil. They will help you understand how to stay healthy. For in understanding the importance of these oils, one must fully comprehend inflammation and its effect on the body.

Inflammation is a chemical fire. That's why it causes redness, swelling, tenderness, and pain. Some fires burn fast and furious and then burn out. That's the kind of inflammation caused by an acute febrile illness, where your fever spikes high and then breaks, or by an accident, where a bruise or injury swells and then heals. Other fires are like a hot bed of ashes, always releasing heat, never quite dying, never bringing down the whole house. That's the kind of response caused by chronic autoimmune diseases like arthritis or asthma.

Inflammation is actually a complex response to some kind of damage to the body—whether it's from bacteria, viruses, toxins, or the waste products of the body's own chemical reactions. And it involves a sequence of reactions and chemicals. The inflammatory process attracts cells called platelets, white blood cells, and macrophages, which are designed to kill bacteria by actually eating them up.

Our immune system needs inflammation in order to help heal wounds and fight illness. However, sometimes the process becomes disregulated or goes awry. This is where the essential oils, and fish oil in particular, come into play. These oils contain essential fatty acids called omega-3s. In the last ten years, nearly five thousand studies have been conducted on omega-3 acids alone. These studies have researched the benefits of omega-3 fatty acids for everything from heart disease to cancer, psoriasis, autoimmune disorders, and even kidney disease. It has long been known that Eskimos suffer very little cancer and autoimmune disorders because their diet is so high in fish, which is a great source of omega-3 fatty acids.

How Can Fats Be Essential?

Fish oils—and their chemical cousins found in plants—are among the greatest nutritional stories of our time. The oils in specific plants and fish are so important that they are called essential fatty acids. Specific fatty acids modify inflammation and help treat such conditions as diabetes, asthma, hypertension, and arthritis. They are even crucial for the development of nerve and brain function in infants. Fish oils are actually absorbed directly into the outer fatty layer of every cell, where they act as a kind of cellular cushion or barrier, protecting each cell from the outside environment—like a moat around a castle.

Recently fat has become a dirty word, but in truth, fats are life's lubricants and energy powerhouses. We need fats for optimal health, and women in particular need fats to build their hormones. However, there are a variety of fats, some good, some bad. Here's a brief guide:

Saturated fats are either derived from animal sources or have been artificially saturated by the food industry. They can promote free radical damage and clog the arteries. In saturated fats—such as those found in meat and cheese—every carbon atom is completely saturated with all the hydrogen it can carry. It is a solid, thick fat, like the yellowy fat you find in chicken and beef. This fat is known to be a major risk factor in raising cholesterol levels.

Trans-saturated fats do not exist in nature (or occur in very small amounts) and are artificially produced. In America, margarine contains trans-saturated fats (in Europe, this is not the case; the trans-saturated fats have been eliminated). Oil is manufactured to harden at room temperature and have a long shelf life, but in the body, it is harmful. It actually blocks your cells' use of essential fatty acids. This fat should be avoided whenever possible. Laws are being enacted to eliminate these dangerous fats from our diets.

Unsaturated fats are found in most oils. They are called unsaturated or polyunsaturated because many of the carbon atoms are "empty" and don't carry hydrogen. Corn oil is a common unsaturated fat, along with safflower, soybean, and other vegetable oils. When used in cooking, they easily become oxidized and create free radicals. High amounts of unsaturated fats were once thought to be healthy, but they are now believed to contribute to a variety of illnesses, including heart disease and cancer.

Monounsaturated fats such as olive oil are good for your health. They contain the fatty acid known as oleic acid. It has 18 carbon atoms and only 16 hydrogen atoms, which makes the fat less solid. It flows easily at room temperature.

Omega-3 and omega-6 fatty acids are unsaturated; they are so important to health that I put them in their own category.

As you can see, overconsumption of the wrong type of fat can cause serious damage within the body by blocking your body's ability to access essential fatty acids. Eating the right amount of fat is a delicate balancing act.

Remember These Numbers: 3 and 6

The body uses omega oils to regulate a wide variety of cellular functions and substances, including the level of prostaglandins, active hormonelike substances that regulate almost every bodily function, including the work of the heart and kidneys, the constriction of blood vessels, healing and repair, immune function, allergy defense, digestion, inflammation, menstrual cramps, body temperature, and pressure in the eyes, ears, and joints.

There are three important classes of prostaglandins: each is made from different fatty acids and is influenced almost entirely by our diet.

The first class, class 1, quench inflammation, and are derived from a fatty acid called dihomogammalinolenic acid (DGLA). This is found in only one substance known to man: mother's milk. However, our body can make its own DGLA from GLA, a healthy omega-6 fatty acid. In turn, our bodies can make GLA from linoleic acid, which is found in nuts and seeds. Many women's problems are triggered or worsened by a single deficiency in GLA or DGLA and the resulting deficiency in class 1 prostaglandins.

Class 3 prostaglandins are also anti-inflammatory agents. They are derived exclusively from omega-3 fatty acids, which primarily come from fish oils. (Our bodies can make EPA [eicosapentaenoic acid] from the oil in flaxseed, which is good news for vegetarians.)

Class 2 prostaglandins are powerfully proinflammatory fire starters. Our bodies make them from meat or from vegetable oils that contain omega-6 fatty acids. Many of these omega-6s are an important linchpin in the inflammatory avalanche.

Our body needs all three classes of prostaglandins, but it needs them in a proper balance. Too many class 2 prostaglandins—fueled by an unhealthy diet—may be an important factor in many chronic inflammatory illnesses.

Where Do I Get My Good Fats?

Two important forms of omega-3 fatty acids come in fatty fish like salmon and mackerel. (Other fish, though offering a healthy form of protein, are not high in omega-3s. These less fatty fish, such as flounder, simply do not provide beneficial amounts.) They are eicosapentaenoic acid (EPA) and docosahexaenoic acid (DHA). Symptoms of EPA and DHA deficiency often include allergies, inflammation, and dry skin. Prolonged deficiencies can lead to serious autoimmune diseases.

Omega-6s have a wide variety of effects. They can trigger or inhibit inflammation, depending on the individual—his or her genes and diet. Unhealthy omega-6 oils permeate every portion of the typical American diet—in corn oil and saturated fat.

An important and healthy omega-6 fatty acid is gamma linolenic acid (GLA), which has been found helpful in menstrual disorders. This omega-6 acid is found in evening primrose oil and black currant oil. I recommend evening primrose because it is very stable and doesn't degrade as easily while sitting in capsules on the shelf.

These days, the dietary availability of omega-3 fatty acids in America is only 20 percent of what it was a century ago. This precipitous plunge is cause for concern. Studies in Eskimos show that they eat an excess of omega-3s and lack the enzymes that convert omega-6s into inflammatory substances. Their genes are protecting them from the potentially harmful by-products of omega-6s, and their high-fish diet is protecting them as well. That's probably why their rates of heart disease are negligible.

Why are omega-3s and -6s so important? Simply because many of the chemical signals that stimulate a cell to act do so by metabolizing and changing the fatty layer of the cell's membrane. The signals that can impact that layer range from adrenaline to histamine as well as powerful neurotransmitters such as serotonin and dopamine. If the fatty layer is deficient or impaired, chemical signals don't have the proper effect, and the body's functions are impaired.

How important are omega-3s? In a study that was conducted in 1970,

FISH OIL AS A BLOOD THINNER

Fish oil not only inhibits excessive inflammation, it can actually thin the blood and work like a kind of natural aspirin—only better. Fish oils inhibit the clumping together of cells called platelets. Platelets have a complex array of functions, including the ability to bind together and help the body heal wounds by clotting blood. When a blood vessel is injured, platelets adhere to the exposed part of the blood vessel, secreting a veritable fountain of chemicals that help promote inflammation. The inflammation seals the wound and keeps bacteria from spreading. It's like when firefighters build a ring of fire around a raging blaze, sealing it off and preventing it from spreading.

Are we getting enough omega-3s? Think of the huge increase in autoimmune and inflammatory diseases today. Half a million people die of heart disease each year. Two million are diagnosed with cancer. More people go to their doctor for joint pains than any other condition. Asthma is now recognized as a national epidemic. Why are these diseases on the rise? Our typical American diet is not very different from the diet of the sick monkeys that were studied many years ago.

Individuals who live in cold climates seem to need higher levels of omega-3 fatty acids. Individuals who suffer from atopic eczema often have a poorly functioning enzyme that makes it hard for them to convert their essential fatty acids into anti-inflammatory prostaglandins. If they are given evening primrose oil, their eczema may clear up.

If your diet is high in nuts and seeds, and in flaxseed oil, and you still suffer from inflammatory disease, consult your nutritionist about eating fish and taking fish oil capsules. But remember, fish oil capsules inevitably become oxidized, or rancid, causing free radical damage. A study of twenty smokers and twenty-two nonsmokers given 10 grams of fish oil daily found that after four weeks, peroxide damage to cholesterol increased by as much as 50 percent in both groups (oxidized cholesterol can be harmful to health). The antioxidant vitamin E, which is fat soluble, can provide partial protection, but it can't entirely solve the problem. Therefore, first try eating fish high in omega-3s three or four times a week, then add fish oil capsules if necessary, and be sure to take vitamins C and E as well.

eight monkeys were placed on a laboratory diet with every essential nutrient and only one fat—corn oil. Within two years, the monkeys all became sick and developed patchy hair loss. Two suffered from severe intestinal inflammation, two began to gnaw obsessively at their own bodies, and four died. That's of particular concern to me because corn oil is such a commonly used oil in the American diet and is often used to deep-fry fast foods.

Fish that Put Out Fires: Some True Tales

Seventy-year-old Bill Richards loved to help others. He owned and operated the largest hardware store in Westchester County. He was an active man, the type of guy who'd run over to a neighbor's house to fix something five minutes after getting the call. His store was fully stocked; if you needed a special part, he had it.

However, all this changed after arthritis struck him down in the summer of 1990. He had trouble moving his hands and difficulty walking and bending his knees. When I saw him, his ailment had been written off as the simple but cruel act of time ("old age," he was told), but I wasn't so easily convinced of that. He'd been healthy all his life and enjoyed swimming and playing racquetball with his friends every week. He was a robust, energetic man who'd always been told he was the picture of health and that he'd never get old. Even though he had a hard time walking, he still gave the impression of strength and vitality. Could it really be that old age had suddenly dealt him this blow?

We ran a lot of tests investigating the possibility of rheumatoid arthritis and other autoimmune diseases. We tested his blood for vitamin deficiencies and took x-rays of his joints. Sure enough, the x-rays of his hip showed significant degeneration, but his knees and shoulders looked clear. He wasn't taking any supplements at the time, but his vitamin levels were normal. His diet, however, left much to be desired. He snacked on pretzels and potato chips and roasted peanuts, and he loved a good hamburger or steak. He told me that cake was his weakness even though it nearly always gave him indigestion.

When I told him that he would need to alter his diet radically, like many patients he looked crestfallen. But he told me that if this dietary change would restore his health and allow him to play catch with his grandson, he would do whatever was necessary. I put him on a diet rich in vegetables, eliminated red meat entirely, and started him on fish four times a week. He began taking six grams of fish oil a day—twelve 500-milligram capsules—along with vitamin E and vitamin C to protect from oxidation.[1] I saw him monthly, over the course of the year, and noticed a steady improvement over time. He, too, could see improvement—he was swimming regularly. His hip, however, did not improve, and the long-term damage done by his lifestyle could not be reversed. He actually decided to undergo hip surgery so that he would one day get back on the racquetball court. A year later he said, "I've never felt this well in my life." He'd lost twenty-five pounds, was fit, had high levels of energy, and told me that he literally felt twenty years younger.

If Fish Is Not for You

Vegetarians may wonder what dietary option they have if they don't eat fish. Flaxseed oil is a plant counterpart to fish oil and an excellent alternative for most vegetarians. It contains the essential omega-3 fatty acids that, when converted by an enzyme in the body, turn into the active eicosinoids found in fish oil. However, I find that most vegetarians eat too little of these essential oils, concentrating instead on the polyunsaturated fats such as those found in corn oil and safflower oil, which can ultimately promote inflammation.

This was the case with May Ireland, a vivacious thirty-seven-year-old homemaker who first noticed her asthma flaring up during a series of brush fires that swept through her hometown in Idaho. These fires sent black plumes of smoke over her home for months at a time. Chronic exposure to smoke wore down her lungs' ability to fight inflammation. She needed a firefighter inside her lungs. May had read an article I'd written about asthma in a magazine, and she flew in from Idaho to see me. She agreed to take fish oil supplements, along with flaxseed oil as a backup—though she staunchly refused to eat fish. She took three grams a day of both, in capsules, along with 400 units of vitamin E to counter any oxidation of these oils. I also put her on my complete asthma program, including magnesium, antioxidants, environmental testing and cleanup, breathing exercises, and dietary changes. Once her condition improved, she was able to wean herself from the fish oil capsules and just keep flaxseed oil in her diet.

I'm not surprised she was helped. Many studies have shown that fish oil helps asthma. A recent study in the *International Archives of Allergy and Applied Immunology* treated twelve asthmatics with a diet high in omega-3s for one year. After nine months, their ability to breathe was significantly improved. Another 1996 study in the *Medical Journal of Australia* found that eating fish more than once a week reduced asthma in children.

Fish for All

Fish oils don't just help asthmatics. They are helpful in combating most inflammatory conditions, of which asthma is just one. Others include lupus, arthritis and other rheumatic diseases, scleroderma (where the skin and organs harden), Raynaud's disease (where the fingers turn purple whenever exposed to cold), and autoimmune thyroiditis (where the thyroid becomes inflamed). In these illnesses, a tremendous amount of inflammation is produced by the body, and it ends up fighting itself. Nobody knows quite what triggers these illnesses, although viruses are possible culprits. Whatever the cause, studies have shown that essential fatty acid levels in patients with autoimmune illnesses are depressed. I recommend fish and/or flaxseed oil in any of the aforementioned conditions, and I have found the results extremely encouraging.

Why Women Need Fish

Fish oils are key nutrients for women suffering from chronic PMS. Rose Crane was one such patient: a twenty-eight-year-old secretary with persistent yeast infections and a history of disabling PMS—cramps, terrible bloating, migraines, and mood swings. Finally, her gynecologist put her on birth control pills to try to balance her hormones and treat her PMS. Unfortunately, while on the birth control pills, her yeast infections increased. She was caught in a pharmaceutical Catch-22.

Rose was frightened because, despite rounds of antibiotics, her condition was worsening. Though she was a beautiful young woman, she no longer socialized or dated.

I immediately placed her on a program to treat her yeast problem, which included changes in her diet. The foods she ate were typical of someone with a yeast problem—lots of bread, cakes, cookies, sweet sodas, pasta, and corn. She admitted that she loved sugar. At the same time, her diet lacked essential fatty acids. Patients with yeast problems and PMS invariably feel better if they include a lot of fish in their diet, because then their body is given the building blocks to fight inflammation. I started her on three grams of fish oil per day, as well as two grams of flaxseed and primrose oil. I added vitamin B_6, a natural diuretic that can help reduce symptoms of PMS, and magnesium, which reduces muscle cramping. I remember Rose looking at me and saying, "There's no way I'm going to be able to take all these pills." I told her to try to stick with it and let me know if she saw any improvement in the next thirty days. She stayed on the program, and she steadily improved. But three months later, after drinking a bottle of wine to celebrate her master's degree, her PMS symptoms returned with a vengeance. "I thought I was cured!" she said, mystified. The truth is, it can take up to a year for fish oils to reach effective levels, so dosages should be maintained for the first twelve months. After that, some patients find they can reduce their intake of capsules, or even eliminate them entirely. And I encourage that, when possible, since oil in a capsule on a shelf is in danger of oxidizing and becoming rancid. That damage is certainly less worrisome than a chronic illness like asthma or disabling monthly symptoms of PMS; however, in an optimal situation, oils should be obtained from the diet. Therefore, I encourage my patients to look forward to a time when their health has returned and they can be maintained with a diet that includes fish at least three times weekly.

Scaly Fish, Smooth Skin

We live in a society obsessed with beauty. Although skin ailments are not life threatening, they can devastate one's quality of life.

Adrienne Austin, a thirty-one-year-old fashion designer, had spent the last decade of her life battling the skin ailments eczema and seborrhea. In addition to her chronic itching and rashes, she experienced frequent headaches and sinusitis. Over the years, she'd been on a number of antibiotics to treat a variety of skin and sinus infections. Adrienne's skin problem alerted me to the possibility of an underlying deficiency in essential fatty acids. Her chronic sinusitis could be brought on by allergies, to

WHERE AND HOW TO GET YOUR OILS

Nature is an abundant source of vitamins, minerals, and nutrients needed for good health, including essential fatty acids, so unless you are trying to combat an ongoing inflammatory illness or heart condition, there's no need to rush to the health food store for these supplements. Three servings of fish a week should be adequate for most people. Fish high in EFAs are tuna, salmon, halibut, bluefish, red snapper, and mackerel. However, you must also eliminate the unhealthy fats that compete with fish oils. You can't continue eating fatty, fried foods and meats every day.

Different diseases require different amounts of EFAs. Inflammatory bowel disease can require as much as 6,000 milligrams per day, partly because the inflamed gut cannot absorb oils as well. Arthritis may require 2,000 to 6,000 milligrams of fish oil a day, perhaps because of the many different sites of inflammation involved in arthritis. Treatments for asthma and lupus generally require 1,000 to 2,000 milligrams of fish oil a day. Most other conditions, such as PMS, skin conditions, or Raynaud's, will usually improve with 2,000 milligrams a day; however, higher doses may be necessary with Raynaud's.

Flaxseed oil can be used as a supplement to fish oil, especially for vegetarians. I recommend 3 grams a day in most illnesses. Otherwise, flaxseed oil can be a healthful addition to salads and can be used instead of butter on baked potatoes, squash, or other vegetables. It should not be cooked, as it easily turns rancid, and it should always be refrigerated, with the cap closed tightly.

which the body was overreacting. Although she had seen numerous specialists and was constantly prescribed creams for her skin and sprays for her nose, nobody had made a connection between these two conditions. I felt that both of these inflammatory conditions could be cooled down with a healthy dose of omega-3 fatty acids.

Unlike some of my patients, Adrienne *did* eat fish, but the fish were not especially high in the omega-3s. She loved flounder and fishsticks made from cod. Both, unfortunately, were not choice fish for replacing essential oils, and frying the fishsticks destroyed any other benefits.

Our first step was to change the kind of fish she ate. That was easy; she quickly began to enjoy salmon, tuna, halibut, and bluefish. I also put her on a supplementary three grams of fish oil a day, in addition to licorice extract. Licorice is a powerful anti-inflammatory herb that boosts adrenal function and is an important part of many Chinese medicinal treatments for skin disorders.

Within three months on my program, her skin improved to the point where she was comfortable wearing short-sleeved shirts again and was confident enough to resume dating.

Our bodies have an almost effortless ability to absorb omega-3s. Every other fat requires enzymes to activate it. This is not the case with fish oils.

However, the secret of omega-3s is that they concentrate and accumulate over time. If your diet has been rich in omega-3s for years, you will have an equally rich store of these essential fatty oils in your cells. If, however, your diet has been deficient, and your body has been forced to use

HOW MUCH SHOULD I TAKE?

For General Health

2-3 6-oz. servings of fish per week, or 1 tablespoon of flaxseed oil daily in salad dressing

Divided doses after meals

Special Conditions

Arthritis	3,000-4,000 mg/day
Inflammatory bowel disease	1,000-8,000 mg/day
Heart disease	1,000-6,000 mg/day
Blood pressure	3,000-4,000 mg/day
Diabetes	3,000-4,000 mg/day
PMS	2,000-4,000 mg/day
Asthma	3,000-4,000 mg/day
Eczema/Seborrhea	3,000-4,000 mg/day
Raynaud's disease	3,000-4,000 mg/day

The above dosages are based on a fish oil formulation containing at least 300 mg of EPA, 200 mg of DHA, and 190 mg of other omega-3 fatty acids, per 1,000 mg capsule. Always purified or pharmaceutical strength.

other fats (and to utilize precious enzymes in an attempt to convert them), you will need time in order to bring yourself back into balance.

Understanding fish oils helps us to peer into the very inner workings of each cell in our body. I feel there is a certain ancient mystery about omega-3s—they are a link in the vast arc of time, a reminder of the change that occurred eons ago when we moved from sea to land yet retained this very important need for this essential oil. Omega-3s are indeed the firefighters from the ancient oceans—they can work marvels, and the only thing they ask of you is patience and time.

5

Isoflavones: Mother Nature's Healing Hormone

Does your food talk to you? Maybe it doesn't audibly yell at you or whisper sweet nothings in your ear; but the fruit, meats, and vegetables that we eat every day have a message to tell us. We are only now beginning to realize what birds, bees, and even other cultures have known for centuries: help for many of our society's most debilitating illnesses can be found right in the flora and fauna around us. In fact, scientists have come to realize that we share much in common with our foods. They are made of the same building blocks we are. Plants, for instance, often contain hormonelike substances that are similar to our own. They, like us, need to protect themselves from predators and to kill bacteria and fungi. They need to reproduce, just as we do.

Did you know that plants can change their nutritional content, depending on whether we're experiencing a feast or famine? Normally, certain plants produce many hormones that enhance the fertility of the animals that eat them. However, when food is scarce in the environment, these plants somehow know to reduce their hormone levels. Research on quail and other birds has shown that their fertility cycles are controlled by the plants they feed on, which are influenced by the wetness or dryness of the season. In this way, the vegetables we consume every day give us a message, a kind of history, of the state of our environment.

Like a silent, ethereal language that unites all forms of life, the earth has developed a remarkable communication system that exchanges information about the state of the seasons and our surroundings, of environmental health risks and hazards. So the crisp lettuce, tender string beans, and tangy red peppers sitting on our plate every night are actually sending us a message that's important news about our own life cycle.

In ages past, people's dietary needs were fulfilled by what they could harvest from the soil and hunt from surrounding animal populations. Today, we live in a global community. Because we have altered our natural environment, and most of us now live in cities where we buy food at supermarkets, we are much less influenced by season, climate, or geography. This is not necessarily a bad thing. With our growing knowledge of the body and its intricate functioning, we can utilize plants and herbs from around the world to balance our hormones consciously. One of the most powerful and fascinating of plant ingredients available today are isoflavone, a plant hormone in the soybean that has been found to profoundly influence our hormone cycles and health. You may be surprised to learn just how powerful and yet gentle plant hormones are. If estrogen has been a failed miracle pill, then phytohormones (plant hormones) are the true miracles, made in nature's own garden. One of nature's most important plant hormones is found in the unglamorous little soybean. Soy contains phytoestrogens, or weak plant estrogens, such as genistein and daidzin. (Some researchers even regard them as antiestrogens because they compete with estrogens in the body, reducing the effects of our own powerful hormones.) These nutrients can reduce menopausal and PMS symptoms. Even more impressive, they can also lower the risk of heart disease, osteoporosis, and even cancer.

Sound too good to be true? Their powers lie in their gentleness and their remarkable ability to adapt to your body's particular needs. Phytoestrogens latch on to the same receptor sites as estrogen from your body and may actually help prevent hormonally linked cancers. Like a light switch, they can both turn on estrogenic effects and turn them off, depending on what your body needs. Not only can this phytoestrogen found in soy repair both the deficiency of estrogen involved in menopause and the excess that causes PMS, but exciting studies like one in the *American Journal of Clinical Nutrition* suggest that it might be an effective treatment against breast cancer. Cultures that consume a great deal of soy suffer far less heart disease and cancer. Consider the women of Okinawa, an idyllic oasis of subtropical islands four hundred miles southeast of Japan. These remarkably healthy females have less breast cancer, heart disease, and osteoporosis than any other population in the Western world. Early menopause is almost a foreign word to them, and PMS is virtually unheard of. In contrast, currently, heart disease is the number one killer of American women over fifty, and it is projected that almost 50 million will suffer from a difficult menopause by the year 2010, one out of eight will get breast cancer in their lifetimes, and one out of three women will suffer from hip fractures due to osteoporosis by the age of ninety. What secret do Okinawan women possess that protects them from the diseases so common to Westerners? The right diet.

It turns out that Okinawans eat an incredibly varied diet, and one of the most important ingredients in that diet is soy. It has the amazing ability to work subtly, without significantly altering our body's machinelike precision, yet powerfully adapting to almost any hormonal problem it finds.

The fact that isoflavones work weakly enough not to overpower our systems yet are versatile enough to both rebalance estrogen deficiencies and excess estrogen is their groundbreaking advantage. Estrogen replacement therapy (ERT) was the most common treatment for hormonally related conditions, from menopausal hot flashes to osteoporosis and heart disease. But for many, synthetic estrogens are too powerful and harmful. Women should not take them.

When I began to examine the literature on plant estrogens, I was stunned. It had to be more than coincidence that allowed us to discover the benefits of plants like soy, just as we were realizing the downsides to estrogen replacement therapy. They appear to solve some problems as synthetic estrogens. Note, for example, that while thirty-two of every one hundred thousand American women die of breast cancer every year, only nine out of one hundred Japanese women claim this fate.[1]

The baby boomer generation has begun to reach its fifties, an age for which the most frequent cause of death is malignant tumors (in 1995, out of the 376,000 people between forty-five and sixty-four who died, almost 132,000—nearly one-third) suffered cancer-related deaths. Yet hormone-replacement therapy, which was most commonly prescribed drug treatment in America and friend to over nine million women, has actually been reported by sources like the *New England Journal of Medicine* to *increase* the risk of breast cancer, not to mention others, such as endometrial or uterine cancer. The synthetic estrogens used in replacement therapy are incredibly strong, bombarding our internal receptors with too many hormones.

Even if you were not on such treatment, the influence of synthetic estrogen is in the fruits we eat, the steaks we grill, the milk we drink, even the plastics we use in objects too countless to name. One of the most potent sources of environmental estrogens are pesticides, which act as powerful pseudohormones in our bodies, disrupting our endocrine systems and even overpowering our own estrogen. We're particularly vulnerable to these chemicals in the United States, where the almost 371,000 tons of pesticides contaminating our food and environment in 1991 crowned us the king of pollution. That's three times the amount of pesticide that Spain, the second worst offender on the pollution list, was guilty of using. Not only do these excess estrogens stimulate cancer growth, but they are wreaking havoc with our fertility by insidiously derailing the natural hormonal balance that we normally maintain. Men's sperm counts have plummeted by nearly 50 percent in the last sixty years, and 10 million American women are currently infertile. Such couples have no idea that the root of their problems might be in the very diet they ingest, the very air they breathe. We can protect ourselves from these poisons. We can avoid synthetic hormones. The new answer: eat foods rich in isoflavones, such as soy milk, soybeans, or tofu, and you, too, can derive the benefits of this subtly powerful phytoestrogen. Isoflavones has been nature's hormone for thousands of years. Maybe it's time we paid attention to it.

The Miracles Soy Can Make

There is an exciting, rapidly growing body of literature on the benefits of soy and its phytoestrogenic powers. Most astounding is the fact that one dietary product can eliminate so many of the well-known, sometimes lethal, diseases that particularly plague women:

Cancer: Soy shows an exciting ability to decrease the risk of cancer. The *Journal of Nutrition*, for example, reported that soy supplements can suppress carcinogenesis and lower cancer-related deaths. An intriguing study in the *American Journal of Clinical Nutrition* shows that soy protein can reduce the frequency of menstrual cycles by increasing the length of the follicular phase. This can decrease the risk of breast cancer, since more menstrual cycles lead to more estrogen production, which in turn promotes the growth of cancer in breast cells to which the hormone has attached. Isoflavones, specifically, packs a pretty powerful estrogen punch: a study from the University of Alabama showed that the plant hormone reduced skin cancer in lab animals by 50 percent. In humans, too, doses of the phytoestrogen have been found to inhibit breast cell tumor growth, reports the journal *Carcinogenesis*, which is devoted to researching the development of cancer and tumors. And a study in the journal *Breast Cancer Research and Treatment* concluded that phytoestrogens could be safely used in place of tamoxifen to treat breast cancer. Finally, genistein can help prevent excessive new blood vessel growth. Cancerous tumors grow by creating a rich network of new blood vessels. By inhibiting this ability, genistein effectively slows cancer down.

Heart Disease: Heart disease is the number one killer of women over the age of fifty. Women seem to lose resistance to heart disease as the years increase, and it kills more women than all the types of cancer combined. A large body of evidence indicates that soy can reduce cholesterol levels, thereby lowering the risk of heart disease. A study in the *New England Journal of Medicine* found that consuming soy protein significantly decreased serum concentrations of triglycerides and

LDL (low density lipoprotein), or bad cholesterol. A recent study of sixty-six postmenopausal females with excessive cholesterol showed that taking soy protein lowered blood cholesterol, thus decreasing risk of cardiovascular disease. Even more promising, a number of clinical studies demonstrate that soy proteins may have other cardiovascular benefits. The *Journal of Nutrition* also reports that genistein may be effective therapy against vascular disease, by preventing damage to special endothelial cells that line our blood vessels.

MENOPAUSE: Menopause today is often called an estrogen-deficiency state. Menopause, a gradual process that usually begins for women around age fifty, is often characterized by hot flashes, vaginal dryness, and sleep disturbances. I consider isoflavones to be the best and safest treatment for such problems. New controlled clinical studies in several countries demonstrate that soy has been effective in controlling negative menopausal symptoms, and a study of nine woman taking soy daily for three months also saw reduced hot flashes as well as other menopausal symptoms.

OSTEOPOROSIS: The seeds of osteoporosis—the thinning of bones—are planted in a woman's teenage years. A diet low in calcium can lead to weakened bones and devastating fractures by the age of thirty-five. The high amounts of caffeine, salt, and carbonated beverages in our diets don't help bone strength, either. Over a million bones are fractured a year in women over the age of fifty-five, and there are 150,000 hip fractures every year. The chance of dying from complications three months after a hip fracture is 20 percent. Encouraging studies in both humans and animals confirm that we can use soy as prevention against bone loss and perhaps as a means of reversing low bone density. In women with low bone mass, preliminary data show that dietary supplements of soy milk seem to promote bone recovery. Isoflavones have been shown to prevent bone loss. In a study of postmenopausal women over a six-week period, soy protein supplements increased bone mineral content and density in the lumbar spine, supporting soy's potential for improving skeletal health in women at risk.

THYROID: The *Journal of Nutrition* reported that genistein was able to increase blood levels of the thyroid hormone thyroxin, in animal studies. This may have implications for patients with thyroid deficiencies and merits more research.

ESTROGEN: FIRST VIOLIN IN THE BODY'S ORCHESTRA

Before I tell you more about soy and the wonders it has worked for some of my patients, I'm going to talk more about estrogen. You need to understand the power and perils of estrogen and just how it works before you, like me, will become a convert to isoflavones.

Estrogen is an essential hormone that we synthesize naturally. Cells in every part of the body contain receptors that attract estrogen molecules floating through our bloodstream. Like a key fitting into a lock, these receptors are specially designed so that only estrogen is able to attach to them. When the hormone and its receptor are bound together, important events are triggered—from the development of breasts and curves at puberty to bone growth and bone density throughout life.

Both men and women utilize estrogen, but women use much more. Estrogen assumes special importance in females because their reproductive process is complex and involved. The miraculous ability to conceive, nourish, and finally give birth to a new life requires a delicate, finely orchestrated balance between hormones, glands, and organs. Hormones such as estrogen, testosterone, progesterone, FSH (follicle stimulating hormone), and LH (luteinizing hormone) all come into play in this orchestral suite. In females, hormone levels rise and fall according to the phase of the menstrual cycle, which ultimately signals the uterus to house and sustain a fetus for nine months of pregnancy. An LH surge is crucial for implantation of the fertilized egg, estrogen is needed for building up the uterine lining, and progesterone is needed to maintain the lining during pregnancy and ultimately to promote the return of the next menstrual cycle.

You may be wondering why estrogen can be a factor in debilitating diseases such as osteoporosis, ovarian cysts, or breast cancer when the hormone is a natural product of the body. How can something we produce ourselves work against our health?

It's the unique intricacy and precision of the female reproductive

HORMONES AND MEN

Although women undergo more complex monthly reproductive cycles, men still depend on hormones to maintain fertility and reproductive function. The hormones FSH and LH are secreted by the pituitary gland and directly affect sperm production. In addition to testosterone, they are important in regulating hormonal feedback cycles in the reproductive organs.

Contrary to popular belief, estrogen is not just a female hormone. Both men and women synthesize and have receptors for estrogen. Estrogen has even been found to prevent prostate cancer. In fact, the unhealthy environmental estrogens that wreak havoc with the female body are just as dangerous for men because they block receptors for the male hormone, androgen, and counteract testosterone's effects. Dioxins, found in pesticides, have been shown to reduce testosterone levels in men who eat foods bearing these chemicals. For this reason, adding phytoestrogens to a healthy diet may be just as important for men as for women.

system that leaves women susceptible to a whole range of illnesses that men don't experience—such as yeast infections, PMS, vaginitis, menopausal symptoms, cancer of the cervix, ovaries, uterus, and breasts—and those men experience less frequently, such as urinary tract infections, thyroid diseases, and even autoimmune diseases like lupus. Many of these illnesses stem from the difficulty in keeping one specific hormone at just the right level—you guessed it, estrogen.

Estrogen: Lifesaver?

Estrogen was at one time the most popularly prescribed drug. Forty percent of American menopausal women were on hormone-replacement therapy, whether conjugated estrogens or synthetic hormones in the form of pills, patches, or creams. Estrogen prescriptions more than doubled between 1982 and 1992. Conjugated estrogen, made from the urine of pregnant horses, was the most common estrogen treatment and

THE LATEST ESTROGEN DISCOVERY

Very recently, estrogen has been thrust even further under the spotlight with a new discovery about its effects. It has long been known that estrogen could be taken up by a certain kind of receptor in our bodies called the alpha receptor. Although these receptors are located on cells all over the body, they tend to be focused in the breasts and ovaries.

Now, however, scientists have determined that there is a second type of estrogen receptor—the beta receptor. Not only are beta receptors found all over the body, they're specifically found in places where alphas are not. This means that estrogen could have effects more far-reaching than we've ever dreamed.

This revelation could give us more insight into estrogen's role in men. Estrogen, for example, has been found to help stem prostate cancer; could the hormone be working undetected at beta receptors, where we hardly expected to look? Could there be a whole new class of drugs that improve men's health by working at these newfound beta receptors? This new discovery has staggering ramifications for the medical community.

the best-selling drug in America. I understood all the excitement. Estrogen strengthened bones, dilates and strengthens blood vessels, and even reduces heart disease, according to the *New England Journal of Medicine*. In a study of Swedish women, hormone replacement decreased the incidence of strokes and reduced blood pressure. In fact, a ten-year study of 120,000 nurses found that postmenopausal women taking estrogen reduced their risk of heart disease by half. Hormone replacement begun at menopause had been shown to cut the risk of hip fractures by up to 50 percent. Women taking estrogen for more than ten years had a 50 percent decreased risk of colon cancer.

With so many health benefits to gain from estrogen, it almost seemed like a crime to ignore its powers. You might have been tempted, after reading about its widespread effects, to run out and ask your doctor to prescribe it. But, buyer, beware. Beneath the attractive data on estrogen-replacement therapy lies more data that was not so pretty. And knowing that data might just have saved your life. Estrogen replacement is a tale of modern medicine gone wrong.

. . . Or Cancer in a Pill?

Conjugated estrogen's status as the best-selling drug in America implied that estrogen replacement therapy must be a safe, accepted treatment for the many ailments that women must face in their lifetimes. That was not so. Estrogen treatment truly had a dark side.

First, estrogen was a long-term prescription. In order to gain some of its benefits, you needed to be on the hormone for years. To help prevent osteoporosis, a woman must take the hormone continuously for years after menopause. But experts agree that hormone replacement may not be enough to avoid the disease. And this preventive action will not necessarily stop a hip fracture from taking place in later years. Estrogen does not replace bone, it simply slows its loss, and once estrogen is stopped, bone loss proceeds at its usual pace. So by the time a woman reaches age seventy-five, when she is most vulnerable to fractures, it may not matter whether she has taken conjugated or synthetic estrogen treatments.

Similarly, estrogen's cardiovascular effects disappeared as soon as you stopped taking them. Up to 90 percent of women are expected to experience some form of fibrocystic breast disease, and they may find that estrogen worsens these conditions as well. And then there's cancer. Studies showed that women taking conjugated estrogen for at least six years have up to a 40 percent increased risk of ovarian cancer; that increase soars to 70 percent when they've been taking the hormone for more than eleven years. And a recent article in the *New England Journal of Medicine* reported that estrogen-replacement therapy significantly increased the risk of breast cancer; according to *Oncology News*, the treatment doubles your likelihood of breast cancer.

The Knight in Soy Armor

You don't want to risk heart attacks, hot flashes, and hips that shatter like glass. On the other hand, you don't want to risk losing a breast or, worse, dying of cancer. Newer anticancer drugs, among them tamoxifen, can be life saving and, in recent, widely publicized studies have been shown to reduce the risk of breast cancer recurrence by 35 percent. Yet tamoxifen has also been reported by the *Journal of the National Cancer Institute* to increase the incidence of colon cancer. A crop of new so-called designer estrogens, which target specific estrogen receptors in the body while leaving others untouched, are now being studied and may offer even greater protection than tamoxifen, with less risk. Even so, we still don't know the long-term impact of such drugs, and they do have side effects.

And, as I stated earlier, common pesticides like pentachlorophenol (PCP) and dioxins contain halogenated hydrocarbons that mimic estrogen's effects on the body. At least 40 percent of the pesticides currently used are suspected to be endocrine disruptors. Fruits like grapes and strawberries, which are imported, are more likely to bear multiple pesticides as well as outlawed pesticides like DDT. Most cattle and poultry are fed hormones to make them fatter and "healthier." Even thalides, which are used to make plastics, can be estrogenic.

Women today are caught in a bewildering whirlwind of statistics and health risks. Here's where soy can come to the rescue. Remember, soy contains nature's plant version of estrogen. It's gentle but effective. And it has helped many of my patients.

Janet Sterling came to me in a state of panic. A fifty-four-year-old freelance writer and mother of three, she was distressed by the literature on hormone-replacement therapy. She already ate a balanced vegetarian diet and enjoyed speed walking and karate in her spare time. Because her mother had had osteoporosis, Janet was worried about her own future health. She asked for a bone density test, and results showed that her density already fell one standard deviation below normal, placing her at risk for bone fracture. Her doctor had been a big proponent of estrogen-replacement therapy and practically insisted that she take a prescription for Premarin, the most popular estrogen treatment. However, breast cancer ran in her family.

"Tell me there's something else I can do," she pleaded. "I've read so many studies on estrogen, and there's no way I can take a pill that may cause me to get cancer. I've had friends with cancer, and they've gone through hell."

She was right to worry about breast cancer. Women on hormone-replacement therapy for five to nine years had a 59 percent increased risk of breast cancer.

Isoflavones were the perfect solution for her concerns while protecting her from breast cancer. I recommended 500 mgs per day. That's the minimum amount needed to make a difference in your physiology. But any amount of estrogen could be dangerous, so we had to be careful. A cupful of tofu is said to contain the same amount of isoflavones, and I recommend generous portions of soymilk and tofu as well, if patients enjoy eating it. Some of my patients love soy products, and make everything from stir-fried tofu to tofu "scrambled eggs" and tofu "whipped cream," while others can't stand the taste of soy and prefer to take the powder alone.

I put Janet on a number of other natural nutrients as well, like boron, calcium, and magnesium, all of which enhance bone health. A high soy diet and phytoestrogen supplements, however, are the stars of my hormone program. A follow-up test one year later showed a definite improvement in her bone density. Now Janet totes a soy drink with her as she goes off to karate class. Her progress has been excellent.

Isoflavones: A Kinder, Gentler Alternative

Soy subtly sways the body into health. Soy-based foods like tofu contain isoflavones, which are thought to be the driving force behind soy's healing effects. When we eat tofu or drink soy milk, isoflavones are converted into weak estrogens by our intestinal flora. Amazingly, phytoestrogens are gentle and sensitive enough to act both as estrogens and as antiestrogens. If there is too much estrogen coursing through your body, the phytoestrogens can balance it out by binding to all available receptor sites. The receptors respond to the phytoestrogens, which exert only a mild effect. Excess estrogen then passes out of the body as waste. On the other hand, if your body lacks estrogen, then phytoestrogens stimulate estrogen receptors effectively but gently. It's the amazing double action of soy that allows it to counteract both the excess estrogen that can hasten breast cancer and the estrogen deficiency that aggravates osteoporosis.

One caveat: although soy is usually beneficial, in some cases it should be regarded with caution. For instance, for someone with an active malignancy such as breast cancer, soy should be used under a knowledgeable doctor's supervision, since it *does* possess estrogenic properties, and people with rapidly progressive tumors that are strongly stimulated by estrogen might choose to limit dietary sources of hormones. Such patients would want to proceed with caution and discuss this thoroughly with their doctor.

The *Journal of the Dietetic Association* notes that the philosophy that foods can be useful beyond their nutritive benefits is gaining acceptance in the medical community. Instead of taking medication for the rest of your life, consider the natural benefits of plants and herbs that can relieve the main diseases facing women today, just by being added to the diet.

How Isoflavones Helped Real Women

The pain of menopause brought Mrs. Pauline Carter to my office. Mrs. Carter was a fifty-three-year-old housewife who absolutely hated going to the

DRINK TILL YOU DROP

Can alcohol affect the level of estrogen in your body? Yes and no. A study in the *American Journal of Clinical Nutrition* reported some fascinating links between alcohol and hormones. When one to two ounces of alcohol is consumed, no changes are found in the levels of estrogens naturally occurring in the body. However, the level of estrogens from birth control pills or hormone-replacement therapy—in other words, estrogens from outside the body—are indeed affected. These estrogens, whether conjugated or synthetic, increase two to three times. I consider that an alarming interaction, and it is probably due to the fact that these estrogens are usually too powerful and do not really replicate the body's own normal hormones. That's one more reason I prefer using natural sources of estrogen, from plants, whenever possible.

doctor. She had finally been forced to see a physician two years earlier, however, when she started experiencing hair thinning as well as menopausal symptoms like acne and hot flashes. This doctor started Mrs. Carter on hormone-replacement therapy, which caused her to gain sixty pounds. Mrs. Carter loved to travel, but her new weight and uncomfortable symptoms turned even the south of France into a painful experience.

I showed Mrs. Carter the results from a group of studies at Tufts University in Boston, which showed a decrease in symptoms over a twelve-week period in women eating a soy bar containing fairly small amounts of phytoestrogen.

The first and most important step in reducing her menopausal symptoms, I told her, would be to change her diet. I talked with her at length about the benefits of natural plant estrogens, informing her about their gentle methods of blocking the excess estrogen from the receptors in her body. Not only would this new diet expose her to milder hormones, it would allow her to lose weight. That, in turn, would lower her own estrogen levels, because body fat is associated with estrogen production in the body.

Mrs. Carter willingly agreed to any program that would help her lose the weight and alleviate her menopausal symptoms. I eliminated bagels, caffeine, and her daily cigarettes and substituted tofu, herbal tea, and soy milk, along with a generous daily serving of genistein in powder form. After a month, Mrs. Carter returned to my office in despair. "I thought this diet would work," she exclaimed. "You promised it would!"

"I believe it will," I said. "But foods need time to exert their influence on your body. Be patient and allow their healing effects to work slowly. Remember, the studies watched women for three months."

Over the next three months, as I predicted, Mrs. Carter finally began to notice the results of her dietary changes. Her hot flashes and mood swings diminished, and she began to feel stronger. I then started her on calcium and magnesium to strengthen her bones, along with a B vitamin, biotin, which is known to combat hair loss. So far she has lost thirty pounds and is feeling much better.

Unlike Mrs. Carter, whose menopause deprived her of estrogen, Kristy Novak had way too much of the hormone in her system. She was on the birth control pill, and she also spent many evenings drinking beer and wine with her friends. A nineteen-year-old college student, Kristy suffered from PMS as well as painful cystic breasts. In fact, during the week before her period, her breasts hurt so much she couldn't wear a bra or sleep on her stomach. Isoflavones seemed the perfect choice for treatment.

It wasn't easy for Kristy to agree to go off the birth control pill. She enjoyed the spontaneity the pill offered in her relationship with her first serious boyfriend. She also found it difficult to turn down pizza and beer most nights, and she told me she was embarrassed when her friends saw her eating tofu. "They say, 'How can you eat that stuff, it's disgusting!'" She didn't mind taking isoflavones in powder form, but sometimes in the mornings she woke late and rushed off to classes and work as a waitress and forgot her good intentions. "It's weird, but I'm not as tired in the mornings. And my breasts don't hurt as much before my period." Impressed with the improvements, she slowly changed her diet, adding more and more soy. She discovered that if she blended silken tofu with cocoa powder, vanilla, and honey, she had a concoction that was almost like ice cream. "A very strange kind of ice cream, I admit," she said. She also agreed to make suitable birth control choices.

Julie Thomas was a fifty-seven-year-old actress who visited my office to rid herself of postmenopausal symptoms. She'd suffered from PMS throughout her life, and she was now experiencing crippling joint pains, stiffness, and alternating chills and hot flashes due to menopause. She also noticed swelling in her legs and ankles. She finally swept into my office one day, tired of the burden these symptoms were placing on her current off-Broadway role, and asked for my assistance.

"I could deal with this thing if it wasn't so unpredictable," she boomed, literally clutching her velvet opera cape around her shoulders. But even as we sat discussing her treatment options, she pulled a Chinese fan out of her purse and started waving it as a bead of sweat ran down one cheek. "See, it's happening now. I'm sick of it!"

Clearly, her estrogen levels were low, and I started her on a varied treatment program to relieve her painful symptoms. I used a group of nutrients to enhance her hormone levels, such as isoflavones, licorice, magnesium, and calcium. I also added the herb black cohosh, which is high in phytoestrogens. Although isoflavones are my favorite phytoestrogens, these other mild plant estrogens offer additional support to balance bodily hormone levels gently and safely. Despite the severity of her problems, this natural program worked well. Julie barely noticed the changes at first. Hot flashes are one of the most common and uncomfortable symptoms of menopause, and studies seem to show that soy products treat them better than other symptoms. A United Kingdom study of twenty-seven menopausal females found that a soy diet caused a significant reduction in hot flashes. Indeed, three months after her first visit to my office, Julie woke up one day and suddenly realized that her symptoms had been diminished for almost a week. The natural estrogens I had given her worked.

"They always say nothing happens when you go to the doctor's office," she told me, "but this time they were wrong!" I never found out who "they" were, but I was happy to accept complimentary tickets to her play, where I saw for myself how phytoestrogens had restored Ida to her dramatic best.

Susan Nicolson, forty-one years old, didn't originally make an appointment with me to talk about hormonal issues. She first came in because of a terrible festering spider bite on her left leg. After I quickly treated her with antibiotics, vitamin C, and topical aloe, her leg began to heal. On her follow-up visit, however, she told me of her ongoing problems with PMS. Susan held a very unique and fascinating job: she organized and performed wedding ceremonies. Couples hired her to locate a meaningful, peaceful spot for the big event. Unfortunately, Susan's PMS caused her aggravating cramps. Her symptoms, she assured me, did not alter her ability to offer words of hope for the future; however, it would be nice to feel better. Susan was already a healthy eater, but I started her on a number of supplements, including isoflavones such as genistein and black cohosh.

Six months later, Susan came back to see me. The scar on her leg was healing nicely, and her cramps had disappeared a while ago, she told me with a smile.

"It was amazing," she reflected. "The other day, I was going through a ceremony and realizing that I hadn't had a PMS symptom in months." Like Julie, Susan's recovery was so natural and gentle that she barely even noticed when it had happened.

Isoflavones and Fatigue

Not every patient who benefits from phytoestrogens comes to me complaining of PMS or menopause. Louise Marsden, a fifty-seven-year-old legal secretary, told me she was always completely exhausted. She was caring for her sick mother and was involved in a turbulent romantic relationship. Work at her law firm was equally tense. She found herself constantly sleeping through her morning alarm, and arriving at work late did not exactly please her demanding boss. "It's just too much," she whispered to me, shaking her head. "Too much."

Louise had a thyroid deficiency—which could very well have caused her fatigue—along with low bone density. Her previous doctor had recommended Fosamax, a medication to stimulate bone repair, but she was adamant about not using any drugs. I told her that many of her symptoms, as widely varied as they were, could be helped by isoflavones. The nutrient has been shown to increase and boost bone density and ease symptoms like hot flashes and fatigue. These supplements appeared to reduce her hot flashes and depression, and her fatigue has decreased, though she still complains of tiredness and stress.

The Realities of Radically New Treatments

It's important to remember that, despite the exciting studies, phytoestrogens are still new to the scientific community. Plant hormone therapies have not been researched as thoroughly as synthetics, and we don't yet know if the noted benefits of plant hormones outweigh the long-term risks. They do seem like safe, effective remedies for the hormone-related diseases that plague modern life. In some cases, I've found that when dietary supplements are not enough, replacement therapy is needed for complete recovery. Even so, I try to stress the importance of natural estrogen replacement therapy over the synthetic or conjugated forms.

June Wharton was one woman who tried dietary phytoestrogens before turning to natural estrogen replacement therapy. A fifty-five-year-old psychologist, June frequently suffered from viruses, sore throats, and muscle aches. She had also been on antidepressants for the last ten years. When menopause had struck three years earlier, several doctors had recommended that she get hormone-replacement therapy. June, however, was very concerned about the risks that such therapy entailed, especially since her father had had colon cancer.

I treated June's fatigue with coenzyme Q_{10} and tyrosine, both of which have been shown to enhance energy. I added isoflavones, dong quai, and black cohosh to help balance her hormones. June was an informed patient: she had already read studies on the Internet like one in the *Journal of Nutrition* showing that in addition to relieving menopausal symptoms, plant hormones are associated with low cancer mortality rates, not only for breast cancer but for colon cancer as well.

Isoflavones: Back to the Future

Since early humans first roamed the earth, plants and herbs have learned how to propagate life and maintain a balance of vitamins, minerals, and nutrients. Although we depend on scientists and laboratories to produce the cutting edge in health treatments and cures, it's important to remember how difficult it can be to improve on nature's genius. Now that we know that hormone receptors are in almost every part of the body and may be far more prevalent and varied than we thought, I am more excited than ever about plants like the soybean. As we learn to join our scientific and nutritional knowledge, we stand at the beginning of an improved new era in medicine. We do have the potential to be healthier than we dare to believe.

HOW MUCH SHOULD I TAKE?

Isoflavones
For General Health
Isoflavones food per day

Daily in the morning
Special Conditions

200 mg-1 gm Per Day
Divided Doses

Note of Caution
Individuals with a history of cancer or a family history of cancer should consult a physician before embarking on a supplement program. Estrogen, whether natural or synthetic, can promote cancer in estrogen-sensitive individuals.

6

Coenzyme Q_{10}: Universal Energy Source

Few supplements have faced such a storm of controversy as coenzyme Q_{10}, which was first discovered in 1957. What is a coenzyme? A coenzyme is technically not a vitamin—it is a substance that enhances the action of other enzymes. And an enzyme is a protein that catalyzes chemical changes in other substances, remaining unchanged by the process. Depending on who you ask, coQ_{10}, as it's more commonly known, is scam or savior. Take the Texas Health Department, for example. For reasons unknown, in 1991, it snatched every single bottle of coQ_{10} out of every health food store in the state—as if it were an illegal drug. Within weeks, however, many angry patients and customers protested to Congress, demanding to know where the nutrient had gone and why it had been taken away. Ultimately, the health department reversed its decision, and coQ_{10} was returned to the shelves, but not before causing an uproar.

At the eye of the storm is a compound found in every cell in the body except red blood cells. Peter Mitchell, Ph.D., won the Nobel Prize in chemistry when he discovered coQ_{10} and its role in each cell's energy metabolism. CoQ_{10} (pronounced coh-cue-ten) has been the subject of impressive studies in Japan and Europe, where it is routinely used as therapy in the treatment of heart disease, especially congestive heart failure. In the United States, however, coQ_{10} has had a far different history. Although more than fifty major medical studies have been published and at least eight international symposia have been held on coQ_{10}, it has somehow escaped mention in most nutritional or medical textbooks. It has been almost completely ignored by the American medical community.

The Japanese currently manufacture all the coQ_{10} in the world, and some people have even argued that trade issues have prevented this supplement from gaining a stronger foothold in the United States. CoQ_{10} has an excellent safety history, and scientific findings suggest that the possibility of further applications should be explored.

The Truth about CoQ_{10}

CoQ_{10} has been described as a biochemical spark plug. It is a naturally occurring substance that our body produces. Every second, energy factories called mitochondria are at work inside each of our 30 trillion cells, turning oxygen into pure energy. CoQ_{10} is instrumental in this process. Not only does coQ_{10} assist in fueling the body, it is also a uniquely powerful antioxidant. In fact, a 1991 study showed that coQ_{10} is better at preventing the dangerous free radical damage caused to arteries by bad cholesterol than vitamin E, an antioxidant known to protect the heart. Like vitamin E, coQ_{10} is astoundingly helpful in treating and preventing all kinds of cardiovascular problems, from arrhythmias to heart attacks, and even congestive heart failure. Karl Folkers, a scientist at the University of Texas at Austin, is the father of coQ_{10} research, and for the past twenty years he has consistently proven in dozens of groundbreaking studies that coQ_{10} protects the heart from failure by keeping its energy levels high. But this nutraceutical doesn't just keep the heart pumping. Through its profound energizing ability, coQ_{10} can help treat illnesses as diverse as diabetes, chronic lung disease, and gum disease. One study even shows that the coenzyme can reduce tumors associated with breast cancer. For those of us who are in good health, coQ_{10} can improve fitness by increasing our exercise endurance.

What CoQ_{10} Can Do for You

CoQ_{10} is ubiquitous. It works everywhere in the body to increase energy and fend off disease:

HEART: If you have any problems with your heart, from angina to coronary artery disease, coQ_{10} is a perfect supplement for you. A study by Dr. Karl Folkers found that 72 percent of individuals with cardiovascular ailments had a coQ_{10} deficiency. This nutrient is particularly noteworthy as a treatment for heart failure, perhaps because a depletion of coQ_{10} may lead to lowered cellular energy and a weakened heart. A 1985 study discussed in *Medical World News* reported that of thirty-four patients with congestive heart failure, 82 percent showed improved cardiac function after taking 100 milligrams of coQ_{10} a day for six weeks.

CoQ_{10} has also been shown to be beneficial for patients taking cholesterol-lowering drugs, such as lovastatin, which actually interfere with the body's coQ_{10} production.

DIABETES: This illness arises from the body's inability to process carbohydrates properly, which can lead to abnormally high blood sugar levels. Japanese researchers have found that coQ_{10} supplements of just 30 to 60 milligrams a day were able to decrease significantly the fasting blood sugar levels in diabetic patients.

BREAST CANCER: A 1994 study in *Biochemical and Biophysical Research Communications* reported that in thirty-two patients suffering from high-risk breast cancer and treated with 90 milligrams of coQ_{10} daily, six had a partial tumor regression. The researchers then increased one patient's dosage to 390 milligrams a day, and within two months, mammography confirmed that the tumor had disappeared. Not only does coQ_{10} have promising implications for breast cancer treatment, but studies show that coQ_{10} can eliminate the heart-harmful side effects of adriamycin, an anticancer drug, without altering its therapeutic benefits.

HYPERTENSION: A 1994 study of patients with high blood pressure demonstrated that taking coQ_{10} in addition to antihypertensive medications over a period of approximately four months reduced the need for such drugs.

PHYSICAL PERFORMANCE: In a study of healthy males twenty years of age and older, 60 milligrams of the coenzyme administered daily for eight weeks significantly improved exercise capacity.

CHRONIC OBSTRUCTIVE PULMONARY DISEASE: A 1993 study in *Clinical Investigations* reported that eight weeks of coQ_{10} supplementation at 90 milligrams a day notably improved respiratory performance in individuals with chronic lung diseases such as emphysema.

PERIODONTAL DISEASE: Low levels of coQ_{10} have been found in the gum tissue of patients with periodontal disease, and similar studies indicate that patients with gingivitis saw a reduction in their condition after taking coQ_{10} at 50 milligrams a day for three weeks.

CHOLESTEROL: When LDL cholesterol becomes oxidized, it creates free radicals, which collide with—and cause serious damage to—the walls of the arteries. CoQ_{10}, a proven antioxidant, protects LDL from this harmful peroxidation process. Moreover, a 1992 study suggests that coQ_{10} can regenerate another antioxidant, vitamin E, which is also particularly good at preventing the oxidation of cholesterol.

CoQ_{10} Keeps the Heart Ticking

Philip Appleton was in precarious health. Although he could still go bowling with his pals, travel with his family, and live a basically normal life, the apparent exuberance of this seventy-four-year-old was misleading. For Philip had a history of high blood pressure and congestive heart failure, and in the past decade he had succumbed to adult-onset diabetes as well. He was also prone to back pain and heartburn.

Because of his serious list of ailments, Philip was on a host of medications, including Vasotec for high blood pressure and Glyburide for diabetes. As if a feeble heart and weakened arteries were not enough, Philip had been hospitalized eight years earlier for appendicitis. Shortly after his release from the hospital, he had developed a sign of heart failure, called pitting edema, in which fluid accumulates in the lower extremities of the body because of reduced circulation. He soon developed palpitations as well, as his heart began to beat a syncopated rhythm. Diabetes can lead to silent heart attacks, in which the typical warning signs of attack—chest pains or tightness radiating down the arm—are muffled by nerve damage. It was likely that Philip had already succumbed to a silent heart attack without even realizing it.

On the Fourth of July, Philip was in charge of manning the grill for the annual family picnic in the local park. As Philip delivered each burger with a bad joke, with orders coming in fast and furious, he began to feel a tingling sensation in his chest. After a few minutes, he grew worried and sat down, asking someone else to take over at the grill. The next day, Philip visited his internist.

An angiogram revealed that two of his arteries were 50 percent blocked. Philip went to several doctors to confirm the diagnosis, but they were all in disagreement on the treatment. One insisted that an angioplasty was the only procedure that would save his life, and another told him he need only follow a low-fat diet that has been proven to reverse heart disease. Philip came to me for another opinion, insisting on a natural approach.

I knew that a combination of diet and specific nutrients designed to treat each of Philip's concerns could both relieve his symptoms—including his backaches, which I suspected could be related to the angina—and eliminate many of his terrifying heart problems.

First, I put Philip on a low-carbohydrate diet to lower his high blood sugar and cholesterol. He'd been eating way too many carbohydrates, which the body metabolizes into sugar and fat. I prescribed essential fatty acids in the form of fish oil, which regulate blood sugar and thin the blood. And I rounded out Philip's program with heart-protecting magnesium, soothing aloe juice for his heartburn. And finally a number of powerful antioxidants to reduce free radical damage to the heart and arteries, including vitamin E and grapeseed extract, one of the healthy antioxidants found in grape juice and red wine.

A crucial piece of the puzzle was still missing: coQ_{10}. A report in *Alternative Medicine Review* confirmed coQ_{10} deficiency in patients with various types of cardiovascular disease. A 1991 Amsterdam study monitored a group of 180 subjects who suffered from congestive heart failure. Half took 100 milligrams of oral coQ_{10} supplements daily, and half were control subjects who did not take the supplement. All of the control patients died within five years, but those patients on coQ_{10} had a much greater rate of survival. Seventy-eight percent of the coQ_{10} patients also showed increased cardiac function. Furthermore, a Japanese study found that, in a group of patients with arrhythmias who were diabetic, coQ_{10} reduced irregular heartbeats by 85.7 percent—significant for the diabetic Philip.

A month after Philip began taking 150 milligrams a day of coQ_{10} in divided doses, he started to notice that his episodes of irregular heartbeat or PVCs (premature ventricular contractions) had diminished. His ankles swelled only occasionally, occurrences he controlled by wearing support stockings. I continue to monitor Philip closely by ensuring that he sticks to a heart-healthy diet of foods like tofu, leafy green vegetables, and fish. It's obvious that he's on the road to recovery: his triglyceride levels dropped 50 percent, from 240 to 120, and his cholesterol has gone down 20 points as well. CoQ_{10} was one of the keys to keeping his heart pumping properly.

Mighty Mitochondria

How exactly did coQ_{10} help Philip? The answer to the puzzle lies in a tiny structure called the mitochondrion, which is the energy powerhouse inside almost every single cell of your body.

When we are tired or lethargic, we often wish for newfound energy to increase our productivity. But energy is not just an amorphous life force that improves mood and helps us through the day. The process of extracting energy from food ensures that cells have the power they need to work effectively.

Aerobic respiration occurs in the mitochondrion. Mitochondria are the primary sites of oxygen use in the body and are responsible for producing most of the energy used by cells. Many cells contain more than one mitochondrion, depending on the need for energy and oxygen in that part of the body.

Certain cells in the body are extremely dense in mitochondria—liver cells contain as many as 2,200 per cell. But the heart has by far the largest number of mitochondria in its cells; 40 percent of the space within each heart cell is made up of mitochondria. This abundance of mitochondria in the heart is no coincidence. The reason? Energy is crucial to keeping our hearts beating, pumping out the steady rhythm by which we live. But the constant functioning of the heart requires an enormous amount of energy. Heart failure occurs when the heart is too weak to work properly.

HOW MUCH COQ$_{10}$ DO YOU NEED?

CoQ$_{10}$ can be found in foods like fish, eggs, spinach, broccoli, red meat, peanuts, and organ meats. Unfortunately, there is no consensus on the optimum dosage of coQ$_{10}$ necessary for good health.

A 1994 report in the *Quarterly Review of Natural Medicine* recommends an average daily dose of 30-60 milligrams a day, although studies using up to 200 milligrams a day have shown no complications. Some studies, such as those in breast cancer patients, have used up to about 400 milligrams a day. Indeed, coQ$_{10}$ seems to be a safe medication at a large range of doses. It also seems to work well in combination with other nutrients and drugs. END BOX

How CoQ$_{10}$ Restored Energy to Real People

Herbalist James Karon advised customers on the uses and benefits of plants and herbs, working out of his Greenwich Village brownstone and growing his products in his own backyard. James was both an avowed plant lover and a vegetarian, and his nutritional know-how kept him looking much younger than his sixty-seven years. When he wasn't preaching the wonders of herbs, he taught music at a local public school. On weekends, James loved to sit on his front stoop and trade stories with his neighbors or stroll to Washington Square Park and join a game of chess. All in all, James led a peaceful and fulfilling life.

Then he mysteriously began to feel exhausted, and the herbal formulas he tried didn't seem to help. He had a peptic ulcer and a history of stomach pains, so when he came to see me, I explained to him that this might be a contributing factor. Once I had conducted some tests and examined him further, more pieces fell into place. He had somewhat elevated cholesterol and triglyceride levels, an enlarged prostate gland, and mildly arthritic joints. I had no doubt that he was nonetheless vital for his age and eating well, and that most likely he was suffering the normal symptoms of aging. Even herbalists can succumb to Father Time.

Because he was facing a variety of issues, I attacked his problem from several different angles. He was already taking the herb saw palmetto for his prostate. This herb has been shown to help reduce swelling and inflammation in the prostate gland. I added the anti-inflammatory supplement glucosamine for his arthritis, and flaxseed powder to provide healthy fiber and keep his intestines functioning properly. Finally, to alleviate his fatigue, I gave him supplements of tyrosine and coQ_{10}.

Oxidative injury to body tissue can be measured by thiobarbituric acid reactive substances (TBARS). Studies show that coQ_{10} supplementation can improve TBARS levels, meaning that dangerous oxidation was reduced. CoQ_{10} has been discovered to deplete with age, so as we get older, we may need to supplement this compound to protect ourselves and feel our best.

Finally, I also advised that James eat small amounts of lean meat to increase his protein levels, which might make him feel stronger. Just two weeks after he started his new nutritional regimen, James called to inform me that he already felt reenergized. Within six months, his stomachaches were gone, and his arthritis was gradually improving. Most important, he felt like he had a new lease on life. He was once again a regular in Washington Square Park, mulling over chess moves and sharing his gift for the clarinet with others.

CoQ_{10} and Asthma

As a little boy, Mark Sherman would sit captivated in front of the TV, watching his DVD collection so many times his parents thought he'd wear out the DVDs. By the age of twenty-nine, Mark, now a production assistant, was on his way to fulfilling his dream of becoming a film director. He traveled all over the world to various location sites, which would have been very exciting had it not been for the fact that his asthma was aggravated each time he visited a new place with new allergens and a change of climate. He was allergic to aspirin (as some asthmatics are) but took it anyway for frequent headaches, and the result would be worsened asthma. On a recent job, shooting a commercial in Los Angeles, Mark experienced shortness of breath and had to take up to sixteen puffs of his inhaler to relieve his symptoms. He was also paralyzed with shakiness, anxiety, and hyperventilation.

When he returned to New York, Mark came to see me, having heard from a friend that I had a special interest in reversing asthma. After all, I'd suffered from asthma myself and reversed it through, a comprehensive approach to healing.

"The first thing you've got to do," I told him, "is cut down on your inhalers." I explained that studies have shown that taking sixteen puffs a day from an asthma inhaler can lead to sudden death. I offer a comprehensive asthma program including breathing exercises that, with practice, facilitate clear breathing. I taught him these deep-breathing exercises.

Next, I asked him to switch to a healthy diet of vegetables, whole grains, fish, lean meat, and fowl. He started taking the supplement NAC, which has been shown to reduce free radical damage that often accompanies asthma, vitamin C, as well as additional antioxidants. Finally, I prescribed coQ_{10} to round out his asthma treatment program.

From what I've observed in my practice, this nutrient helps patients control their asthma.

Mark worked so hard to follow my asthma program that within two months he was down to four puffs a day on his inhaler. He has maintained this success. With the added energy granted him by coQ_{10}, Mark even found the determination and stamina to start his own production company.

Drinking Can Make You Tired

The social hub of office culture is usually the water cooler, where people gather to gab about last night's sitcom episode or the latest office romance. Lindsey Cooper, a forty-year-old secretary, was often found at the cooler, but not because she liked to gossip. Lindsey was plagued with unquenchable thirst, and she was frightened that it might be a sign of incipient diabetes, which ran in her family.

Not only was Lindsey chronically thirsty, she was chronically fatigued and suffered from sinus congestion. I decided to address the easiest symptom first: her stuffy nose. I suspected that she had allergies; sure enough, tests revealed allergies to molds.

Luckily, Lindsey was about to move to a newly renovated apartment, and we seized the opportunity to make her home an allergen-free zone. Making sure that everything in the house was new and dry, plus giving her a dehumidifier as a housewarming present, ensured that no molds or mildew would aggravate her allergies. Within two weeks of her move to a mold-free new apartment, Lindsey's nose was clear, and she was breathing easily. More important, she began to feel hope that she might reverse her other health problems. Because she wasn't sleeping well, I used the hormone melatonin to reset her body clock, telling her to take one-half milligram a day one hour before bedtime for just a month, since the long-term effects of this circadian rhythm adjuster are still unknown. The herbs valerian and passionflower are calming and soothing, and I hoped that these would also lull Lindsey to sleep more easily. I asked her to stay away from alcohol temporarily, since alcohol has a profound negative effect on our sleep. The worse your sleep is at night, the more fatigued you are during the day, and the effects of frequent sleeplessness can quickly accumulate to lower cognitive ability and mood.

Finally, coQ_{10} revitalized Lindsey and eliminated her fatigue. At first, at 90 milligrams a day, Lindsey noticed little effect on her energy level. After I increased her daily dosage to 180 milligrams, however, Lindsey started to feel much more alive. In fact, she began to experience such an improvement in mood that her snappy temper started to mellow into a happier frame of mind. Energy is such a subjective quality that I can't be sure that coQ_{10} was the sole cause of Lindsey's new outlook or that it will work exactly the same way for everyone. For Lindsey, though, it definitely worked some mood magic.

"I wouldn't stop taking coQ_{10} for the world," she told me emphatically.

One of Lindsey's big health risks was her alcohol intake, and coQ_{10} has been shown to protect against alcohol's effects, especially in combination with a nutrient called L-carnitine. A 1993 study from Italy found that taking coQ_{10} and L-carnitine together could reduce the damage induced by chronic alcohol poisoning. It's my feeling that coQ_{10} helped Lindsey by shielding her from the effects of frequent drinking.

Quality of Life

Most of my patients wish for more energy. Our heart has long been fabled as the source of passion and emotion, and now we know that this muscle holds much of the sustaining life force that we call energy. The heart, indeed, is far more than a pump. It is actually a kind of orchestra conductor, sending out electrical signals throughout the body that keep all our cells functioning in harmony with each other.

Unfortunately, we are all susceptible to fatigue. CoQ_{10} can be very

HOW DO I KNOW COQ_{10} WORKS?

Doctors use coQ_{10} in different ways. I prescribe it for an energy boost when fatigue takes its toll on daily life. Yet energy is a very subjective concept and therefore difficult to measure, so I must rely on the testimonials of my patients to ensure that this nutraceutical is working. Cardiologists, however, use it very effectively to heal the heart, and they have more objective means by which to gauge results. Dr. Steven Sinatra, a pioneering cardiologist at Manchester Memorial Hospital in Connecticut, has seen thousands of patients with congestive heart failure in the past twenty years. Inspired by a book on coQ_{10} by Dr.

Emile Bliznakof, entitled *Miracle Nutrient* CoQ_{10}—which listed study after study in which coQ_{10} has been proven a safe and effective treatment against heart diseases like hypertension, angina, and especially heart failure—Dr. Sinatra has treated over ten thousand patients with the nutrient, and he's extremely happy with it. Dr. Sinatra even believes that coQ_{10} can be used as an aid to weight loss. This makes sense in theory, since perhaps weight gain stems in part from an inability to use energy efficiently. CoQ_{10} could facilitate energy production, thus making weight loss much easier.

Currently, the use of such nutraceuticals in hospitals is rare. Dr. Sinatra, however, is taking a stand and trying to spread the word that natural therapies can be extremely valuable adjuncts to conventional treatments, with minimal risk.

instrumental in helping almost anyone restore their vitality. Normally, we have an abundance of this nutrient, but in stressful situations, we may need to replenish our stores of coQ_{10} to recharge our bodies. Everyday pressures, common colds and viruses, and life-threatening disease all take their toll on the body, draining us of the energy needed to live. CoQ_{10} has the potential to increase quality of life and keep us at our best. CoQ_{10} works particularly well with other nutrients such as tyrosine or L-carnitine. It is time that we begin to further investigate this essential nutrient that appears to play such a vital role in keeping us energized, day in and day out.

HOW MUCH SHOULD I TAKE?

For General Health
30 mg/day (optional)
Divided doses before meals

Special Conditions

Congestive heart failure	120-180 mg/day
Angina	120-180 mg/day
Diabetes	60-120 mg/day
Chronic obstructive pulmonary disease	60-120 mg/day

Periodontal disease	60-120 mg/day
Hypertension	60-180 mg/day
Fatigue	60-180 mg/day
Asthma	60-120 mg/day

CoQ10 can be increased to 300-400 mgs per day. Consult with your physician.

7

Milk Thistle: The Liver's Best Friend

You are being poisoned. Every day your body is assaulted by countless toxins and pollutants—from the fumes of chlorine in your morning shower to foods laden with pesticides, hormones, and additives, to thousands of airborne pollutants in the air of the city or suburb where you live. The water in your shower is chlorinated and releases chlorine in the hot steam. The chemical used in dry cleaning, perchlorethylene, can cause liver damage and is so potent it has been found in apartments ten floors above dry-cleaning establishments. New cars outgas numerous toxins, which are often sealed in by drivers who close the windows and turn up the heat or air-conditioning. Vinyl chloride, a chemical used in plastics manufacturing, is known to cause liver cancer. The conveniences you take for granted every day can invisibly and relentlessly compromise your health.

And the poison isn't just coming from the outside. Bacteria in your gut and free radicals spewed out in the normal process of living poison you daily as well.

But most of the time, you hardly notice. That's because your liver, which may be the single most important organ for good health, detoxifies this constant flood of poisons. It is vital in removing parasites, bacteria, and viruses from the bloodstream. Every minute—every second—special cells in the liver are waiting to pluck out toxins from the bloodstream and destroy them. But if too many toxins are storming its castle, your liver telegraphs its stress the only way it knows how. Acne. Rashes. Itching. Headaches. Aches and pains. Fatigue. Gas and bloating. Even autoimmune disorders.

Overstressed livers are present in at least 40 percent of my patients—and often they don't know it. The liver is implicated in a much wider array of diseases than we once thought, from cancer to lupus, arthritis, Parkinson's, and some of the signs associated with aging. In fact, 80 percent of all cancers are thought to be triggered by carcinogens in the environment—carcinogens that the liver must detoxify in order to protect us. Proper liver support is crucial in any chronic illness. The good news is that your liver responds quickly to help and is the one organ in your body that can regenerate itself, even if it has been terribly damaged.

Many doctors and their patients don't recognize the profound connection between the liver and even the simplest ailments. Cybil Stevens had no idea that her adult acne was connected to liver dysfunction. A graduate student in art history at twenty-three, her face had become an unsightly battleground, pocked with acne pits and flaring up with cystic pimples that took weeks to go away. Cybil's dermatologist had prescribed Minocin, an oral tetracycline drug, for the last six months. She took 200 milligrams a day. He also gave her a topical antibiotic called Cleocin T, as well as Retin-A cream. Although these drugs helped initially, the antibiotics made her more vulnerable to yeast infections, and she still suffered from frequent breakouts. Finally, her doctor prescribed Accutane, a drug that can cause liver toxicity and is known to concentrate in tissues and remain there for years. It is an extremely potent acne medication, a last resort. In addition, her dermatologist warned her that Minocin could cause her to be photosensitive, and that she shouldn't spend much time in the sun.

It was June, the semester had just ended, and Cybil had been planning a summer out on the Jersey shore with her family. At that point, she came to me.

They say that the skin is the mirror of the soul, but the truth is, the skin is the mirror of the liver. When the liver is weak and fails to perform efficiently, toxins can pass into the bloodstream. These toxins can easily cause skin problems. I explained to Cybil that her face was like a morse code being sent out by her liver, and the code kept repeating the word "help!" The liver is the largest organ in the body, and it is involved in almost all metabolic processes. It filters a Herculean two quarts of blood every single minute. The liver is as crucial to our continued health as the heart, kidneys, and lungs. When I asked Cybil to think back about the time when her acne had first begun, she instantly said, "It was when I began graduate school two years ago." She had moved in with her boyfriend, and the relationship was stressful and punctuated by arguments. She recalled coming down with bronchitis that winter and being given three courses of antibiotics before she finally got well. In addition, she'd begun to adopt his way of eating—ordering in pizzas and downing a couple of beers each night.

The puzzle pieces began to fit. First, high levels of stress. Then, a month of antibiotics that had disrupted the balance of flora in her gut. Frequent yeast infections. Add a poor diet and nearly a year of prescription drugs. No wonder Cybil's liver was unable to do its job.

A poor diet is a frequent cause of excess stress to the liver. Any toxins that leave the gut are transported almost instantaneously into the liver, almost as if they'd been beamed up by the starship *Enterprise*, right through a special vein called the portal vein. The liver immediately has to detoxify this material. The liver produces bile, which is crucial for emulsifying fatty acids. It even produces special substances that stimulate blood clotting. The liver, along with the kidneys, acts as a superb filter for any substance that might be hazardous to the body, from drugs to chemicals, solvents, and pesticides, and even our own hormones and inflammatory chemicals.

I explained to Cybil that today, more than ever, our liver faces a hugely difficult task. And that is where milk thistle, the liver's best friend, comes into the story.

A Little Help from a Daisy

Milk thistle is a North American weed, a member of the daisy family that grows all over the United States. It has shiny dark green leaves with spiny edges and reddish purple flowers. Known as *Silybum marianum* (milk thistle), it is an extraordinary herb that powerfully protects, assists, and even regenerates the liver. In the words of Joseph Pizzorno, ND, founding president of Bastyr University in Washington State, "Milk thistle is possibly the most potent liver protective agent known. It is so effective that in experiments with mice, if milk thistle is administered within a few minutes of ingestion of the deadly *Amanita phalloides* mushroom, death is not only prevented, but little liver damage is found!"

Traditionally, when liver disease strikes, such as after an infection with hepatitis B or C, most patients are told to take medications like alpha interferon, which can cause numerous side effects, including bone marrow suppression. When steroids have been used against hepatitis, they have often proven ineffective and damaging to the immune system. Liver transplants can be life-saving; however, reinfection of the new liver usually occurs. Although not a cure, milk thistle, on the other hand, has been found to be not only rapidly effective but also safe and free of debilitating side effects.

This is why milk thistle is my centerpiece in restoring the healthy functioning of this organ. It not only protects the liver from damage, it actually stimulates the growth of healthy new cells. Amazingly, studies have shown that this humble herb can reverse liver damage, protect against hepatitis and cirrhosis, speed recovery from jaundice, and even protect laboratory animals from kidney toxicity normally caused by a potent drug. A fifteen-year study in Sweden showed that the active ingredient in milk thistle, called silymarin, protected against potentially fatal mushroom poisoning. Silymarin is now a standard part of emergency room treatment for mushroom poisoning in Europe. Another study of over 2,600 patients with liver disorders found remarkable improvement with daily doses of milk thistle extract. After two months, 63 percent of patients reported that their symptoms had completely disappeared. They no longer suffered from nausea, itching, bloating, lack of appetite, and fatigue. Laboratory tests found that elevated liver enzymes, a signal that the liver is inflamed, had decreased by an average of 40 percent. Other studies have shown equally impressive results and have confirmed the improvements with actual liver biopsies. Silymarin can protect the liver from a wide range of potential poisons, from alcohol to mushrooms to prescription drugs (without interfering with the drugs' potency).

Not surprisingly, an herb this potent has long been known to folklorists and has been in use for thousands of years. Research into its liver-protecting properties began three decades ago in Germany when the active ingredient, silymarin, was first discovered. I sometimes think of silymarin as a Secret Service agent taking a bullet for the president, because the compound binds to receptors within the liver that are vulnerable to toxins, thus preventing their damaging effects. Silymarin has been used to treat cirrhosis, hepatitis, gallstones, and skin disorders like psoriasis and acne. In fact, herbalists find it useful in any chronic illness that stresses the liver.

Silymarin in Practice

Milk thistle was a key to healing Cybil's skin. My experience has been that acne can be a sign of poor liver detoxification. Liver problems may not manifest themselves in the liver at all. Instead, they may show up in other parts of the body, where toxins congregate—like escaped convicts. One reason adolescents break out so often is because their livers are not yet accustomed to sudden hormonal surges. Cybil's physician was trying to quiet the erupting fires in her face, without understanding their source. Cybil was shutting off her security system, while the toxic bandits robbed her of essential nutrients, depriving her of her health.

I wanted to wean Cybil from her drugs, treat her for the yeast that was incubating in her gut because of constant doses of antibiotics, and support her liver function.

First, I placed her on a weeklong detoxification diet. Day one consisted entirely of vegetables; on day two, she could add rice; on day three, fruit, especially lemons as juice or on salads; and on the fourth, fish. On day five, she substituted beans for her vegetables, and on day six she was allowed to eat all the foods.

"Doctor," said Cybil, "this diet sounds like hell. Why do I have to do it?"

I explained that this short detoxification program would lay the foundation for recovery of her liver. On day one, we were removing any foods to which she might be allergic. On day two, rice would help absorb water and toxins in her gut, so the lining would not be irritated. On day three, fruits and lemon would stimulate detoxification in her liver. By day four, she was adding back protein, and on day five, fiber and vegetables like broccoli and beets, which also stimulate liver detoxification. Each day, she should consume one teaspoon of flaxseed powder in an eight-ounce glass of water. Flaxseed helps bulk up bowel movements and absorbs bacteria and toxins. It also contains healthy omega-3 oils (see chapter 4) and fibers called lignans, which are known to reduce the risk of cancer.

"All right," she agreed. "I'll tough it out."

After the weeklong detox, Cybil followed a maintenance diet that eliminated fried and excessively fatty foods, which are often hard for the liver to handle. I literally "prescribed" daily doses of the vegetables and fruits that are known to support liver detoxification, including lemons, beets, and broccoli (see Box: Phasing Your Foods). I asked her to stop consuming beer, pizza, and sugars, all of which stimulate yeast and were a staple of her diet.

Finally, and most important, we addressed Cybil's liver directly. Vitamin C, at 2,000 milligrams a day in four divided doses, was important as an antioxidant and general detoxifier. B complex, zinc, and magnesium were added because the liver needs these nutrients in order to function well. N-acetyl cysteine (NAC), a special form of an amino acid, is a powerful liver protectant, because it stimulates the liver's most powerful antioxidant, glutathione. I suggested Cybil take 250 milligrams four times a day. Most important, however, was silymarin. I prescribed 400 milligrams daily.

The rest of her story is short and sweet. She improved steadily over three months. My receptionist, Amy, didn't recognize Cybil the last time she came into the office for a consultation. Her complexion was smooth, almost flawless. She looked wonderful, thanks to silymarin, which had helped her liver to help her.

A Short Primer on the Liver

I never prescribe silymarin without addressing the liver's general health and changing my patients' diets to support liver function. Here's why:

About one-quarter of detoxification in your body occurs in the intestines. The other three-quarters occurs in the liver, and it is a stunningly complex cascade of events. The explanation that follows will probably seem complicated, but it is actually as simplified and streamlined as I can make it.

Your liver clears 99 percent of all bacteria and toxins from the blood before it enters general circulation. This is done by liver cells called Kupffer cells and hepatocytes. The Kupffer cells are actually specialized macrophages—immune system cells that engulf and destroy toxins. Kupffer cells are high-speed warriors that sit at the portal vein of the liver and engulf bacteria in less than 0.01 seconds. They release powerful inflammatory chemicals as they do so, which need to be mopped up by antioxidants. The liver's primary antioxidant is glutathione. Hepatocytes are like escorts that shuttle away small molecules not destroyed by Kupffer cells, taking them into the bile ducts. Hepatocytes are the target for most common liver viruses, including hepatitis A, B, C, D, and E, as well as Epstein-Barr, the virus responsible for mononucleosis.

When this process of liver detoxification is not functioning properly, toxins and bacteria are released back into the bloodstream, where the immune system forms antibodies to them. High levels of these antibodies have been measured in the blood of patients with hepatitis.

The liver has other weapons in its detoxification arsenal. It creates and secretes one quart of bile each day. Bile is sent to the intestines, where it is absorbed by fiber and feces and then excreted. This powerful substance also helps break down fats so they can be absorbed, increases peristaltic movement, and retards putrefaction in the elimination process. A diet high in fiber is necessary so that bile, with its river of toxins, can be bound up in feces. Otherwise, the toxins floating in bile may simply be reabsorbed into your system.

Finally, the liver uses enzymes in two powerful phases of detoxification. In phase I, many poisons and toxins—along with hormones, histamine, and other inflammatory chemicals that your own body produces—are attacked. Phase I enzymes either neutralize these compounds or break them down into other forms. These other forms are processed by phase II enzymes.

Remarkably, the liver is unique among all organs in its ability to regenerate itself. It can recover completely, even after severe damage.

A Short Guide to Phase I

Phase I detoxification involves a stunning fifty to one hundred selective enzymes, which have all been grouped together under the name cytochrome P450. Each enzyme has special gifts for detoxifying certain types of chemicals, but all the enzymes can act as pinch hitters for each other. All of us were born with different strengths and weaknesses in our P450 system. Poor nutrition and environmental toxins weaken this system. Yet some lucky individuals are born with a very strong P450 system; they are probably the ones who can, for instance, smoke a pack of cigarettes a day for decades without getting lung cancer.

Detoxification, like war, is not a benign process. Casualties mount up. When a P450 enzyme attacks a toxin, it must chemically neutralize it, or make it water soluble so the kidneys can excrete it, or temporarily convert it to an even more active chemical that can then be attacked by phase II enzymes. Just remember that every time the liver metabolizes a toxin, free radicals are generated. If the onslaught of toxins is high, so are the free radicals that are spewed out. These free radicals can damage the liver. That's how poisonous mushrooms kill you: the liver is working so fast and hard to detoxify the chemicals in the mushroom that it actually destroys itself with free radicals.

As I mentioned, the most powerful antioxidant and free radical fighter the liver has is glutathione. The liver uses glutathione in both phase I and phase II detoxification. A lack of glutathione inevitably means liver damage.

A Short Guide to Phase II

Those toxins that phase I enzymes converted into even more active chemicals—in order to prepare them for destruction by phase II enzymes—are often incredibly toxic. They can actually be carcinogenic. They must be immediately removed from the body by phase II enzymes.

Phase I and phase II must work in perfect synchronization, like acrobats on a circus trapeze. As you may have guessed, this doesn't always happen. In many of us, either phase I or phase II is overactive or underactive. In some of us, both phases are askew.

Do you wonder about the health of your liver? One key to a sluggish phase I is caffeine intolerance. Does a cup of coffee keep you up at night? An overactive phase I system will tolerate huge amounts of caffeine, so that you can drink several cups of coffee and still sleep soundly. On the other hand, if you cannot process the sulfur-containing molecules in drugs and foods well, your phase II may be underactive. Do you have trouble eating garlic? Do you react badly to sulfite food additives in wines or commercial salad bars? Suspect phase II sluggishness.

Most people are too fast in phase I and too slow in phase II. That means their own body is generating potent and damaging toxins. I utilize some simple tests that show me how strong an individual's phase I and phase II systems are. One test measures how quickly you clear caffeine from your body; caffeine is neutralized by phase I enzymes.

How to Orchestrate Phase I and Phase II

Milk thistle has potent antioxidant ability and increases the amount of glutathione in the liver. Research has indicated that silymarin has a much greater activity within the liver than vitamin E, increasing glutathione levels by over 50 percent.

Foods and other substances can also powerfully influence the liver's detoxification system. Alcohol, nicotine, drugs like phenobarbitol and steroids, the fumes from exhaust and paint, and pesticides all kick phase I into action and use up precious liver enzymes in that phase. Tranquilizers, antidepressants, antihistamines, some antacids like cimetidine, an antifungal drug called ketoconazole, and bacterial toxins all upregulate phase II and use up precious liver enzymes as well.

You may have read that broccoli helps prevent cancer, and you may have wondered how. Broccoli and other foods in the *Brassica* family stimulate detoxifying enzymes in the gut and the liver. That helps protect you against many carcinogens. Curcumin, the substance in the spice turmeric, also helps prevent cancer, although in a different way. This spice inhibits phase I enzymes and stimulates phase II enzymes so that they can clean up toxins faster. Oranges and tangerines contain limonene, a nutraceutical that can prevent and reverse cancer in animals. Limonene stimulates phase I and phase II.

As you can see, a diet rich in phytochemicals from fruits and vegetables can "cover the waterfront," supporting the wide range of detoxification enzymes that your liver deploys every moment of your life.

PHASING YOUR FOODS

Here's how you can upregulate sluggish phase I activity: eat more cabbage, broccoli and brussels sprouts, oranges, tangerines, and protein. To slow down a hyperactive phase I system, eat grapefruits, drink fresh grapefruit juice, and take the herbs turmeric and chili pepper.

To upregulate a sluggish phase II system, eat cabbage, broccoli, brussels sprouts, and fish and fish oils and take the nutrients N-acetyl cysteine, methionine, glycine, vitamin B_6, glutamine, and the herb milk thistle. All these nutrients will enhance glutathione production.

To slow down a ballistic phase II system, eat a low-protein diet.

And Our Winner: Milk Thistle

Now that our short course in molecular biology is over, you understand the miraculous functions your liver performs and the absolute necessity of eating a proper diet to support liver function. Let's turn back to milk thistle and see it in action.

When Jeff Walker, a sixteen-year-old with mononucleosis, came to see me, he was completely exhausted, and his liver enzymes were alarmingly elevated. He'd been bedridden for three weeks, and his doctor had advised him to take off the last semester of high school, which meant delaying his entrance to Yale University in the fall. Needless to say, Jeff was crushed. After three weeks on silymarin, his liver enzymes returned to normal, and he felt well enough to return to school. This was one of the most dramatic cases of recovery from mononucleosis I had ever seen. I told Jeff to stay on silymarin for another few months to continue offering protection for his liver. It was a clear example in action of silymarin's ability to protect the liver from free radical damage and to help it regenerate. As I mentioned, silymarin has been used to treat both acute and chronic viral hepatitis—hepatitis can be a complication of mononucleosis.

If a patient comes in to me with a long list of health problems, especially skin disorders, allergies, fatigue, or frequent infections, I immediately suspect liver dysfunction. That's because this organ is so crucial in boosting immunity and combating infection related to toxins invading the body. External conditions, like acne, might mask an internal hormone imbalance. It may be that hormones are not being broken down properly by the liver so they can be excreted.

Marissa Canderra was one such case. A thirty-five-year-old restaurateur who had suffered for many years from digestive problems, she'd been diagnosed with giardia, a parasite that is asymptomatic in some people but can cause disabling discomfort in others. Though she had taken several rounds of an antibiotic, metronidazole, the infection kept returning. She also suffered from fatigue, acne, insomnia, and herpes breakouts. I knew that milk thistle would help her, not only because her liver was surely overloaded but also because the herb is anti-inflammatory and useful in conditions like acne and herpes breakouts. A 1996 British study showed that the active ingredient in the herb is a potent inhibitor of inflammation.

Detoxification was the first key to improving Marissa's health. First, I placed her on a modified fast that used a powdered rice drink, rice, and vegetables. I suggested she eat organic foods that weren't laced with pesticides, and I took her off her herpes medication. Instead, I prescribed lysine, an amino acid that has been shown to inhibit the herpes virus. I added herbs that are antiparasitic, including goldenseal and *Artemesia annua*. My intention was to give her liver and digestive system a rest.

When I tested Marissa for food allergies, I found she was sensitive to both chicken and wheat. Her allergic response to these foods meant that her body was producing inflammatory compounds that needed to be detoxified by the liver. This is where silymarin came to the rescue. The liver can be damaged by the action of potent inflammatory compounds called leukotrienes. Silymarin is a powerful inhibitor of the enzyme that allows leukotrienes to be formed. Liver toxicity, like heart disease, may take years before it is apparent.

Milk of Goodness

Milk thistle can protect against chemical poisoning. The results are profound in the case of alcoholism, a disease that can ravage and destroy the liver. Even in livers that are severely scarred and cirrhotic, silymarin is beneficial. It can extend the life span of such patients. In a two-year study of one hundred seventy patients with cirrhosis, eighty-seven patients—forty-six of whom were alcoholic—received milk thistle extract. Another eighty-three received placebos. After an average of three years, eighteen of the milk thistle group had died of liver disease, while thirty-one of the placebo group had died of liver disease.

Other studies on cirrhosis and alcoholism are equally astonishing. Another study of sixty patients with cirrhosis found that milk thistle lowered liver enzymes in just one month. And studies of red and white blood cells in patients with cirrhosis found that milk thistle protected the cells from free radical damage and increased levels of glutathione.

Silymarin protects against chemical poisoning in the workplace as well. In one study of two hundred workers exposed to the toxic compound toluene for up to twenty years, silymarin had amazing benefits. Forty-nine of the workers, or almost one-quarter, showed abnormal liver function tests, as well as abnormal blood cells. Thirty of those forty-nine were treated with milk thistle. All their tests improved significantly. This shows that even after decades of abuse, silymarin can help the liver restore itself.

Heather Michaelson was a forty-four-year-old traffic controller who had worked the night shift for twenty years. She suffered from irregular periods, depression, hot flashes, inexplicable rashes, and allergies. I theorized that she had a problem with phase II detoxification. Therefore, I put her on a detoxification program and diet, emphasizing lemons and broccoli, along with natural progesterone to balance her hormones, and silymarin. This treatment helped her tremendously, and most of her symptoms abated.

Then there was a massive fire at her job, leading to smoke exposure—and later, when the office was quickly rebuilt and renovated, she was exposed to the outgasing of toxic paints, plastics, and chemicals such as formaldehyde. This chemical exposure overwhelmed her liver once again, throwing both phase I and phase II out of whack. The fact that she worked a night shift added to her stress. Our internal cycles, known as circadian rhythms, are thrown off balance when we work all night and sleep during the day. Our body clock usually times functions like digestion and energy release to occur during sunlight hours, while nighttime is meant to promote healing and detoxification.

When Heather returned to her detoxification program, her symptoms slowly improved again. However, she now has to be conscientious about her diet and supplements, or her symptoms begin to return.

Milk with a Twist

Although I often prescribe silymarin alone, new research indicates that a special combination form of milk thistle may be even more beneficial. This form binds silymarin to phosphatidylcholine, a component of common lecithin, and a key fatty acid in cell membranes. Studies show that silymarin seems to be absorbed better in this form. In a 1990 study, nine healthy volunteers were given a single dose of regular silymarin and a dose of silymarin-phosphatidylcholine complex. Tests showed that blood levels of the special form were higher. In another study of patients with chronic hepatitis, doses of phosphatidylcholine-bound silymarin (ranging from 80 milligrams twice daily to 120 milligrams three times daily) were given for two weeks. The supplement significantly lowered the levels of bilirubin in the blood—a marker for hepatitis and jaundice—after only two weeks.

Milk Thistle and Psoriasis

Studies show that silymarin can help treat psoriasis. I believe this is because, as I mentioned, it is anti-inflammatory. It has been shown to lower the risk of skin cancer in laboratory animals and to reduce sun damage in skin when it was applied topically, according to a study by the National Cancer Institute in 1997. One patient of mine, Jason Samuels, was a dentist plagued by the constant itching and flaking of his skin. His psoriasis had started a decade earlier, and his liver enzymes had become elevated five years earlier. I put him on a detoxification diet emphasizing vegetable juices, rice, supplements of silymarin, fish oils (for their anti-inflammatory impact), and N-acetyl cysteine, for its help in boosting the liver's antioxidant, glutathione. It always amazes me how quickly the body can respond—yet sometimes the symptoms of a disease take time to reverse themselves. A blood test only three weeks later showed that his liver enzymes had begun to drop. Even so, his psoriasis took a while to clear up, and it was a full year before his skin was entirely normal again.

Looking Out for Your Liver

As you can see, milk thistle is helpful in treating dramatic diseases like hepatitis, but it is also effective against common ailments like acne. And because the liver has the incredible ability to regenerate, there is almost always hope where liver disorders are concerned. Our liver is the ultimate recycler—extracting what might harm us, and sending on what will nourish us. It's designed to work at top efficiency, safely processing and disposing of toxic substances. But it needs our steady care and support.

While researching this chapter, I became fascinated with the importance

LIVER STRESS TEST

Answer these questions:

1. Do you smoke?
2. Do you live or work with someone who smokes?
3. Are you often exposed to fumes and pollution?
4. Do you live or work in a building that contains new carpeting, furniture, or paint that might be slowly releasing toxic chemicals?
5. Do you drink alcohol more than once a week?
6. Have you taken prescription drugs more than twice in the past year?
7. Do you often eat fried or fatty foods?
8. Do you have chronic skin problems, sinus problems, or allergies?
9. Do you often feel fatigued?
10. Do you often suffer from gas, bloating, or poor digestion?
11. Do you suffer from bad breath or foul-smelling stools?
12. Do you often have headaches?
13. Does your skin itch, or do you suffer from acne or rashes?

> If you answered yes to four or more of these questions, there is a good chance your liver is not functioning efficiently and needs support.

of liver health. Luckily, there are many nutrients that promote liver function and protect it from harm. Vitamin C is a detoxifier and an immune booster, and it allows the liver a rest. Lemon in hot water is a key to detoxifying the liver and can be used as a morning wakeup call instead of coffee. Most important, silymarin is the liver's most powerful herbal friend, more than a guardian, even more than a protector. It actually stimulates the liver to regenerate itself.

As we learn to protect our environment, to keep our rivers and forests clean, to recycle our bottles and newspapers, remember that the liver is nature's original recycler, and if milk thistle is the liver's best friend—well, the liver is your best friend.

HOW MUCH SHOULD I TAKE?

For General Health
70 milligrams a day (optional)
Divided doses before meals

Special Conditions

Adult acne/Liver dysfunction	140-280 mg/day
Alcohol poisoning	280-560 mg/day
Cirrhosis	280-560 mg/day
Psoriasis	140-560 mg/day
Mononucleosis	140-280 mg/day
Fatigue	140-280 mg/day
Chemical toxicity	140-560 mg/day

8

Probiotics: Protecting the Digestive Tract

One spring day, when millions of Americans were enjoying crisp, supposedly healthful summer salads, sixty-one citizens of Connecticut, Illinois, and New York fell sick from eating these very greens. One was a young three-year-old girl whose food poisoning was so devastating that it put her in intensive care for almost three months and left her with damaged vision. The reputed cause? The bacterial strain *E. coli* 0157:H7, found in cattle feces, which may have contaminated the produce.

Later that same year, a sixteen-month-old child fell tragically ill after drinking apple juice, with a condition that caused her kidneys to fail and her little heart to give out and ultimately led to her death. Again, investigators believe that bacteria tainted the fruit used in the drink.

Nationally publicized food scares such as these are at the root of America's current obsession with scrupulous hygiene practices and products. But not all bacteria are harmful—in fact, some are crucial for keeping our digestive tracts clean, obliterating harmful infections, and protecting us from systemic illness.

Long before the discovery of antibiotics, scientists knew that bacteria caused disease. Louis Pasteur, for example, taught us how the very organisms that thrived in our intestines were causing many of the most ravaging medical problems of the twentieth century, such as tuberculosis and blood poisoning, and led the way to revolutionary new medicines—like antibiotics—to treat and prevent them.

Inside our intestinal tract reside four to five hundred different species of bacteria. In this diverse bacterial universe, microbes both foul and friendly coexist. Nature provides the human gastrointestinal tract with a healthy balance of different types of bacteria. Although bad bacteria can overwhelm the good, leading to the infections we fear so much, beneficial bacteria exist that improve our well-being in ways that we are just beginning to realize. These potent healing bacteria—these tiny "probiotics," as they are known—can reverse the disease-causing effects of their toxic counterparts.

What can probiotics do? Believe it or not, probiotics have the ability to prevent and reverse urinary tract, vaginal yeast, and some systemic infections while also manufacturing vitamins and nutrients necessary for our well-being. Ensuring that probiotics flourish within us is especially important in this day and age, as more and more people grow resistant to antibiotics due to frequent usage. Meanwhile, the increasingly poor American diet (low in fiber, for example, which bacteria need to survive), not to mention environmental and societal stressors, have created a need for healthy bacterial supplements that were unnecessary in the past. Luckily, we can replenish our bodies with good, healthy bacteria by taking daily doses of probiotics, the little housekeepers that keep our systems strong.

It All Began with Yogurt

Probiotics are as naturally beneficial to our health as their very definition—"for life"—suggests. At the turn of the century, a scientist named Elie Metchnikoff proposed that yogurt was the elixir of life because it contained a strain of bacteria known as *Lactobacillus* that purportedly cleared the large intestine of toxins. We now know that two particular species of probiotics, *Lactobacillus bulgaricus* and *Streptococcus thermophilus*, are the primary cultures in yogurt, and they make this dairy treat a supremely healthy food by combating certain bad bacteria and improving lactose tolerance. These two strains work together and combine their unique powers to defend the gut from potentially harmful bacteria.

Probiotics have proved, in numerous studies, to be indispensable in keeping us healthy by cleansing our intestines of excess pathogens, thus preventing allergies, yeast infections, diarrhea, gas, bloating, and digestive problems. Findings from a long-term study on mice in *Nutrition Review* suggest that probiotics may even alleviate inflammatory diseases such as rheumatoid arthritis and colitis.

Consider this chapter an introduction to the most potent healing strains: *L. acidophilus*, which produces its own natural antibiotics; *B. bifidum*, which crowds out unhealthy yeast and bacteria and assists the liver; and *L. rhamnosus*, which defends against food allergies.

How Probiotics Heal

A key characteristic of healthy bacteria is their ability to antagonize unhealthy, or pathogenic, bacteria. Pathogenic organisms are dangerous because they either cause infection or release harmful substances as a by-product of their natural digestive processes. Probiotics work in a variety of ways to keep unhealthy bacteria in check. Some crowd out nasty bacteria by competing with them for the same nutrients; others produce substances like peroxides or lactic acid, which can kill pathogenic bacteria by virtue of their respective detergentlike and acidic properties. Probiotics can sometimes absorb excess minerals that pathogens use for growth. Some probiotics form a defensive barrier around the walls of the intestines to protect against damage and can even release their own natural antibiotics, such as acidophilin.

Probiotics may sometimes be safer and more effective than antibiotics, since man-made antibiotics are so lethal that they kill not only bad bacteria such as *E. coli, Salmonella, Klebsiella*, and *Staphylococcus*, but also the good strains. When healthy strains are killed, any harmful bacteria that have survived the antibiotic onslaught adapt to resist the medication and reproduce, so the next time this antibiotic is used, it is rendered useless against the strengthened, "smarter" pathogens. Increasingly antibiotic-resistant bacteria have caused recent epidemics of tuberculosis and meningitis reminiscent of ancient scares. Unlike antibiotics, natural probiotics have smaller, more selective targets.

Good Bacteria: Their Secret

Probiotics produce enzymes that help us digest our food. They are even responsible for manufacturing B vitamins in the process of metabolizing nutrients. By cleaning up the gastrointestinal tract, probiotics reduce embarrassing symptoms like bad breath, gas, and diarrhea stemming from digestive problems. They also treat more serious conditions like vaginal and yeast infections, and even some food allergies. Exciting research in humans and animals alike shows that probiotics may bolster our immune system. One study even indicated that *L. acidophilus* can help combat HIV. This research has been published in journals such as *Immunopharmacology and Immunotoxicology* and the *International Journal of Immunotherapy*.

How Probiotics Helped One Woman

Suzanne James was a forty-five-year-old stockbroker working in her hometown of New York City. Her job was fast paced and competitive, and between long days in the office and nights of homework, Suzanne was completely overwhelmed. She also had a history of urethritis, a condition which can be associated with vaginal burning and frequent urination. She was constantly running for the bathroom, often at inopportune times. Lately, too, she had been experiencing severe exhaustion, frequent yeast infections, and intestinal upset.

When Suzanne first came to my office and listed her complaints, I knew that one treatment was the clear choice: probiotics. Any time I see a patient with recurrent yeast, vaginal, and intestinal infections, I suspect that unfriendly bacteria have overtaken the gut, permeating the intestinal lining, spewing toxins, or otherwise leaving the patient susceptible to infection and symptoms like diarrhea, exhaustion, and gas. A 1996 study in the respected *Journal of the American Medical Association* (*JAMA*) evaluating the use of microorganisms in treating vaginal and intestinal infections deemed probiotics useful not only in establishing a healthy microflora to treat these infections but also in preventing acute infantile and antibiotic-induced diarrhea.

Because of the severity of Suzanne's distress, I prescribed supplements of healthy bacteria to be taken both orally and as a vaginal suppository.

"In order to protect your urinary tract with the proper microorganisms," I explained, "we have to get them as close to your urethra as possible to combat infection. Oral supplements of probiotics such as *L. acidophilus* have been found to ameliorate vaginal infections, but vaginal suppositories allow healthy bacteria to get closer to the source of the problem."

I asked her to use an *L. acidophilus* suppository once a week and to take a teaspoon of refrigerated acidophilus powder (storage in a cool place helps preserve these bacteria) in a glass of water three times a day. I also prescribed cranberry extract and bilberry supplements, which are beneficial against urinary tract infections; cranberry in particular has specific compounds that bind to harmful bacteria before they get a chance to adhere to the lining of your bladder and cause inflammation.

Suzanne took her supplements religiously, even the suppositories. The effort was worth it. After three weeks, the burning and frequency she had experienced diminished and finally disappeared. Soon, she was feeling more refreshed and alert than she had in months, and it showed in her work. When she arrived at my office for a follow-up visit six months after beginning her course of probiotics, she was proud to tell me that she had slowly but surely increased her productivity so much that she recently won the Stockbroker of the Month award at her firm. Even better, her infections have not recurred.

What Probiotics Can Do for You

Diarrhea: Diarrhea is often a symptom of gastrointestinal distress caused by bacteria. Probiotics normalize bowel function by neutralizing infectious microorganisms. A study of Pakistani children with acute diarrhea reported that only 31 percent of those treated with the probiotic strain called *L. acidophilus* continued to experience diarrhea, as opposed to 75 percent of the nontreated group.

Urinary Tract: Although antibiotics are usually prescribed for urinary tract infections, studies indicate that probiotics might be the most effective preventive treatment. In a study of forty-one women with urinary tract infections, just 21 percent of subjects taking probiotic supplements had recurrence of the illness, while up to 41 percent of subjects on antibiotics experienced future infection.

Yeast Infection: Yogurt is an excellent source of probiotics, and one study showed that consuming it daily could prevent recurrent yeast infections, a nagging health concern for many women. Subjects in a 1992 study who ate yogurt every day for six months displayed a threefold decrease in vaginal yeast infection.

Dermatitis: Whether you have allergic skin rashes, otherwise known as eczema or dermatitis, or even psoriasis or acne, chances are that probiotics can be part of your program. When intestinal bacteria are unhealthy, the lining of the intestines can become inflamed and permeable. Toxins can be released into the bloodstream and result in skin eruptions. A 1996 study of *L. rhamnosus*, a good bacteria strain, showed that the probiotic significantly improved atopic dermatitis.

Food Allergy: A study proved *L. rhamnosus* effective in treating food allergies. Researchers from Finland noted that infants with cow's milk allergy demonstrated significant improvement of symptoms when taking this probiotic.

Lactose Intolerance: The gas, bloating, and bowel problems some people experience when they eat milk and cheese—more technically known as lactose intolerance—is often caused by deficiency of the enzyme lactase, which helps digest dairy products. Because probiotics actually produce significant quantities of lactase, they are extremely beneficial to those who want to eat dairy products without experiencing painful symptoms.

Immune System: The *L. casei* strain of healthy bacteria was found in one study to stimulate production of secretory IgA, a chemical weapon used by our immune systems against invading pathogens. Another study showed that sixty-eight adults who consumed live cultured yogurt for four months displayed a fourfold increase in gamma interferon, a sign that probiotics in the yogurt had boosted immune function.

Good and Evil in the Gut

Most of the microorganisms that reside in our bodies coexist in the intestines, which contain more bacteria than there are cells in the body. The intestinal flora is a garden bearing different varieties of bacterial growth. Maintaining many diverse types of bacteria is important, so that one particularly noxious strain cannot take control of the gut, or one particularly beneficial strain cannot be singled out for damage. At birth, the human intestine is sterile, with no microorganisms dwelling inside. Upon delivery, however, the intestinal tract becomes colonized; its initial dose of bacteria is picked up as a child passes through its mother's birth canal and inhales all the microbial inhabitants through its tiny screaming mouth. A substance that protects against bacterial infection, lactoferrin, is actually transferred from mother to child during breast-feeding. This is one reason why breast milk is preferable to formula when feeding infants.

The intestinal world is a complex ecosystem. Some bacteria are truly ruinous to our health and can release toxins, mutagens, carcinogens, or tumor promoters as natural by-products of life processes. Many increase the permeability of the intestinal lining, allowing infectious agents and allergens to pass through. Bacterial secretions can directly affect the cytochrome 450 detoxification system, by which the liver purifies the blood of harmful chemicals that are both inadvertently created by the body and ingested from the environment. Tampering with this cleaning system can increase the risk of cancer in the liver and other organ systems by producing carcinogens. An ammonia by-product of bacterial activity can disturb normal brain function in high doses. Several studies have shown that inflammatory diseases like Crohn's, rheumatoid arthritis, and colitis may be provoked by improper intestinal bacteria.

Harmful bacteria can saturate the intestine in severe situations, seeping through the intestinal lining to cause disease or overstimulate the immune system. For instance, chronic arthritis can be induced in rats by injecting them with fragments of anaerobic bacteria, the type that most heavily populates the gut. One bacterium in particular has gotten a lot of bad press as a dangerous one to watch: *H. pylori.* This pathogen causes ulcers in humans and animals alike, which can lead to serious disease. *Salmonella* is another famously infamous bacterium often found in infected chickens. Studies show that poultry fed health-promoting bacterial strains, like *L. acidophilus* or *B. bifidum*, are protected against *Salmonella*.

One unfriendly microorganism has even inspired a namesake infection, *Clostridium difficile*. It occurs when you use too much of a broad-spectrum antibiotic—such as penicillin—and can lead to the development of enterocolitis, the painful and obstructive inflammation of the colon's lining. But perhaps the most feared strain of bacteria is *E. coli*, which can contaminate the red meat we buy at the grocery store and hamburgers sold at local fast-food joints around the country, sometimes rendering unsuspecting consumers ill.

Probiotics, on the other hand, are a group of gut-friendly bacteria. Also known as lactic acid bacteria (LAB), so called because when they ferment sugar to make food for themselves they produce lactic acid. They make up just a small subsection of the vast spectrum of microorganisms occupying our intestines. (The same lactic acid that can cause muscle cramps after exercise if the body doesn't get enough oxygen works in the intestines to zap unfriendly bacteria.) Lactic acid bacteria are stationary, meaning they tend to park in one permanent area of the gut for life, and anaerobic, meaning that they don't need oxygen to thrive. Four genera, or categories, of these bacteria are typically used in the probiotic supplements and food products we can buy in stores: *Lactobacillus, Streptococcus, Enterococcus*, and *Bifidobacteria*. Each of these genera contains a host of related bacterial strains.

As we age, pathogenic bacteria become insidiously more prominent within us, perhaps due to a progressively weakening immune system, stress, years of poor diet, or lifetime overuse of antibiotics. So which ones are the good guys, and how do they work? Here's your guide to the best and brightest of the probiotic team.

Lactobacillus Acidophilus: The best known—and most extensively researched—of all healthy bacteria, this strain is so ubiquitous in probiotic supplements that other types of microorganisms are often described by this name. *L. acidophilus* is the most abundant bacterium in the small intestine and probably the most effective. Also found lining the vagina, cervix, and urethra, it protects the gut by inhibiting the actions of pathogenic bacteria, keeping them from multiplying and colonizing. *L. acidophilus* also produces its own natural antibiotics, such as lactocidin and acidophilin, to blast harmful organisms out of the digestive system.

Lactobacillus Rhamnosus: A hardy, ever-abundant little microorganism, *L. rhamnosus* resists the caustic bile salts sloshing through the gut and adheres to the mucosal cells of the intestinal lining. As it colonizes the mucosa with probiotics, *L. rhamnosus* protects the intestinal tract from the invasion of harmful bacteria. Studies suggest that this bacterium decreases the severity of symptoms such as intestinal inflammation and sensitivity due to food allergy and eczema. It also produces the enzyme lactase, which digests lactose more fully and may thus reduce the symptoms of lactose intolerance such as gas, bloating, and bad breath.

Lactobacillus Casei: A close relative of *L. acidophilus, L. casei's* greatest claim to fame is that it activates white blood cells and secretes a substance called peptidoglycan, thus enhancing our immune systems; it also has tumor-inhibiting properties.

Lactobacillus Bulgaricus: *L. bulgaricus*, unlike *L. rhamnosus*, is transient in the intestinal tract and does not implant in its walls but plays a key supportive role in the bacterial drama unfolding in the gut. This probiotic strain is most famous as one of the two main active cultures in yogurt; it not only ferments the yogurt but also ameliorates the environment for acidophilus and bifidobacteria, which grow in and clean up the intestines. The main dangerous bacteria it fights are *Staph, Salmonella, Shigella*, and *H. pylori*.

Streptococcus Thermophilus: *S. thermophilus*, another strain found in yogurt, is thought to alleviate lactose intolerance problems because lactase, the enzyme it produces, efficiently breaks down dairy products for easy digestion.

Bifidobacterium Bifidum: Bifidobacteria are among the most populous lactic acid bacteria in the human intestinal tract. *B. bifidum*, in particular, prefers the mucus membrane of the large intestines and vaginal tract. Attaching to the intestinal wall, this strain of bacteria staunchly protects the gut from harmful, invading organisms by crowding them out and depriving them of the nutrients they need to survive. Another of its sly tactics: producing lactic and acetic acid, which lower the intestinal pH and keep pathogens from growing, preventing cancer.

Bifidobacterium Longum: *B. longum*, concentrated primarily in the large intestine, acts much like *B. bifidum*, its bacterial cousin, by lowering gut pH to kill harmful organisms, crowding out the ones that do live, and ultimately reducing the frequency of gastrointestinal disorders such as diarrhea and nausea during antibiotic use.

Enterococcus Faecium: For those prone to the diarrhea-causing diseases common in underdeveloped nations, *E. faecium* is a wonder probiotic. It has been proved effective against viral, bacterial, and fungal microorganisms in the intestinal tract. While some claim that this is a controversial bacterium that may produce harmful enterotoxins, these statements have not been substantiated. Meanwhile, the World Health Organization has researched *E. faecium* extensively for use in Bangladesh, where diarrhea is a serious health threat.

DDS-1: Once called the superstrain of all probiotics, DDS-1 is a powerful form of *L. acidophilus* that was developed in a laboratory for the express purpose of being the ultimate in healthy bacteria. Although we now know that a variety of strains, each helpful in its own way, are needed and a lone superstrain cannot be enough, DDS-1 is still useful in conjunction with other probiotics. One study found that eating milk products containing DDS-1 led to a 16 to 41 percent reduction of cancer proliferation in animals.

FRUCTOOLIGOSACCHARIDES (FOS): These are not bacteria, but they actually promote the growth and activity of friendly bacteria in the gut. A naturally occurring compound found in fruits and vegetables, FOS is a noncaloric substance that is not broken down by the digestive tract. It passes through us easily, inhibiting the growth of pathogens like *Salmonella* and enhancing the growth of healthy organisms like bifidobacteria all the while.

Waging War on Yeast

Although vaginal yeast infections are incredibly common in women, they often aren't viewed as a serious health threat. When coupled with stress and job concerns, and a generally discontented life, as they were for twenty-eight-year-old Alison Berlitz, however, they can be a source of intense aggravation. Alison had been riddled with yeast infections her whole life, plagued by painful and persistent vaginal discomfort, burning, and itching. She began to shy away from sexual intimacy with her boyfriend, straining their already tenuous relationship. Despite a secure job as a hotel industry executive, Alison was frustrated because her true career goal was to be in musical theater, and her physical discomfort made her days both physically and emotionally difficult. Worst of all, none of the many medications Alison took to eliminate her infections was effective.

When she came to see me, Alison was perplexed and felt defeated by the failure of these drugs, which would relieve her symptoms only temporarily. I explained that most medications zap yeast without introducing healthy bacteria to keep it from reappearing. By taking probiotics, Alison could not only cleanse pathogens but replenish her system with natural organisms that would work constantly to keep yeast out for good. Because some women seem to have allergies, sensitivities, or other reactions to foods that promote intestinal yeast growth, I put Alison on a special yeast-free diet. All breads, wine, and beer were removed from her menu, plus moldy foods like cheese, other sugars, fermented foods, and carbohydrates. Certainly, this was a severe dietary change for a young woman whose dietary routine included sugary muffins for breakfast and drinks on Friday nights to celebrate the end of a boring workweek.

Alison's road to recovery was far from easy. Yeast can be tenacious, and effective treatment would take time. For months, Alison's condition fluctuated between radically better and then worse again. Finally, however, her determination and faith in probiotic supplements paid off. Alison has not had a recurrence of her yeast infection in a whole year—the first time in ten years that she's been infection free. Not only are her painful symptoms gone, but her quality of life has improved significantly. When she visited my office to inform me that her pain and irritation were gone, I saw her smile for the first time since she'd been my patient. She had smoothed things over with her boyfriend, and her newfound health left her in better spirits each day—and gave her energy to go on auditions so that she could one day leave the hotel for the stage.

Running Out of Gas

Millions of Americans each year are afflicted with uncomfortable gas and bloating caused by irritable bowel syndrome. Unfortunately, how the bowel got so cranky is often a mystery. Was it allergies? Infection? Sensitivity to certain foods? In many cases, such a condition can prove difficult to treat, but the story of Louise Marsden, fifty-seven, shows that intestinal distress can be relieved naturally and effectively.

When we first met Louise, in chapter 5, she'd had a host of medical concerns, including hot flashes and low bone density. Another complaint of hers was seemingly less serious but still a source of embarrassment to her: halitosis. Thinking this might be the nasty trick of bacteria whose unpleasant by-products can cause bad breath, I took a stool sample to monitor any growth of dangerous microorganisms in her intestine, plus possible overgrowth of yeast or parasites. Louise came up strongly positive for an overabundance of yeast. I asked her more questions about other symptoms, looking for clues that intestinal dysbiosis was a trigger for some of her symptoms.

"Bacteria may have caused your halitosis," I told her, "but it can also cause other symptoms. Have you experienced any gastrointestinal disorders, like diarrhea, gas, or bloating?"

This poised legal secretary turned a warm shade of crimson.

"I do have gas," she admitted. "It's pretty bad. I just didn't mention it because I was ashamed."

"Well, it's a good thing you mentioned it, because now we can correct it," I said.

One of the most common causes of gas and bloating is too much bacteria lining the gut. Bacteria and yeast emit carbon dioxide and methane gas as natural by-products of respiration. Luckily, there are a number of natural remedies with antibacterial effects to reduce these embarrassing symptoms.

Furthermore, I learned that she had been ingesting high doses of fiber because she thought it was good for her. While fiber is a necessary ingredient in any diet, it can also promote gas because it stimulates the growth of good bacteria, and even good bacteria pass gas.

I recommended the following substances for Louise: garlic, caprylic acid (grapefruit extract), and goldenseal. I also prescribed a wide range of healthy replacement bacteria to cleanse her gastrointestinal tract, including *L. acidophilus* and *B. bifidum*. An antiyeast diet would also go a long way toward alleviating her symptoms. Not only did I ask her to junk the junk food she guiltily loved to eat, but I recommended that she eat yogurt regularly, and I lowered her fiber intake.

During the first week of treatment, Louise's gas and bad breath persisted. As the weeks went on, however, and she learned to enjoy yogurt and yeast-free foods, she noticed that she felt much healthier, and her mouth felt fresher. Free of the tyranny of her uncomfortable symptoms, she felt like a new woman.

Scoring with a Team of Antibiotics and Probiotics

True or false: antibiotics are a miracle of modern medicine. Actually, it's a trick question. Certainly, antibiotics have made great strides in healing patients who have fallen victim to debilitating, sometimes fatal, bacterial infections, not to mention wiping out epidemics like tuberculosis. But what many physicians and most antibiotic users fail to realize is that the medications nonselectively kill not only insidious pathogens but health-promoting probiotics as well, leaving us vulnerable to any bad bacteria that manage to live or resist medication. This was the dilemma facing Kimberly McCarthy.

Kim was just sixteen years old, and quite a dynamo. She was loud and boisterous, with a laugh loud enough to be heard in five area codes, and a gregarious personality that put everyone who met her at ease. She was an A student at her tony private school, but she was best known for her exploits on the soccer field, where she was a rough-and-tumble goalie. Unfortunately, as her junior year began, Kim was sidelined with chronic sinusitis. Even worse, when her physician put her on the antibiotic amoxicillin to counter her sinus allergies, she experienced severe diarrhea the very next day caused by a serious medical condition called pseudomembranous enterocolitis. This occurs when a harmful bacterial strain called *Clostridium difficile* creates a false membrane of dead bacteria cells across the colon, trapping in and protecting the bacteria. Her doctor prescribed her yet another course of antibiotics, this time of Flagyl, to repair the bacterial overgrowth caused by the first course. This Band-Aid relieved Kim's intestinal symptoms and her sinusitis for a few weeks, and she happily resumed soccer practice, until her nasal pain and congestion flared once more. Again, she went through the ordeal of taking amoxicillin, having uncontrollable diarrhea, and then using Flagyl to fix the mess. This time, Kim's diarrhea was so grueling that it forced her to miss days of school and left her dehydrated and exhausted.

In an effort to bring her star goalie back to health, Kim's coach referred her to me, hoping that a natural approach to her infection would do the trick. My first action was to determine the cause of her diarrhea episodes; I took a stool sample to rule out any other conditions such as parasites or yeast. My plan of attack, then, was to treat the sinusitis without spurring the bad bacteria into action. First, counterintuitive as it may seem, I had to put Kim back on antibiotics. Understandably, she was wary.

"Isn't there some natural treatment you can put me on, instead of the amoxicillin again?" she asked, eyeing me skeptically. "I thought antibiotics were the problem in the first place."

As I explained to Kim, antibiotics can be a boon, the best ammunition we have against infection, if we make sure to take them along with probiotics that replenish the useful microorganisms that antibiotics can accidentally sweep away. I convinced her to try antibiotics once more, but this time taking a good mixture of probiotics heavy on *B. bifidum*, which is especially good at counterracting *Clostridium*, before the course to cleanse her system. Kim agreed to this plan, and she began her forty-eight-hour probiotic purging, taking two full teaspoonfuls a day in a full glass of water each time. She continued on the probiotics during the amoxicillin regimen, taking them two hours after a dose of antibiotics (so they would have time to establish themselves in her intestinal tract before being temporarily diminished by the drug).

Kim was amazed to find that she made it through the entire ten days of medication without a single episode of diarrhea. Not only did the clostridial diarrhea disappear, so did her sinus allergies. I asked Kim to continue her probiotic supplements for at least a month, which she did willingly, amazed that her nose was finally clear without the trade-off of diarrhea. Her gut clean, her sinus quiet, Kim played soccer through her senior year in high school and did so well that she was recruited to play for a prestigious northeastern university on athletic scholarship.

Bacteria and the Bowel

While Kim experienced bouts of diarrhea, a fate common to many who take antibiotics, thirty-two-year-old Sally Kutzer had the opposite response: constipation. Prone to upper respiratory infections, Sally had been prescribed various antibiotics, but with a single dose of the drugs, she would immediately get constipation so bad that it often lasted a month. Sally lived with a genuine health dilemma: Should she forego antibiotics and suffer racking coughs, sore throats, and sinus pain? Or breathe easy and learn to live with the stomachaches that stemmed from her constipation?

At first, I decided to try eliminating antibiotics by substituting an arsenal of natural nutrients with antibiotic properties. A combination of mushroom extract, zinc, selenium, and vitamin C successfully treated Sally's mild respiratory complaints and seemed to prevent further infections. One weekend, however, Sally was on a plane returning from Maine, and it seemed as if every person on her flight was hacking away or sniffling loudly. Soon afterward, she came down with her infection, only this time we were unable to treat it with the usual supplements. It was time to turn to antibiotics. Sally was terrified, even in her congested, weakened state. Constipation would just make her condition worse, she felt. But just as I gave my patient Kim a course of probiotics to balance out any diarrhea-causing bad bacteria, I prescribed a large dose of healthy bacteria, especially acidophilus, for Sally to take before and during her antibiotic rounds. She had little choice but to trust me, and now she's glad she did, for taking several days of probiotics before beginning antibiotics—and taking them for several days after ending them—kept her free of constipation and infection.

Bacteria and Arthritis?

The case of fifty-eight-year-old Peter Francis has to be one of the strangest I've seen in my years of practice. Although Peter had suffered from arthritis for a number of years, which is odd at his age, we could find no reason why such joint pain should strike so early in his life. At the young age of thirty, Peter began experiencing stiffness in his hands. As time passed, arthritis had spread from his fingers into his arms and legs, until it got so painful that he could hardly work anymore. Known especially for his quick and intricate carving and attention to detail, Peter's claim to fame dwindled as the arthritis took over, leading to fewer customers and less income. The worst part of this scenario, however, was the depression he felt at losing his woodworking talent.

I was determined to uncover the secret of Peter's premature arthritis. I tested all the usual suspects: allergies, rheumatoid arthritis, as many medical conditions as I could. Peter was negative for every single culprit. Then I read a study in the *Lancet*, a well-respected medical journal, proposing an intriguing hypothesis about enterometabolic disorders—that is, disorders of the intestines. The hypothesis, posited by J. O. Hunter, stated that the intestines affect human health so profoundly that their increased permeability or overgrowth of harmful bacteria can lead to serious conditions in other distal parts of the body. As I read that seemingly simple idea, Peter Francis appeared in my mind's eye. Perhaps a proliferation of bacteria was causing his arthritis!

The next day, I called him in for a stool test. My hunch proved correct: his gut was so flooded with pathogens and so devoid of healthy bacteria like lactobacillus that it seemed a quite possible cause of arthritis, according to Hunter's hypothesis. I told Peter the good news but warned him that recovery from a condition as far gone as his might take a large amount of time and commitment.

"I'm willing to try practically anything at this point, Doc," he told me. "I can't face going through the rest of my life getting worse and worse, or the possibility that one day I won't even have the strength to lift a hammer to nail. Tell me what to do."

First, I wanted to purify Peter's intestinal tract as well as I could after years of abuse from bacterial toxins. I asked him to refrain from eating milk, wheat, nightshades, junk foods, and greasy snacks. Peter also had a terrific sweet tooth and was constantly munching on the delicious baked goods his wife concocted. These, too, had to go. In their place came fiber, flaxseed, and supplements of glutamine, aloe, and zinc, all designed by Mother Nature to soothe the damaged intestinal lining and guard it from future attack. For two weeks Peter dutifully stuck to his strict diet and varied regimen of pills and tonics, but he did not substantially improve. Perhaps, I thought, administering probiotics might prove powerful enough to solve not only his intestinal problems but also the accompanying arthritis. Peter, ever the good sport, agreed to begin taking a complete bacterial replacement program composed of all the major different types: *L. acidophilus, L. rhamnosus, B. bifidum*, the works.

It may sound too good to be true, but within two months, Peter arrived in my office with a beautifully built solid oak chair. As he placed it in front of my desk, I sat speechless.

"It's for you," he cheerfully explained. "Hard to believe, but my joint pains are going away! My hands have more movement now than they did when I was forty."

Peter's arthritis never completely vanished, but it was much alleviated. Could replenishing his gut with healthy bacteria really improve a condition that took its toll nowhere near the intestines? Did probiotics alone do the trick? I honestly think so.

Have a Healthy, Happy Gut

Like any city or neighborhood, our intestines are inhabited by a diverse variety of organisms, some dangerously insidious, others virtuously good. Nature provided us with a balance of bacteria both healthy and harmful, allowing them to coexist peacefully as long as the helpful type remain in the majority. Although people have long thought of yogurt as a life-sustaining food and feared strains like *Salmonella* and *E. coli*, few realize the importance of specific bacteria in our gut for our health and well-being. The truth is, the symbiotic relationship between these tiny species and our bodies knows no parallel and ultimately produces a wide range of major health benefits.

I recommend probiotics to everyone, even healthy individuals who have no digestive problems. They can be taken in the form of yogurt (or, for those allergic to cow's milk, soy or goat's milk yogurt).

TAKING IT

> The question of when to take your probiotics is a matter of debate. These supplements work best when the stomach isn't excessively acidic (when you haven't eaten for a long time) or alkaline (when it's filled with neutralizing food). Most people tend to take them before meals. Studies using yogurt cultures show that probiotics that work well may not stick to the intestines for long periods, so daily use is most beneficial. In general, keep your bacteria in a cool environment, refrigerating them especially in the summer. Statistics on bacterial survival during storage indicate that within six months of purchase, over half the microbes will be destroyed if kept at 70°F.
>
> Even if you don't take daily probiotic supplements, there are other measures you can take to avoid unhealthy bacteria. Washing your hands frequently with soap is a simple but extremely effective method. Trying to drink tap water that is filtered and eat produce that has been well washed or cooked is another route of precaution. Some foods, while not bacteria laden, have natural antibiotic effects and will steer pathogens clear of your intestines; these include garlic, oregano, and turmeric.

Supplements taken a few times a week can also be beneficial. The most potent probiotic supplements usually come in powder form and are kept refrigerated. During illness, a full teaspoon can be taken in water on an empty stomach in the morning. As a maintenance dose, an eighth of a teaspoon in a glass of water, or three capsules containing 1 billion bacteria per capsule, should be sufficient. Probiotics that are put on the shelves of health food stores can lose some of their potency over a period of months. Probiotics are especially useful when traveling, to prevent diarrhea; they are also a necessity whenever you take antibiotics.

A clearer understanding of probiotics is essential, particularly in this modern age of medicine, where antibiotic resistance is hindering our ability to heal the ill. By forging a relationship with probiotics and entrusting them with the health of our guts, we can face infection with new ammunition: our little friends, working night and day to keep our systems clean and disease free.

HOW MUCH SHOULD I TAKE?

For General Health

Through foods, such as yogurt (1 4-oz. cup a day)

Divided doses after meals

Special Conditions

Yeast infection	1-2 billion organisms/day
Vaginal and intestinal infections	1-2 billion organisms/day
Intestinal dysbiosis	1-3 billion organisms/day
Halitosis	1-2 billion organisms/day
Diarrhea	2-6 billion organisms/day
Gas/bloating	1-2 billion organisms/day
Urinary tract infection	1-2 billion organisms/day
Constipation	2-4 billion organisms/day
Parasites	2-4 billion organisms/day
Arthritis	1-4 billion organisms/day
Dermatitis	1-4 billion organisms/day
Food allergies	1-4 billion organisms/day
Lactose intolerance	1-2 billion organisms/day

9

Glutamine: Food for Your Gut

Imagine for a moment that you're a football quarterback and your life's dream is just within your grasp: your team is about to win the Super Bowl. You're on the fifty-yard line, facing down the enemy and about to launch the winning pass. Those guys are rushing at you like a human avalanche, and you raise your arm as high as you can to hurl that ball as hard as you ever have. The last thought in your head—but maybe the first thought in mine—is that that star quarterback fifty yards from the end zone is looking at the surface area of his own intestines.

There are literally trillions of microbes along the fifteen feet of your intestinal tract. That football field is the area that the immune system must constantly defend from bacteria, viruses, or harmful microbes that threaten to intercept your health. There are more bacteria in one centimeter of intestine than there are stars in the known universe. The world within us is in some ways greater, more infinite, and more fascinating than the world beyond—and this is particularly true of the intestinal world.

I believe physicians have been shortsighted about the importance of intestinal health. It's here that the body must recognize what is an "enemy" to be flushed out as waste and what is the bedrock of life, the nutrients that bring vital nourishment to every cell in the body. Thirty percent of our immune system is located around the lining of the intestine, constantly working to protect the intestinal lining and prevent toxins from entering the body.

Healthy digestion is one of my patients' greatest concerns. And they're not alone: a recent children's book explaining the wonders of intestinal health, *My Poop*, actually became a surprise best seller. Adults were buying the book not only for their kids but to satisfy their own curiosity. People are fascinated by the mysterious demons and gremlins that lie within the digestive system. Why does our stomach growl? What causes constipation or diarrhea? How can all those colonies of bacteria live inside us? Just how does the intestinal wall act as a barrier, protecting us from potentially fatal toxins, even as it absorbs and digests our food?

Intestinal disease can be the source of many disparate conditions, from arthritis to allergies and fatigue to skin eruptions. If the intestine becomes eroded due to infection, inflamed due to allergies, or damaged due to toxins, we will become subtly malnourished and our well-being will surely suffer.

A complete nutritional program is crucial for patients with compromised intestines, but no nutrient is more important than glutamine for our intestinal health. That's because it's a primary fuel for the intestine, and it helps heal the intestinal lining. Only by keeping your intestines healthy can you further repair your body with other nutrients. In fact, a 1993 study in the *Lancet*, one of England's most important medical journals, showed that out of twenty patients receiving intravenous nutrients, only the ten who were treated with glutamine preserved the mucosal cells that comprise the intestinal lining. Damage to the mucosal lining is a common problem associated with intravenous feeding. Glutamine prevented infectious bacteria living in the intestines from leaking through the intestinal walls into the bloodstream.

What Is Glutamine?

Amazingly, glutamine was once termed a "nonessential" nutrient, and so its incredible potential was obscured by that benign description. Glutamine is anything but nonessential. It's easy to see, though, how it earned this reputation. Although synthesized and primarily released by skeletal muscle, every organ actually contains glutamine and is capable of releasing it. It is the most abundant amino acid in the body, and the amount that we manufacture on our own—without obtaining any from the food we eat—is usually enough to fuel important metabolic processes, like the rapid growth of cells and tissues. As an amino acid, glutamine is an important building block for many other amino acids, proteins, and nucleotides. It also regulates protein synthesis in muscles and glycogen synthesis in the liver, both of which preserve muscle mass. But most important, glutamine is crucial as an energy source for our bodies. In fact, it is the primary fuel of the upper intestinal tract.

If the body is running smoothly, then, like other nutrients, glutamine goes about its business quietly, an unassuming but necessary member of the backstage crew. When the body is stressed, however, glutamine transforms itself and becomes a show-stopping star. A study in the *Journal of Parenteral Enteral Nutrition*, which is dedicated to researching the role that nutrition plays in our health, found that the concentrations of this nutrient decrease when the body is fighting disease.

Glutamine, then, is at times *extremely* essential: we need extra amounts of it if our systems are stressed by sickness and depleted of this amino acid.

The typical American diet offers about 3.5 to 7 grams of glutamine per day. More glutamine is needed during stress infections, trauma, inflammation, allergic reactions, or chronic illness. Under these conditions, an extra 1 to 3 grams of glutamine per day may be needed just to maintain normal intestinal structure and function! That's a huge increase; but glutamine is virtually nontoxic even in very large quantities. It is rapidly metabolized.

I find glutamine supplements key to repairing damage to the intestines from diseases like colitis, irritable bowel syndrome, celiac disease, and any condition affecting digestion. In fact, the *Journal of Surgical Research* found that a glutamine-enriched diet appears to be effective in maintaining a healthy intestine in critically ill surgical patients.

I like to think of glutamine as a carpenter, rebuilding all the doors that toxins and detrimental bacteria have knocked down in the intestinal walls. Simply put, glutamine keeps the intestines healthy and helps ward off ailments as diverse as impotence, arthritis, and allergies.

Elizabeth Whitaker, a thirty-five-year-old vice-president of a major New York advertising agency, can attest to the protective powers of glutamine supplements. She had suffered constipation, painful gas, and bloating for more than five years. Her biggest nightmare was riding the crowded elevator to her office on the thirty-eighth floor. Elizabeth's medical history quickly revealed the source of her problem: As a child, she had suffered many allergies to foods like milk and wheat. There is a strong link between allergies and bacterial infection; a study conducted at George Washington University showed that food allergies were present in 80 percent of children who had ear infections. Elizabeth had also been on many antibiotics, after which she experienced diarrhea in addition to her usual gas and bloating.

I wasn't surprised when she tested positive for gluten sensitivity, so I helped her to remove gluten, which is a main component of wheat, from her diet. Gluten is not only found in wheat, barley, and rye but is also hidden in foods such as pasta, canned soups, and processed foods. I also gave her flaxseed powder, a gentle and healing fiber source that absorbs toxins and bulks up the bowel to stop diarrhea (see chapter 10). As an added benefit, acidophilus (see chapter 8) thrives in the presence of fiber like flaxseed. Most important, I prescribed her 3 grams daily of glutamine to repair the abuse and allergy damage to her intestines. All three worked together to help repair her intestinal lining as quickly as possible.

Intestinal Fire

As I explained to Elizabeth, an inflamed intestine can be the source of a startling range of problems. Normally the intestines are selective barriers, preventing toxic compounds from entering the bloodstream and allowing admission only to digested food particles. However, when the intestines become injured by infectious bacteria, excess alcohol, drugs, or other offending chemicals, they can become inflamed. This inflammation increases the permeability of the intestines, allowing allergens and toxins to sneak through the intestinal lining. The immune system declares war against the new influx of bacteria or food particles leaking into the blood; and the resulting battle can lead to symptoms like chills, fatigue, or fever.

Too much exposure to antibiotics can disrupt the health of bowel flora by killing off not only the bad bacteria but also the good, beneficial bacteria that protect the huge intestinal surface area. Elizabeth's gluten sensitivity only worsened the condition, since gluten is a known disease-causing substance. (Celiac disease, triggered by a component of grain called alpha gliadin, is one such illness.) Normally our intestines are lined with branches of fingerlike villi, which help us absorb our nutrients and exponentially increase the intestinal surface area. Gluten sensitivity can destroy the villi, leading to a form of malnutrition. In response, the immune system attempts to destroy the gluten but eventually ends up attacking its own intestinal lining. All this because of an innocent little grain of wheat!

Within two months of starting on her gluten-free diet, Elizabeth had significantly less pain and constipation. Meanwhile, daily doses of glutamine were repairing her intestinal lining. Within four months, her gas had virtually disappeared. She continues to avoid wheat, and she is feeling better than she's felt in years.

Glutamine Keeps the Body Together

Glutamine is an amazingly effective intestinal glue, reducing porosity and the inflammation caused by toxins or disease that allow harmful bacteria access to the bloodstream. Many studies show that glutamine is key to maintaining the health and mucosal structure of the digestive tract. It is actually the principal fuel used by the upper intestinal tract. Most of the illnesses that benefit from glutamine stem from problems with intestinal permeability or inflammation. Examples follow.

Immune Function: Numerous studies on lab animals have shown that glutamine can enhance immune function during severe infections and trauma from burns or surgery. In humans, glutamine is also crucial in maintaining the immune system. As just noted, the most important part of our immune defense is located in the digestive tract. Glutamine, the main source of intestinal energy, preserves the immune system by preventing pathogens from leaking in and overwhelming the system.

Inflammatory Bowel Disease: Glutamine is critical in treating colitis and Crohn's disease, two of the most prevalent and devastating digestive diseases. These illnesses are often treated with powerful steroids or chemotherapy drugs and sometimes result in surgical removal of whole sections of inflamed intestines. A study from the *British Journal of Surgery* showed that glutamine improves conditions similar to inflammatory bowel disease in lab animals by significantly decreasing the permeability of the intestinal lining as well as bacterial translocation, which is caused by permeability. This occurs when bacteria from the lining gets into the blood and migrates to areas of the body, like the heart or lungs, where they can cause systemic infections.

Arthritis: Inflammatory arthritis and intestinal permeability may be linked. A review of a number of studies on permeability in *Clinical and Experimental Rheumatology* concludes that several rheumatic diseases are triggered in part by pathogens crossing the intestinal barrier. A report in the *Lancet* also linked intestinal infections to arthritic conditions like Reiter's syndrome. This painful illness is characterized by arthritis, conjunctivitis, and urethritis, which might be caused by a variety of intestinal infections, like *Shigella* or *Salmonella*. Although it's still unknown how antigens escaping the intestines actually irritate the joints, glutamine can often heal a leaky intestine and may play a role in the treatment of arthritis.

Food Allergies: Again, by healing the intestinal lining, glutamine keeps food particles out of the bloodstream. When the intestines are more permeable, incompletely digested food and other large molecules can enter the bloodstream in larger amounts than usual, causing some people's immune systems to become sensitive to this unexpected onslaught of allergens. Studies like one in the journal *Contemporary Surgery* have shown that glutamine can repair the mucosal cells that make up the intestinal lining, prevent the immune system from going on red alert, and prevent it from overacting to foods and microbes.

Muscle Strength: Glutamine can actually preserve muscle, preventing it from being broken down for use as a primary fuel in wasting syndromes such as cancer, where the body is in need of extra energy. This amino acid increases the ability of muscles to store sugar, and it even stops them from atrophying.

AGING: Glutamine also increases growth hormone, which can help preserve muscle mass and provide antiaging benefits. A study in *Nutrition Science News* suggests that glutamine might effectively slow the effects of aging by not only maintaining muscle mass but also by reducing fat accumulation. By around age thirty, growth hormone begins to decline, taking with it muscle tone and leaving behind signs of aging and weight gain. The study, explaining that glutamine can boost growth hormone levels by 43 percent, supports glutamine supplements as protection against aging.

HORMONAL IMBALANCE: Impotence, breast cancer, prostate cancer, and menstrual abnormalities are all medical conditions that can be caused by irregular hormone levels. When the intestines become too permeable, excess hormones meant to pass out of the body as waste are allowed to remain or return to the body. Glutamine can prevent estrogen and other hormones from reaching harmful levels in the body by containing discarded amounts in the digestive tract.

THE GLUTAMINE/CANCER CONNECTION

The role of glutamine in tumor cells is a source of controversy. A number of new studies suggest that glutamine may be a potent cancer therapy because it increases levels of the powerful antioxidant glutathione. A study in the *Annals of Surgery* showed that glutathione may increase the effectiveness of antitumor drugs by sensitizing cells to chemotherapy; it may also lead to decreased tumor growth. The *Journal of Parenteral Enteral Nutrition* reported that glutamine decreased the rate of tumor growth by promoting activity of natural killer cells. Similarly, a study in the *Journal of Surgical Research* suggests that glutamine can overwhelm tumor growth. Unlike other cells in our bodies, which require oxygen to live, tumors are anaerobic and use glutamine as their fuel. To get the food they need, tumors are equipped with glutamine traps, which literally wait for glutamine to float by so they can grab it. If tumor cells consistently sap our natural stores of glutamine, our body will run out, and the tumors will demand more. This causes muscle wasting. An obvious solution for this is to use glutamine treatments to stop the wasting and stimulate the body's natural killer cells. However, herein lies the controversy: glutamine may actually *promote* tumor growth as well. Tumors feed on glutamine, among other nutrients. Replacing disappearing stores of glutamine with more of the nutrient may just lead to further depletion and wasting. Despite glutamine's potential role in alleviating the growth of tumor cells, the danger of the opposite result leaves scientists wary. Still, the beneficial possibilities warrant further research.

A Magical Mystery Tour of Digestion

The intestines are a huge part of the digestive system, a finely tuned biological machine designed to process the world outside us so that we can take it in and convert it into energy to fuel the body's infinite functions. Digestion begins at the first bite of food, when your teeth grind the food so that its fibrous membranes can be released easily. Just the delectable presence of the morsels in your mouth stimulates salivation, which lubricates the throat and helps form food into a ball—called a bolus—which makes chewing and swallowing easier. Sugars are broken down by enzymes in the saliva and travel to the stomach, where acids literally strong enough to burn a hole through car paint begin to process this food.

The miraculous process doesn't stop there. Enzymes released from the pancreas in r[illegible]onse to stomach acid begin to break down proteins and allow food to be pas[illegible]mall intestine. When healthy, the intestine allows only the smallest ba[illegible]s amino acids, sugars, and fats through its elite walls, a[illegible]stream for the first time for nourishment. Bile in the [illegible]ts so they can be passed on to the liver through the [illegible]en finally delivered to the doors of cells throughout [illegible]ardian, the digestive tract keeps harmful bacteria and [illegible]s flexible, protective walls until they emerge from the b[illegible]

The Invisible Enemies Within

You may be wondering just how your intestinal tract knows which substances passing through its spiraling loops are beneficial and which can endanger health. After all, not only do the foods we eat contain harmful chemicals and allergens, but the very bacteria that normally live in our intestine can turn against us and damage our intestinal filter. We now know, for instance, that a bacterium called *H. pylori* can live in the stomach and cause ulcers and even trigger cancer through constant inflammation of the stomach lining. If one microbe living in the lining of the stomach can cause serious problems, then the trillions of bacteria that live in the intestines would seem to pose an infinitely greater risk. Indeed, if too many harmful bacteria exist, they can form a membrane that seals them onto the intestinal surface like Saran Wrap and protects them while they attack the intestinal lining.

Unfortunately, we still do not understand exactly how our intestines know which particles to absorb into the blood and which to discard as waste. It is clear, however, that whenever the mysterious intestinal code is broken by clever microbes, our immune defenses become overwhelmed. Our intestines become compromised, and our health is at serious risk.

HOW DO WE TEST FOR PERMEABILITY?

One test for intestinal permeability checks to see if the intestines are still keeping larger particles from leaking out. It uses mannitol and lactulose, both nonmetabolized sugar molecules. Mannitol, a small sugar, normally is free to pass through the intestinal lining. Lactulose, on the other hand, is usually not. First, patients drink a mixture of mannitol and lactulose. Then, six hours later, a urine sample is taken and analyzed to see how much—and which—of the sugars got through the intestines and went through the body. If both sugars are present in levels greater than they're normally found in our urine, then we know that the size of the "pores" in the intestines has stretched, becoming more vulnerable to bigger, and potentially harmful, molecules. The sugar potion can also inform us about decreased permeability. If the urine tested has low levels of mannitol, then it means that even small nutrients are being shut out of the bloodstream, which can lead to malnutrition. This syndrome is informally known as "leaky gut syndrome" among many alternative practitioners. There is increasing scientific and medical interest in the leaky gut syndrome and its links to chronic disease such as allergies, psoriasis, and arthritis.

The Leaky Intestine and Immunity

A leaky intestine is especially dangerous in immune-compromised patients, such as people who are undergoing chemotherapy or those who are HIV positive. Many systemic infections contracted by patients with HIV occur because of bacterial translocation: bacteria or yeast travel from the intestines to the bloodstream and cause infection. It's like a kind of blood poisoning.

That same blood poisoning goes on in a much milder version in those of us who suffer from leaky gut syndrome. Studies on patients with inflammatory bowel disease have shown dramatic increases in intestinal permeability. Drugs like ibuprofen, or Advil, or substances like alcohol exacerbate the problem by inhibiting prostaglandins that normally protect the intestinal lining. Although these medications may protect one part of the body from pain, they hurt another part of the body—the intestines.

SEVEN SIGNS OF INTESTINAL PERMEABILITY

Do you have leaky intestine syndrome without even realizing it? If you have at least several of the following symptoms, then you may be experiencing a permeability problem:

1. Joint pain, particularly after eating
2. Frequent gas and bloating
3. Chronic fatigue
4. Frequent intestinal problems like constipation or diarrhea
5. Headaches, especially after eating
6. A large number of allergies
7. Adverse reactions to many foods

Healthy Handyman: How Glutamine Helped Real People

Lona Hass was a fifty-three-year-old self-made millionaire. She had started her career as one of the first female stockbrokers in history and gone on to become the president of her own investment company. She was responsible for a huge corporation, so it was particularly terrifying to her when she started developing a host of ailments, including crippling fatigue coupled with weight gain, intestinal bloating, back pain, constipation, and irritable bowel syndrome. Strangely enough, Lona had also developed sensitivities to a number of random substances, including talcum powder, newspapers, perfumes, and pineapples. The most frightening problem that she was experiencing, however, was partial memory loss. Lona recalled, sadly, that she once used to stroll around her beautiful flower-strewn backyard, mulling over hundreds of ideas about her life and her company. Recently, however, she could barely remember the details of her daily schedule or recent past. Like a candle that flickers brighter and darker by turns, Lona held on to memories some days and lost them the next. How was she supposed to negotiate big deals and manage a whole company in this condition?

When I first saw Lona, I could tell that she was a bit puzzled by the questions I asked about her medical history. Sometimes, though, the most important clues for a proper diagnosis are ones that are best hidden.

"Lona," I asked, "are you having problems with gas at all? Any bloating?"

"Wait," she interrupted. "I'm telling you about how I can't wear perfume or even touch a newspaper anymore. I'm constantly exhausted, and you're asking about gas? That's the least of my problems!"

"Well, symptoms like gas and bloating can be very important signals of illness, especially when paired with fatigue and allergies," I explained.

"Actually," she conceded, "I have had bloating for years. It's kind of embarrassing; some days I can feel my belt buckle straining, about to pop open, right in the middle of a meeting!"

After further quizzing, I also discovered that Lona seemed to have most of the seven symptoms (see box on page 122) that I associate with intestinal illness, especially the chronic fatigue and random allergies. Whenever I notice one of my patients suffering from a list of seemingly unrelated complaints, I look at several sources, including a sluggish liver (see chapter 7) and a leaky gut. Intestinal permeability, I guessed, may have predated Lona's many symptoms.

After administering allergy tests and a permeability test, I found her positive for both intestinal permeability and multiple food allergies. Still skeptical of my diagnosis, Lona shook her head when I described her treatment program.

"No other doctor has ever cared about my intestines," she said.

"Maybe that's your problem," I said.

As I explained to Lona, excessively permeable intestines allow potentially dangerous particles to enter the body, which erode the intestinal villi, generate bacterial overgrowth, and exhaust the immune system (which must combat all these new toxins). In order to repair this damage, we first normalized her intestines with digestive enzymes, allowing them to once again process food into small particles that could safely permeate a healthy intestinal lining without being attacked as foreign antigens. To repair her leaky gut, I prescribed glutamine. I also gave her a combination of nutrients for her fatigue and antiyeast supplements for her intestines.

Once on this treatment program, Lona felt more energetic, and she returned to work. The first symptoms to completely disappear were her muscle aches and pains. Lona does have to watch her diet, and she is careful not to eat pineapple and gluten-based foods, to which she still has a strong reaction. However, as her health improves, she is able to sneak the occasional pineapple wedge or bagel into her diet. As her intestines continue to heal, she will gradually be able to increase the number of foods she can safely eat.

Allergies, Arthritis, and Glutamine

Janice was a thirty-six-year-old redhead who came into my office complaining of severe headaches, joint pains, dry skin, and hair loss. She worked as an artist in Soho, where she crafted beautiful pieces of jewelry. Lately, however, it was becoming increasingly difficult for her to move her hands. She had a complicated medical history that included bulimia, numerous yeast infections, menstrual irregularity, and problems with irritable bowel syndrome. Yet except for slightly elevated cholesterol levels, she was in good health. What was causing her distress?

Janice had also been feeling exhausted and off balance. This fatigue was especially frustrating for her, since she'd been jogging daily for years to stay in shape. Now, Janice was a member of the running wounded. It seemed that any time she ate certain foods she became sick with cold and flulike symptoms.

The numerous doctors that Janice had visited before me had considered many possible underlying conditions, like thyroid disease or chronic fatigue syndrome; every test, however, came back normal. At some point, a physician determined that she did have arthritis and prescribed the anti-inflammatory drug Motrin. Beyond this ailment, though, Janice's previous doctors were baffled by the seeming lack of a cause for her many symptoms.

"I can't live this way any longer," she told me bluntly.

I suspected that these arthritic and coldlike symptoms were due to intestinal permeability. The idea that rheumatoid arthritis and intestinal health are linked has become increasingly accepted in the medical world. Several studies, including two from the *Clinical and Experimental Rheumatology* journal, show that patients with this form of arthritis have increased intestinal permeability. Furthermore, a *Lancet* study reported that improvements in rheumatoid arthritis may actually be due to a reduction in intestinal permeability. This led me to guess that Janice might be a victim of ailments related to leaky intestine syndrome.

When tested for allergies, Janice was found to be allergic to practically every food and substance. When I see a patient who is allergic to everything, I suspect that her intestines must be too permeable, letting through all kinds of foreign molecules and toxins and causing the immune system to react indiscriminately to these countless "invaders." I had quite a bit of work to do with her.

I put Janice on a program of acidophilus to replenish her intestinal flora; digestive enzymes; an herb called artemisia, which clears out parasites; flaxseed powder, a gentle and healing fiber to help absorb toxins from the bowel; and the herb dong quai, which gently rebalances estrogen levels. Finally, I prescribed both glutamine and zinc to enhance the healing of her intestines.

A yeast-free diet was also important for Janice's recovery; in patients with compromised immunity, heightened yeast sensitivity, along with yeast overgrowth, is common. Indeed, a positive skin test indicated that Janice had both. Because yeast is naturally found in the intestine, people with these sensitivities may be reacting to substances in their own bodies. A diet that does not feed yeast at all is the only way to avoid antigens that might adversely affect the body. Initially, Janice, like most people on such a diet, was frustrated. Eliminating yeast meant no wine, beer, bread, or sugar, and very little fruit.

But it was worth the sacrifice. Within three months, her fatigue and joint pains improved. She felt less toxic. When I tested her again for allergies, they were now reduced by half. She continues to eliminate allergies steadily by adhering strictly to her treatment. Triumphant because she has finally identified her mysterious disease, Janice said recently, "I knew I wasn't crazy! I knew I wasn't imagining everything!" Best of all, she's back to creating the intricate rings and bracelets she—along with millions of Soho visitors—loves so much.

Glutamine's restorative power can actually put food back into the diets of highly allergic people. Dina Lupone also arrived at my office in despair, informing me that she was allergic to everything. This fragile, ethereal-looking young woman subsisted on a minimal diet of rice, water, steamed vegetables, tofu, and a few other grains. Amazingly, Dina was making sure to stay actively involved in other aspects of her health, like exercising regularly, usually by racewalking or bicycling. More than most patients I see, she had a sense of which foods would work for her and which would not.

Dina's extreme allergies suggested to me that her intestines might be drastically eroded, so I prescribed aloe in addition to glutamine. Many people think of aloe only as a lotion to be applied to a sunburn, but the plant also has intriguing internal benefits. I ask patients to drink anywhere from 1 to 4 ounces of aloe juice per day; the powerful anti-inflammatory qualities that are so beneficial to burned skin seem to help internally as well.

Dina's healing began slowly, but when she walked into my office a month later, she had noticed a big change in her health.

"Dr. Firshein," she said, "my headaches are gone."

I was skeptical. Dina's case had been quite extreme. "You used to have them every day."

"Well," she repeated, "they're gone. And I can eat more foods now too!"

In the real world, recovery programs do not always run according to plan, and such was the case with Dina's. Another month went by, and Dina was back, this time without the smile. She lamented that some of her "allergic" symptoms had returned. Healing is not always linear; it can occur in cycles, and sometimes there are relapses that we don't quite understand. Patience and persistence will almost always pay off, and I encouraged Dina to keep taking the 3 grams of glutamine and watch her foods even more carefully. Finally, six months later, she can eat much more freely, and without the pain and irritation that had been inextricable parts of her life.

Glutamine's Restorative Effects

Many of my patients devote themselves to maintaining their health and fitness. I love to see people educating themselves about the benefits of different nutrients, vitamins, natural foods, and disease prevention. It's very important to be aware of which foods and supplements can keep you feeling great and which are insidiously loading your body with chemicals or toxins. Sometimes, however, despite the best intentions, the nutritional program you choose may indeed be healthy—but not for you.

One patient, Charles Foster, is a perfect example of someone putting in the time, effort, and research necessary to improve his health. A fifty-two-year-old high school teacher, Charles was disabled by fatigue and impotence and numerous intestinal complaints. Determined to cure himself without expensive doctors or synthetic drugs, Charles read all that he could on foods and supplements that would boost his energy and his libido.

First, he told me, he took yohimbe, a suspected aphrodisiac that has been found to help some men with impotence. Charles then began a new nutritional program: he gave up meat and switched to a vegetarian, soy-based diet, thinking that it would reenergize him. When he finally came to me, however, not only were the impotence and fatigue still bothering him, but he had developed anxiety attacks. By this point, Charles felt defeated. He couldn't understand how he could be suffering in this way; he saw his entire life in decline.

"I am literally going straight downhill," he told me. The worst problem, in his mind, was the loss of his youth and masculinity. Although his wife never complained, he felt sure that she was disappointed by his impotence and sluggishness. To make matters worse, although he had started exercising and lifting weights more often, his muscle mass was diminishing rapidly. Charles felt like he was disintegrating, despite his best efforts to the contrary.

Charles's symptoms did seem rather unrelated. However, I felt that there had to be some unifying factor in all his problems. I kept listening closely to the clues in his life and history. First of all, I knew that yohimbe has been shown to cause blood pressure elevations in some men; this was probably leading to his anxiety. I also knew that soy contains natural plant estrogens, which can reduce the testosterone levels necessary to maintain libido. Charles's inability to retain muscle mass was also a classic sign of testosterone deficiency. His vegetarian, soy-based diet probably increased his fatigue, because it was deficient in vitamin B_{12}, which is contained in meat and is important for energy. I saw a possible link between the increased estrogen levels and intestinal permeability. If Charles had a leaky gut, it's possible that it might have been reabsorbing estrogenic compounds from the soy into his bloodstream, leading to the impotence.

In this case, all roads led to glutamine as the perfect treatment. Not only would it heal an eroded intestine, it would preserve muscle mass. A recent study showed that glutamine may reduce the rate of muscle breakdown compared to the rate of muscle growth. Last but not least, exercise has been shown to deplete stores of glutamine, which also could have contributed to Charles's fatigue and loss of muscle mass. Compelling recent research indicates that glutamine treatments may have a very important role in physical fitness. As when the body is struggling against disease, strenuous exercise demands more glutamine than the body can make. In fact, one study showed that seven healthy athletes who did intensive anaerobic and aerobic exercise lost 45 percent and 50 percent, respectively, of their natural glutamine levels. (No wonder glutamine is a primary component of all those muscle-building supplements in health food stores.) Some of the runners still had depressed glutamine levels six days after the experiment ended, suggesting that they needed more glutamine than their bodies were providing. Glutamine can also be helpful to athletes because it stimulates bicarbonate production, which alleviates the muscle soreness and fatigue that can come from weight lifting or other exercise. A study in the *Journal of Parenteral Enteral Nutrition* found that glutamine supplements can minimize muscle pain after long, hard workouts. The same study showed that people taking glutamine supplements burned fat faster than those not taking it.

Would my glutamine theory of Charles's health hold up? I took him off his soy-based diet and placed him on a fish and vegetable diet, which helped detoxify his body of extraneous estrogens and cholesterol. I supplemented his new eating habits with glutamine, to repair intestinal permeability, and ginseng, which has been long prized in Asian cultures as an aphrodisiac. Not surprisingly, he did show a B_{12} deficiency, so I gave him weekly shots until he stabilized, and then put him on oral supplements.

Now, Charles boasts of greater energy, and feels he's maintaining good muscle mass. His impotence has improved, though it hasn't disappeared completely. We're now exploring other issues that may further alleviate this problem, including other herbs like ginkgo, which improves circulation (see chapter 13).

Glutamine Repairs Drug Damage

Faith Capra, a fifty-two-year-old floral designer, was experiencing joint pain, headaches, dizziness, tingling and itching, and weight gain. Her doctors had placed her on daily doses of anti-inflammatory drugs. She had also been to numerous diet centers. Like many of my patients, she'd been on a decades-long roller coaster of weight loss and weight gain. An inability to keep the pounds off had seriously diminished Faith's sense of self-esteem.

Then she developed a skin rash that would not go away. Her itching, swollen ankles, and back pain intensified. As is typical for patients with these seemingly random symptoms, Faith's lab tests were all completely normal. However, Faith was taking daily doses of Motrin for her backaches, and she was on a popular diet drug for her weight problem.

We immediately discontinued her use of the diet drug, since I thought a drug reaction might be causing the ankle swelling. Mostly, though, I suspected intestinal permeability as the source of many of her problems. Even her back pain could have been due to an inflamed intestine, though no doctor before me had made the connection. I've actually found that some back problems are derived from intestinal cramping, which then causes back muscles to cramp in a kind of sympathetic spasm. Her problems were stemming predominantly from frequent use of Motrin, which, like aspirin and any anti-inflammatory drug, can actually increase intestinal permeability!

I sat down with Faith to discuss her medical condition. Although many of her symptoms predated her Motrin use, some of her symptoms had actually gotten worse since she started taking it, and as her pain increased, she had increased her dosage significantly. It was crucial that she stop taking Motrin, yet she argued tearfully that it was the only thing that could stop her pain.

The relationship between arthritis and intestinal inflammation has been well established. There are a number of rheumatic diseases related to intestinal pathogens traveling across the intestinal barrier. It is ironic that the drugs prescribed to treat arthritis can actually worsen intestinal permeability and may contribute to the actual cause of the disease. I recommend that any patient with a rheumatic disease see a forward-thinking gastroenterologist or nutritionist as well. These patients need to address the health of their gut linings along with the pain in their joints and muscles.

I started Faith on a treatment program of glutamine, as well as glucosamine sulfate, an anti-inflammatory nutrient that is amazingly helpful in arthritis, along with zinc, aloe, and milk thistle to help her liver, which had been stressed by trying to detoxify high doses of drugs for such a long time (see chapter 7). Her joint pains began to improve after approximately three months.

Happy Intestines Mean a Happy Ending

Glutamine is available in most health food stores as a supplement and often comes in 500-milligram doses. The doses I prescribe my patients range from 1,000 to 3,000 milligrams a day. However, these doses need to be monitored by a knowledgeable physician.

It might seem strange that glutamine can exert so many effects merely by keeping the intestines in good health. But sometimes good things do come in small packages. Unlike over-the-counter drugs that can actually aggravate the ailments we expect them to alleviate, glutamine supplements are a natural way to improve problems related to the digestive system.

HOW MUCH SHOULD I TAKE?

For General Health
100 mg/day (optional)
Divided doses before or after meals
Special Conditions

Constipation	500-2000 mg/day
Inflammatory bowel	disease 1,000-4000 mg/day
Leaky gut syndrome	1,000-4000 mg/day

10

Flaxseed: A Gentle Cleanser

Many of us are lucky enough not to suffer from a specific problem with our eyes or heart or lungs. We're more concerned with the big picture and prevention of illness. But even the most healthy of us have days when we feel a bit sluggish and less energetic.

Patricia Ferris, forty-eight years of age, was suffering from just such a case of the blahs. She came to my office to get to the bottom of several seemingly unrelated health concerns such as constipation, respiratory allergies, and chronic depression. Ironically, Patricia was a motivational speaker who frequently lectured at business conferences and office retreats. She always had an optimistic word and an encouraging smile for her audiences, but her congestion and gastrointestinal discomfort turned her into a walking contradiction. As time passed, she grew more and more frustrated, especially since she couldn't pinpoint the source of her discomfort.

She tried acupuncture, hoping that its gentle balancing action would heal her vague complaints, but it didn't help much. Patricia then attempted to cleanse her body by eating a vegetarian diet and avoiding dairy and wheat products, which, she had read, could cause food allergies and sensitivities, but again she found little relief.

When I hear that someone is constipated, mildly fatigued most of the time, and burdened with seemingly random symptoms, I have one word for them: detoxify. Patricia needed to detoxify her body. She had sensed that—thus her visits to the acupuncturist and her vegetarian diet—but she hadn't hit on the right way to truly cleanse her body.

Surprising as it may sound, she was able to do so using a foodstuff that is already well-known to us as a dietary way to keep us regular: fiber. One form of fiber, in particular, can not only relieve constipation but can also reduce high cholesterol levels and balance an excess of hormones that lead to uncomfortable PMS symptoms. This ancient fiber source is the seed of the flax plant.

Flaxseed has actually been a part of the human diet for thousands of years and has a rich history of use. Four thousand years ago, in southern Mesopotamia, citizens constructed irrigation systems primarily for the growth of flax, and the plant was cultivated in Babylonia circa 3000 BC. The famed philosopher-physician Hippocrates used it to relieve intestinal discomfort. Flaxseed has been known as an important gastrointestinal cleanser for so long that the eighth-century king Charlemagne even passed laws governing its farming and consumption.

Today, we're learning that this ancient fiber has three major health benefits. First, flaxseed contains essential fatty acids in the omega-3 family, in the form of alpha linoleic acid. While the most common source of these important fats is fish, flax is a great vegetarian way to load up on omega-3s, which are lacking in the Western diet. These fatty acids are extremely useful in reducing coronary heart disease, blood pressure, and inflammation of bodily tissues (see chapter 4). A study in the *British Journal of Nutrition* found that subjects consuming flax for four weeks not only increased their levels of omega-3 fatty acids but also reduced their cholesterol by 9 percent and their blood glucose by 27 percent.

Flaxseed is also the richest source of lignans, a type of phytoestrogen (a gentle plant hormone) that is key in maintaining healthy bones and preventing cancer. At high levels, estrogen can actually promote tumors, but flaxseed can balance the hormone in the body. Countless studies have proven that people who consume fiber-rich diets have a lower incidence of hormone-related cancers like breast, endometrial, and prostate cancer.

There are two types of fiber available in food: insoluble, which reduces bowel transit time, is good for constipation, and allows fecal matter to be expelled from the body more rapidly; and water soluble, which helps regulate blood glucose and reduces cholesterol levels. Flaxseed is two-thirds insoluble fiber and one-third soluble fiber, so it carries both benefits.

When I tell patients that they need to detoxify their bodies, I mean that they need to reduce the presence of harmful compounds—like excess hormones, toxins, and waste products—that can ultimately cause serious illness. Eating flaxseed is like cleaning out a pipe so that it can function smoothly, free of obstruction. Because of its cleansing action, flaxseed is a star of my detoxification program.

Cleanse Your Insides

By the time Patricia came to see me, she was pessimistic about how any treatment would improve her health, having been let down by her own efforts at alternative treatments.

"I'm busy with work, and I've felt mildly sick for years," she told me. "I'm coming here because I feel I should make an effort to improve my health, but I doubt it'll help."

Knowing that she would never make any progress unless she changed her attitude, I remarked, "For a motivational speaker, you don't sound very motivated to me."

She seemed surprised; then she said, "You're right. I need to listen to my own lectures more closely. Tell me what to do."

And I did.

I tested Patricia for sensitivities that, when triggered, might be causing her problems. I found that she was allergic to yeast, which is plentiful in foods like bread and pasta. In order to reduce her symptoms, I began with a complete detoxification program that started with a rice-based, hypoallergenic, high-nutrition powder formula called UltraClear. Allergic patients can usually consume this formula daily without triggering allergic symptoms. Anti-inflammatory supplements like quercetin (see chapter 17) and stinging nettle also relieved her allergies. For her mild depression, I suggested St. John's wort, a plant that has gained popularity as nature's answer to Prozac. To soothe and enhance her digestion, I prescribed aloe vera juice. Finally, to cleanse her body thoroughly of toxins and allergens, I asked her to take 1 tablespoon of flaxseed powder daily in 8 ounces of water.

In just a few days, Patricia noticed that her bowel discomfort was gone. A few weeks later, she started feeling more energetic—proof that when you treat one part of the body, other areas will respond as well. After six months of her detoxification regimen, her symptoms had completely disappeared.

"I'm shocked, thrilled, amazed at what I'm feeling," Patricia enthused.

One of the main lessons we can learn from Patricia's case is that you can't become healthy by looking at and treating only one part of the body or one symptom. Flaxseed—in combination with a host of complementary nutrients—was the perfect treatment for her malaise because it helped so many of her symptoms.

Many Functions for Flaxseed

"Detoxification" is a word thrown around quite a bit these days, but to me it means ridding the body of any harmful substances that don't belong in us, from excess cholesterol to high levels of estrogen to toxins from free radical damage to undigestible parts of food we eat. Flaxseed eliminates such waste from the body, helping ease a wide range of conditions, including the following.

LUPUS: Lupus is a seriously debilitating inflammatory condition similar to arthritis; young adult women are particularly susceptible to this illness. A study in the journal *Kidney International* showed that lupus patients consuming 15 to 45 grams of flaxseed daily for four weeks had improved kidney function, helping to clear their blood of toxins more readily.

HEART DISEASE: Hypercholesterolemic atherosclerosis, or the deterioration of blood vessels due to excessively high cholesterol levels can lead to heart disease if left untreated. According to a study in the journal *Atherosclerosis*, modest amounts of a dietary flax supplement reduced cholesterol.

Two of the risk factors for heart disease are high blood sugar and high fat content, and flax fiber has the power to reduce both. Fiber regulates our blood sugar by slowing our body's absorption of carbohydrates. Many studies also show that populations with a high dietary fiber intake have lower incidence of heart disease—a valuable lesson for those of us in America, where heart disease kills more people than any other illness each year.

CANCER: Although estrogen is a natural hormone that is crucial to female development and reproduction, too much of it can cause tumors. Because flaxseed contains phytoestrogens, gentle plant hormones that counteract excess estrogen, it is thought to have an anticancer effect. One study, in the journal *Carcinogenesis*, found that recurrent mammary tumors in women with breast cancer were reduced by 50 percent when flaxseed was administered to patients for 13 weeks. Flaxseed's tumor-reducing factor may be due in part to its high content of alpha linoleic acid, an omega-3 fatty acid.

Fiber is particularly effective at preventing colon cancer since it allows waste to be expelled with shorter transit time, which means there's less time for the carcinogens in our fecal matter to come in contact with our colons. It also makes our stool bulkier, diluting the concentration of carcinogens.

CONSTIPATION: Constipation not only is uncomfortable but can also lead to bowel obstruction and a variety of symptoms such as fatigue, achiness, and irritability. The *American Journal of Clinical Nutrition* reported that subjects in a study who took 50 grams of flaxseed daily for four weeks increased their bowel movements by 30 percent each week.

Immune System Dysfunction: One of flaxseed's most potent components is alpha linoleic acid, an omega-3 fatty acid that is deficient in many people's diets. Essential fatty acids are crucial to healing the body and soothing the inflammation associated with diseases like rheumatoid arthritis, psoriasis, and diabetes. Studies show that flax enhances our immune response, by inhibiting the production of proinflammatory compounds.

What Is Fiber?

Flaxseed is a supernutrient because it works with a triple punch to fight three big health concerns: constipation, cardiovascular disease, and cancer.

As I said, flaxseed's fiber is an important component of its healing potential. Fiber comes from a part of plant walls that is indigestible to humans but digestible to the good bacteria thriving in our guts, which use it for energy. Fruits like apples and strawberries and citrus are particularly high in pectins, a common form of fiber. Another type of fiber, cellulose, a compound used to give plants their structure, can be found in bran, peas, and root vegetables like sweet potatoes. Guar and other gums are common ingredients in prepared foods, and a good source of fiber—they can be found in oatmeal and legumes.

The principal metabolites of the bacteria that digest fiber are short chain fatty acids, one of which is a compound called butyric acid. This fiber by-product promotes healthy cell proliferation in the distal colon, which is key to maintaining intestinal health. People with low levels of butyrate in their colons are at higher risk for inflammatory bowel disease and colon cancer. The microorganisms on the intestinal surface digest fiber, using it as cellular fuel. More fiber means more healthy bacteria in our intestinal flora. The bacteria produce short chain fatty acids like butyric acid, which lower the pH of the colon, further inhibiting the normal breakdown of bile acids in the gut that promote cancer.

Flaxseed is the richest source of lignans. Present in most vegetables, albeit in small quantities, lignans are converted by our gut bacteria into active forms of phytoestrogens. It is believed that lignans protect the body from the most potent forms of estrogen, which can promote cancer. Studies show that populations around the world with diets that are high in fiber and lignans, such as the Japanese and Chinese, tend to have lower incidences of hormone-driven cancers. Vegetarians also seem especially likely to reap the benefits of lignans, since studies show that urinary levels of this fiber are higher in them than in omnivores.

Another disease-fighting component of flaxseed is alpha linolenic acid. This omega-3 fatty acid boosts immune cell response and reduces inflammation in the body. It does this by changing the composition of cell membrane phospholipids and markedly reducing the production of inflammatory compounds that flare up when we fall ill or get injured. This may allow flaxseed to be used as a treatment for autoimmune diseases such as lupus or even for common allergies.

Flaxseed is truly a wonderful supplement. However, if you're not a regular fiber eater, you should add it very gradually to your diet, since fiber in high doses can actually cause gas, flatulence, and intestinal blockage. Also, be sure to drink lots of water when consuming fiber, since its stool-expelling power comes from water it draws from the gastrointestinal tract. The National Cancer Institute recommends eating 25 to 30 grams of fiber a day, and most of us get only 15 to 20. For people attempting to reap heart-healthy benefits, I suggest working up to 50 grams a day of fiber.

Weight Watcher

Cindy Patton was a woman who, like many, had battled with her weight for years but never seemed to make much progress in controlling it. For Cindy, avoiding obesity was of the utmost importance for her health. First, she had a family history of high cholesterol, elevated triglycerides, and diabetes. Her mother had exceedingly high cholesterol levels and adult onset diabetes, and it now looked as if history would repeat itself. At the age of forty-four, Cindy had experienced a recent weight gain, and as the pounds went up, so did her triglycerides. They had risen to a dangerous level—over 300. Her cholesterol, at 250, was also high. Cindy seemed mystified by her inability to remain at a healthy weight and attributed it to her family legacy. I knew, however, that something in her life was triggering her problem. One of the first things I ask my patients about is their diets, since this one area of life can make or break their health.

"I have a sweet tooth," Cindy admitted. "I can't make it through the day without having at least a few chocolate chip cookies or a piece of cake or something satisfying like that. But I've been on all kinds of diets, from high-carbohydrate, low-protein regimens, to high-protein, low-carb regimens, and nothing will help me lose fat."

Cindy told me that she had whittled her daily food intake to nuts for protein, lots of bread ("Low fat!" she chirped), maybe a piece of fruit or two, and six or seven cups of decaffeinated coffee.

"It's low calorie, fat free, and caffeine free," she informed me, "so it's a great drink for a weight-loss hopeful like myself."

Unfortunately, I told her, she was at risk for heart disease, and her excessive coffee intake wasn't helping matters. A study of thirteen thousand Finnish subjects found that coffee drinkers—even those who drank only decaf—had the highest levels of homocysteine, recently highlighted as the one of the greatest risk factors for cardiovascular disease. Added to her high carbohydrate intake, the fat she was getting from nuts, and her family history, Cindy was headed down a hard road. Most notable was the increase in triglycerides caused by her low-fiber, high-sugar diet. Triglycerides are composed of three sugars combined to form a dangerous, heart-stopping fat. They can also stimulate the liver to produce cholesterol and reduce the body's ability to produce good HDL cholesterol. In short, they are a major risk factor for heart disease.

"But I'm eating more bread and less cheese and sweets!" she protested.

"It's the bread that's causing your problems," I told her. "Overeating carbohydrates can hike up your blood sugar."

Cindy was a victim of syndrome X, a constellation of symptoms first noted by Gerald Reaven, MD, which is often a precursor to other diseases. While she had the beginning signs of diabetes, such as a resistance to insulin (hyperinsulinemia) and an inability to handle blood sugar, as well as impaired wound healing, she did not have the disease itself; hence, the mysterious name for a mysterious condition. I knew we'd have to treat Cindy with a comprehensive list of nutrients and natural supplements designed to change her eating habits.

First and foremost, I put Cindy on a plan my patients like to call Dr. Firshein's Park Avenue Spa Diet Program. This is a high-fiber, low-carbohydrate diet that unfailingly helps people reduce their blood sugar, their triglycerides, and their weight. To help neutralize her sweet tooth, I gave her an Ayurvedic herb called *Gymnema sylvestre* (a mild appetite suppressant) to control her cravings. But the crux of the spa program is fiber in the form of flaxseed, starting gradually and adding more as the days pass. At first, she doubted the power of fiber.

"What will this do for me that other foods won't?" she asked.

"Flax will make the difference in your weight-loss, triglyceride-lowering plan," I explained. "It has bulk, which takes up space in your gut, making you feel too full to eat excessively large portions. The essential fatty acids in flax makes the body more sensitive to sugars, keeping them from turning into fat. It helps produce acids in the intestines that interfere with an enzyme that promotes cholesterol production in the liver. Plus, fiber can improve the health and appearance of your hair and skin."

Cindy did remarkably well on this diet; after one week on the program, she had already begun to shed pounds. And as the weight dropped, so did other risk factors, especially those triglycerides: they rapidly decreased to a normal level, about 140. She ultimately lost twenty pounds and has maintained her new weight. She feels healthier, more energetic, and more confident than ever, knowing that she has been able to conquer her family history and her persistent sweet tooth. She still sneaks in a cookie here and there, but making sure fiber plays a huge part in her diet keeps her heart healthy and her body slim.

Beat Breast Cancer?

Like Cindy, forty-seven-year-old Laura Mantle had a family history of disease, but weight gain and cholesterol had nothing to do with the legacy she'd received. Laura, a ballet teacher, was actually a wisp of a woman and, enviably, had no problem with resisting sweets. However, both her mother and her sister had breast cancer, and she was desperate to avoid the same fate. Laura had always experienced menstrual irregularities, and she grew up in an area of Long Island, New York, that has an unusually high incidence of breast cancer. Not surprisingly, she was extremely concerned about her risk of cancer and was absolutely convinced that she was genetically predisposed toward it.

Women with breast cancer—or at risk of developing it—tend to have high estrogen levels, but Laura's were fine. Upon questioning her on her medical history and lifestyle, however, I found that she was at high risk for other reasons. Not only did her female relatives have the disease, but she drank about three glasses of wine every night (alcohol is known to raise hormone levels and increase the risk of breast cancer). Because she so strictly controlled her food intake to preserve her dancer's figure, wine was both her way of relaxing and her single vice. Furthermore, she had her first child at the late age of forty, a factor known to slightly increase breast cancer risk. Finally, despite her healthy diet and regular exercise, tests showed that she had low levels of healthy gut bacteria and butyrate, both of which are linked to increased risk of cancer.

I explained the dangers of daily alcohol to Laura. I asked that she eat as much soy as possible. The isoflavones in soy have estrogenic effects, much like the lignans in flaxseed, which balance out our own more potent estrogens. Finally, I suggested that she consume flaxseed powder daily. A study in the *Journal of Clinical Endocrinology* found that flax not only decreases risk of cancer in women but helps regulate the menstrual cycle by lengthening the luteal phase—which occurs just after the egg has been released.

We can't be sure that Laura will be spared breast cancer, but at this time she shows no signs. And she has already seen improvement in her menstrual cycles, which came sporadically but have resumed with monthly regularity. Beginning a prevention program was the best thing Laura could do to ensure a safe, healthy future. She knows she is doing her best to avert illness.

Hearty Diet

Joe Delantoni was a sixty-five-year-old retired pilot. Although his faithful fighter jet was no longer soaring, his cholesterol levels were. Recently diagnosed with heart disease, Joe was experiencing chronic chest pain, excessive hair loss, hyperthyroidism, and insomnia. His cholesterol wasn't the only risk factor flying high: his triglycerides, homocysteine levels, weight, and iron levels were also at the outer limits. Joe's father had died of a heart attack, and with Joe's risk factors and the spare tire around his sedentary middle predicting a similar demise, I knew we had to get him help, fast.

Joe's diet emphasized hamburgers, fries, grilled cheese sandwiches, and hot dogs. I knew that his diet and his high iron levels (iron is believed to be a risk factor in heart disease) had to be controlled if his health was to improve. Joe told me he knew that heart-healthy diets were severely restricted in fat and that he had to cut his cholesterol intake, but he couldn't bring himself to stop eating fried, fatty treats. Meanwhile, all the chemicals from these fiberless, greasy foods were leaving him constipated. He visited the bathroom constantly, straining to push stool out in what's called the Valsalva maneuver (yes, this has a name). The maneuver actually puts pressure on the heart, aggravating Joe's already serious condition.

Fiber was one solution. Not only can fiber decrease cholesterol production, reduce sugar release, and cleanse the body, it also binds with iron and safely ushers it out of the body. Iron in the blood binds with vitamin C and oxidizes, where it can cause serious free radical damage to blood vessels. Studies show that blood donors and menstruating women have a lower incidence of heart disease than the average male because they lose iron as they release blood. (Although we need iron for our red blood cells to be healthy, too much iron can cause a problem.) I told Joe to take fiber in the potent form of flaxseed powder, stirring it into juice or fruit shakes for easy consumption. I also gave him niacin, which works in the liver to suppress cholesterol production, and vitamin E, which is known to be a heart tonic, along with B_{12} and folate, which counteracts high homocysteine levels (known to be a risk factor in heart disease). Finally, I persuaded him to cut processed foods and carbohydrates out of his diet and boost fruits and vegetables.

I do not believe that cholesterol is as crucial a risk factor in heart disease as we once imagined, but high levels serve as a fairly good indication of a potentially serious problem.

Joe was enjoying retired life, staying home with his wife and preparing for the arrival of grandchildren, so he was determined to do whatever it took to rescue his heart. The blood test I took during his first visit to my office told me that his heart was in serious need of repair. But by his very next blood test, three months later, Joe's cholesterol had dropped from 260 to 190, and his homocysteine levels (see chapter 11) had also dropped significantly. Statistics show that for every cholesterol point you lower, you reduce your risk for heart disease by 2 percent.

Joe's levels still aren't optimal, and despite changes in his diet and lots of fiber, that spare tire around his stomach hasn't totally disappeared. He's lucky he hasn't been urged to undergo bypass surgery; two of his arteries are dangerously narrowed, and surgery may be recommended if three are completely blocked. In the meantime, he is amazed and content with the improvement that he's derived from flaxseed and its supporting cast of nutrients; indeed, his chest pain has disappeared. For Joe, powerful nutraceuticals have been enough to fend off the often-fatal consequences of heart disease. I will continue to monitor Joe in the hopes that further use of these supplements will steer him farther away from the danger zone.

Cleansing Cure?

The story of Paul Moore is one of the strangest and most remarkable I've ever seen. At the young age of twenty-six, Paul was hospitalized with an involuntary muscle seizure disorder. A computer scientist, Paul had always been healthy, until one day in 1991 when his hand started shaking spasmodically. From that day forward, Paul's body was wracked with seizurelike episodes that attacked without warning, took over his bodily control, and shook him to extreme fatigue. His muscles began to weaken so much that he eventually lost the strength to walk, and even when his limbs weren't jerking out of control, he felt numbness and tingling in his extremities.

Paul drove himself crazy trying to understand why this had happened to him; he worried that he had multiple sclerosis. But doctors found no neurological deficits, vitamin deficiencies, electroencephalogram (brain wave) abnormalities, or signs of Lyme disease. Specialists prescribed him a long list of drugs, from phenobarbitol for what they thought were petit mal seizures to Paxil for depression and Elavil for sleep disorders. Meanwhile, brilliant Paul had been confined to a wheelchair and was highly susceptible to colds and flus, even as his apparent seizures continued. When hospital staff couldn't pinpoint his disease, they released him. Back at home, he attempted to continue his passion, computer programming, which led to carpal tunnel syndrome, since he was already so weak and chronically fatigued. This led to the loss of the use of his hands.

It was in this tragic state that he came to see me, seeking some natural respite from his bizarre illness. To be honest, I didn't know what to do with him. Whenever I encounter anyone with such a diverse panoply of symptoms, I begin with an attempt to return the body to its healthiest state through detoxification. Paul himself had considered the benefits of cleansing the body; he had used enemas in the past, but I wanted to start him on a much more comprehensive approach.

First, we'd have to put him on the purest of diets. He still clung to fatty foods like french fries and ice cream, as though he were defying his bad health or perhaps seeking comfort in them. Tests for food allergies showed that Paul was reacting to a number of substances, including gluten, which is found in wheat products. Perhaps this gluten sensitivity had triggered his numerous ailments. We eliminated every possible allergenic food from his daily diet.

Vitamin C and magnesium were two of the first supplements I prescribed for him, since they are known to boost the immune system. A stool analysis revealed severe intestinal dysbiosis, an imbalanced flora with many harmful bacteria. Paul's gut lining was severely impaired, letting toxins and undigested food molecules pass through the now permeable gut lining into the bloodstream.

THE CONSTIPATION QUESTION

Constipation causes most people concern—and often causes physical discomfort as well. It is true that constipation may be a warning sign of internal toxicity, as in the stories told here. But skipping a day or two of "number two" doesn't mean you're unhealthy or that you require serious treatment. In fact, too much stool can mean the loss of important minerals from the body. Regular bowel movements are the optimal way to ensure that you're expelling toxins from the body. If you're eating healthily, exercising, and drinking lots of fluids, however, don't fret if you miss an occasional trip to the toilet.

Once they were there, the immune system reacted to these foreign proteins and toxins as invaders and launched an attack. Symptoms that Paul had always had but were overlooked for their relative innocence, including acne, urinary frequency, canker sores, and gas, made sense if his gut wasn't functioning properly. Metabolic markers also showed that Paul was low in short chain fatty acids like butyrate and proprionate.

In order to heal his inflamed intestines, I gave him a host of nutritional supplements, like fish oils, silymarin, and glutamine, glucosamine for his joints. Finally, I asked him to take 1 tablespoon of flaxseed powder daily.

After only three weeks, Paul told me that he was already feeling more energetic and in control of his health. The first major proof that the natural approach was working was revealed in small ways: his acne began to disappear, his fatigue started to dissipate, and his allergies spawned fewer symptoms. A few months later, however, Paul's seizures miraculously ceased. His health improved so dramatically that he soon felt good enough to apply to the famed Wharton Business School at the University of Pennsylvania. He was accepted. Paul had gone from being almost completely incapacitated to being at the top of his game.

We'll probably never know exactly what hit Paul so hard. It's been a few years since his curious symptoms improved, and we cannot tell yet whether he'd have reached this remission on this own. But his recovery was so complete that I've got to believe that this nutritional approach worked in his favor.

HOW MUCH SHOULD I TAKE?

For General Health
1 teaspoon daily
Special Conditions

Constipation, High cholesterol/ triglycerides, Detoxification, Heart disease, Syndrome X, Hormonal imbalance, PMS, Menopause	1 teaspoon-2 tablespoons/day

11

The B Vitamins: Cardiovascular Healers

It's time to rethink what we know about cardiovascular disease. While certain fats are certainly associated with high risk of heart disease, and while high cholesterol certainly increases the risk of arterial damage, there is a new story unfolding about the heart—a story whose discoveries may help us truly cut the risk of America's number one killer as well as a host of other conditions.

One and a half million heart attacks strike Americans each year, and half a million people die of heart disease annually. Cardiac disease will continue to ring out its death toll until we accept the whole truth, which is that high cholesterol alone is not the root of heart disease. In fact, many people die from heart attacks and coronary artery disease with normal or low cholesterol levels.

Meanwhile, a special derivative of an amino acid called homocysteine lurks in the shadows, letting cholesterol take the blame as it stealthily sabotages our arteries. Homocysteine is derived from an amino acid called methionine. Methionine is found in many foods, like garlic, onions, legumes, fish, eggs, and meat. A process called transsulfuration turns methionine into homocysteine.

Physicians who practice natural therapies are not the only ones taking note of homocysteine's dangers: a study in the *New England Journal of Medicine*, one of the most respected journals in traditional medicine, confirms that increased plasma levels of homocysteine confer an independent risk of vascular disease. This means that even if you are a healthy person with normal cholesterol levels, no family history of illness, and good eating habits, high levels of homocysteine in your body can predispose you to heart disease. And this predisposition to heart risk is powerfully increased if you smoke or have hypertension.

As a pathologist at Harvard Medical School, Kilmer McCully made a series of intriguing observations about homocysteine and our hearts. Two children had died of a genetic disorder called homocystinuria, which is commonly associated with elevated homocysteine levels. Strangely, autopsies showed that these youngsters had a severe degree of arteriosclerosis, or hardened arteries—a condition normally seen only in much older individuals. McCully hypothesized that this arterial damage was caused by excess homocysteine and might also occur in other people who had elevated levels of the amino acid but not the genetic disorder. This was such a radical departure from the accepted cholesterol theory of heart disease that it got him thrown out of Harvard. He ended up working at a small veteran's hospital in Rhode Island.

The discovery might have halted there, but in 1976, two Australians named Bridget and David Wilcken published the first study linking homocysteine and heart disease. Now the homocysteine theory of heart disease has come to the forefront of medicine. Study after recent study confirm that homocysteine is key to determining your risk of heart disease. Years after his brilliant hypothesis was scorned and rejected—and Kilmer McCully was denied tenure, a truly unfortunate turn to his career—he has been vindicated.

A close look at studies of homocysteine shows that this amino acid is present in elevated levels in an alarming number of those suffering from chronic conditions, ranging from arthritis to cancer. It may well be that homocysteine is a marker for—and a key player in—many chronic illnesses. High homocysteine might be an indication that your body's detoxification abilities are failing, putting you at risk for a wide range of disorders. Let me explain why.

Getting to the Heart of Homocysteine

As I explained, homocysteine is created from—and related to—several quite innocuous compounds, like the amino acid methionine. It can be changed in two directions: it can use vitamin B_6 to change into two other important amino acids, cysteine and taurine, or it can use vitamin B_{12} and folic acid to return back to its methionine form. In a normal, healthy body, homocysteine is just a brief intermediate step between methionine, cysteine, and taurine.

But in as many as one in four victims of heart disease, that step is not so brief. If our levels of vitamin B_6, B_{12}, or folic acid are low, then homocysteine cannot be transformed back into these safe substances; and it accumulates to dangerous amounts. Some individuals may have a genetic predisposition to elevated homocysteine levels and may need extra B vitamins.

Homocysteine causes damage to the lining of the arteries and any low-density lipoprotein (LDL) cholesterol that might be found there. And this is why LDL cholesterol—often known as "bad" cholesterol—is so harmful: not because it is the root of coronary artery disease, but because, when oxidized, it causes free radical damage and makes arterial disease worse. Homocysteine may well be the root of much coronary artery disease. Think of homocysteine as the creator of potholes in the walls of the arteries, and when fat or cholesterol surrounds these potholes, they clumsily plug up the hole, further aggravating the damage.

The current mainstream treatment for heart disease includes coronary bypass surgery, literally a chest-splitting procedure; angioplasty, which inflates your vulnerable arteries like balloons to deflect cholesterol plaques; and numerous potent medications with various side effects.

Keeping homocysteine low, however, is often a matter of one simple, natural tool: the dietary supplement. High homocysteine levels have been linked to deficiencies of three crucial vitamins: B_6, B_{12}, and folic acid. Even back in the 1960s, our friend Kilmer McCully observed that homocysteine levels increase as a direct result of deficiencies of these three vitamins and that its levels decrease when they are consumed. With just the help of the basic B vitamin capsule, high homocysteine could be wiped out and the frequency of heart disease lessened. In fact, folic acid is so important to our health that the FDA called for folate fortification of all breads and grains by January 1, 1998. In this country, where we are blessed with a wealth of nutritional knowledge and an abundance of food, it is shocking that so many people lack these vitamins. Simply by bolstering our diets with the right nutrients, we could control homocysteine.

Homocysteine: Not Just a Heartbreaker

Although the big news is that homocysteine, and not just cholesterol, is a major independent risk factor for cardiovascular disease, there are many other ways that this amino acid exerts its harmful effects. Heart disease is just the first.

Heart Disease: An amazing number of conclusive studies clearly demonstrate that high levels of homocysteine can increase your risk of heart disease, including myocardial infarctions and coronary artery disease. A recent report in the journal *Arteriosclerosis, Thrombosis, and Vascular Biology* stated that for every 10 percent increase in homocysteine levels, heart disease risk increases by the same amount. Similarly, a study in *JAMA* showed that, of one thousand five hundred men and women, the ones in the top 20 percent of homocysteine levels had double the risk of heart disease. However, a study in the journal *Circulation* showed homocysteine levels were not found to be an independent risk factor for coronary heart disease. More research will be necessary.

PERIPHERAL VASCULAR DISEASE: Even outside of the precious heart, our veins, capillaries, and arteries are vulnerable to excess homocysteine, leading to killer diseases like atherosclerosis, claudication, and thrombosis. In study of forty-eight patients with peripheral atherosclerotic vascular disease, a whopping 50 percent had abnormally high plasma levels of homocysteine. Researchers in a 1997 study went so far as to assert that individuals with elevated levels of homocysteine face four times the risk of peripheral vascular disease than people with normal homocysteine levels.

BRAIN: Homocysteine is also a neurotoxin, meaning that it kills neurons and their protective myelin sheath. Many diseases of the nervous system have been correlated with high levels of homocysteine and low B vitamin levels, including depression, schizophrenia, multiple sclerosis, Parkinson's disease, Alzheimer's disease, and cognitive decline in the elderly. Another study confirms that deficiencies of B_{12} and folic acid are dangerously common in older individuals, leading to subpar mental functioning.

DIABETES: While individuals with type I diabetes tend to have decreased stores of homocysteine, a study reports that many sufferers of type II noninsulin-dependent diabetes mellitus develop macrovascular disease in relation to hyperhomocysteinemia (too much homocysteine), which also seems to be a risk factor for diabetic retinopathy.

ARTHRITIS: In a study, plasma homocysteine levels were found to be 33 percent higher in patients with rheumatoid arthritis than in healthy subjects. Another study reported 20 percent of patients with rheumatoid arthritis having homocysteine levels above the normal range.

KIDNEY FAILURE: Because homocysteine—like all other substances passing through the body—passes through the kidneys, chronic renal failure can trap excess homocysteine in the body, leading to serious health risks. In a study of 176 patients with end-stage kidney disease, 149 had abnormally high levels of homocysteine.

ALCOHOL INGESTION: Frequent drinking and alcoholism interfere with our natural process of metabolism, which explains the results of a study in the *American Journal of Clinical Nutrition* showing that chronic alcoholics had twice as much homocysteine in their blood as nondrinkers. Alcoholics have not only higher serum levels of homocysteine than normal individuals but also significantly lower folate concentrations.

Osteoporosis: Osteoporosis, which can lead to the painful weakening and possible shattering of bones, is most common in elderly, postmenopausal women. A study in *Indian Pediatrics*, however, found that the condition afflicted young children with homocysteinuria, which produces unusually high amounts of homocysteine. Although there is no evidence that elevated levels of homocysteine lead to postmenopausal osteoporosis, such a connection seems worthy of future research.

Cancer: Cancer patients are frequently noted to have vitamin B_{12} deficiencies and high homocysteine concentrations. In patients with breast cancer, the common medication tamoxifen has been reported to lower homocysteine levels—this may account for some of the protective effects that the drug has.

Birth Defects: Pregnant women are especially vulnerable to homocysteine's dangers, particularly because it is associated with a deficiency of folic acid, which is crucial for normal development of a fetus. This deficiency has been associated with neural tube defects, low birth weight, premature delivery, and spontaneous abortions of the fetus. Numerous studies document that low folate intake increases the risk of delivering a baby with neural tube defects and that taking supplements of B vitamins will enhance not only birth weight but the child's scores on cognitive and mental aptitude tests.

The Diet Woes

Gary Wilbur's wife, Sheila, tried her best to be helpful. He knew she loved him, and he knew that was why she was constantly on his back about his health, his food, and his exercise habits. This was because no matter how hard Gary tried, he could not stick to the sensible diet they both knew could spare him from heart disease. He would start each day with a healthful bowl of cereal and fruit and feast on baked potatoes and grilled chicken for lunch, but by dinnertime, his heart-smart enthusiasm had waned. Gary would ultimately submit to nightly cravings for a juicy steak or salty fries, and it drove his spouse wild with fear. Sheila loved Gary so much that she refused to take any chances with his health, especially with all she had read in the papers about the dangers of heart disease, and she eventually forbade him to eat any fats or oils. With bread, Gary and Sheila ate margarine, but butter never touched their lips. Similarly, low-fat dessert treats were allowed sparingly in the house, but real ice cream and cake were mere childhood memories. Sheila thought all was well with this new diet, until she found some crumpled wrappers of Big Macs and Whoppers stashed in the garage. Enraged, she turned to me to take her side.

"Gary is killing himself, and he doesn't even realize it!" Sheila fumed to me in my office. "He's a smart man, he knows that fat and oil will destroy his arteries, and still he downs junk food like there's no tomorrow!"

Sheila was making a mistake that is all too common in America. In her crusade against heart disease, she had failed to identify the real culprit. Although too much saturated and unhealthy, hydrogenated fats can clog arteries, everyone needs a small amount of good fat in their diets to stay healthy. Her "no fat, no oil" campaign was a little too strict. Meanwhile, the "low-fat" substitutes she was using may actually have been more lethal than their high-fat alternatives. Margarine, while lower in saturated fat than butter, contains trans-saturated fats, which have recently been deemed even worse for heart disease than butter's saturated fats (see chapter 4). Also, Gary ate a lot of breads and carbohydrates as part of his low-fat regimen, and too many carbohydrates were depriving him of the nutrients and vitamins that only fruits and vegetables yield.

I asked Gary if he would submit to some tests, to alleviate his wife's anxiety. He agreed, hoping to prove to Sheila that he was in tiptop shape. Gary's cholesterol levels were admirably low. His homocysteine levels, however, were shooting through the roof. While a normal level of homocysteine falls below 12, Gary was at 25. Clearly, despite the lack of fat in his diet, he was at serious risk of heart disease, probably because of a vitamin deficiency. Besides, your body turns about half of the "no fat" carbohydrates in breads, pastas, potatoes, cereals, and other starches into fat, anyway. Gary was eating death on a roll.

It may seem impossibly simple, but I gave Gary supplements of folate and B vitamins to take daily. I also instructed him to eat less carbohydrates and greater amounts of varied fruits and vegetables. That's all. In four weeks, his homocysteine levels were hovering around 12, low enough to satisfy even Sheila. Granted, this is no promise that Gary will not succumb to heart disease. And while high levels of homocysteine have been widely recognized as a major risk factor for arteriosclerosis, it remains to be seen whether lowering these levels will reduce risk of stroke. The best way to use the knowledge of homocysteine is to keep levels low, preventing them from rising dangerously. By just altering his diet, Gary was able to do his best to protect himself against heart disease—much to his loving wife's relief.

The Historic Origins of Arteriosclerosis

How did the cholesterol theory seize hold of the public consciousness, and why is it so hard to dispel?

In the mid—to late nineteenth-century, a scientist named Rudolph Virchow virtually introduced microscopy to the field of pathology. In doing so, he observed the details of arterial damage. First, he found, the artery wall degenerated. Next, fatty, lumpy, cottage cheese-like substances called atheromas might enter and invade the arteries, leading to the condition known as atherosclerosis. Sometimes, arteries burdened with atheromas harden. Or the arteries might harden at once without any fatty padding; this was known as arteriosclerosis. Although we now believe that homocysteine may cause arteriosclerosis, and perhaps atherosclerosis, Virchow was convinced that they stemmed from some internal infection.

By 1908, English doctors had noted a link between heart disease in upper-class citizens and the high-fat diet they consumed. Upon feeding rabbits similar foods, the physicians realized that abundant meat and dairy products seemed to cause hardened arteries, much like those of the Brits with arteriosclerosis, and with no infectious agents in sight. The doctors surmised that dietary protein was causing the damage. A researcher named M. A. Ignatovsky, however, replicated the rabbit results and concluded that cholesterol, not protein, was the real root of the problem. In 1925, Dr. Harry Newburg looked back at these rabbit experiments and was fascinated by the effects that dietary manipulations could have on arterial damage. Like his predecessors, he decided to monitor the effects of food on rabbit health; he found that the more protein the bunnies ate, the swifter and more severe was the arteriosclerotic damage.

Newburg then tested the relative effects of different proteins on rabbit arteries by injecting various amino acids into them. He determined that cystine was quite harmful to health. Unfortunately, Newburg never tried homocysteine. If he had, perhaps we would have understood the connection between homocysteine and heart disease sooner.

By the end of the twentieth century, the focus on cholesterol and fat as important risk factors for heart disease intensified, especially as heart disease rose to the top of the list of America's greatest health dangers. Because cholesterol was found in the plaques that plastered arterial walls, it was deemed the true marker of arteriosclerosis. The medical establishment soon came to regard cholesterol as the root of all evils. Few, however, considered the possible role of proteins or amino acids, not to mention homocysteine, in the heart disease equation. Evidence shows that most heart disease victims *don't* have extremely high cholesterol levels.

Heart Attacks with Low Cholesterol?

Isn't that shocking? Let me repeat it. Evidence shows that most heart disease victims don't have high cholesterol levels. In the *American Journal of Medical Science* in 1990, Dr. Kilmer McCully reported that in a study of 194 consecutive autopsies of mainly male veterans, only 8 percent of those with severe arteriosclerosis had total cholesterol levels greater than 250 mg/dL, and the mean blood cholesterol level in the group with the severest disease was 186.7 mg/dL. While this study did confirm a positive correlation between the severity of arteriosclerosis and cholesterol levels, two-thirds of the patients with severe arteriosclerosis had no evidence of elevated blood cholesterol, diabetes, or hypertension. Meanwhile, the amount of evidence pointing toward homocysteine as a risk factor for heart disease has exploded of late. For the first time, people are realizing that lacking vitamins can be absolutely ruinous to good health. Every day, studies like one in the *Journal of American Cardiology* are revealing that high levels of homocysteine are a major risk factor for heart disease and that deficiencies of B_{12}, B_6, and folic acid are at fault.

This is not to say that high cholesterol is good or that you now have license to indulge in nothing but high-fat fare. In fact, cream, butter, french fries, burgers, cake, whole milk, doughnuts, and all deliciously fried and fatty foods are devoid of the vitamins that keep homocysteine levels low. Think of homocysteine as the first link in a potent chain reaction or as the spark that sets the fire, initiating damage to the arteries. LDL cholesterol, which is promoted by foods high in saturated fats, becomes oxidized in the arteries, adding insult to the injury homocysteine has already provoked. Free radicals then aggravate the arterial damage, and your body lays down plaques made of cholesterol and fat to try to stop the process in its tracks. But by then it's too late: the damage has spread like wildfire. When cholesterol is oxidized, it is lethal. But it is probably homocysteine that makes the arteries vulnerable to this oxidation. The emerging story of heart disease confirms that number of risk factors from C-reactive protein, LDL (bad cholesterol), elevated iron, ferritin and poor levels of HDL (good cholesterol) also play a crucial role.

Extra, Extra: Homocysteine Heightens Heart Disease

Many news journalists will tell you that their job is their life. Hopping from story to story, from scandal to scoop, leaves little time for romance or family—not to mention eating or sleeping. Steve Greenberg was the highly paid, highly acclaimed, highly stressed producer of a popular New York TV news program. This pressure cooker of a job granted Steve little sleep. He was constantly getting up early to make it to the studio before anyone else so that he could organize the day's show and staying later than everyone else to clear up last-minute glitches for the next morning's session. This meant that he had little time to worry about his diet. Although Steve was constantly grabbing snack foods on the run, he did earnestly try to eat "healthier" foods. As a major player in the news circuit, he needed to look and feel his best while making deals and connections. He swore off burgers and fries completely, and every day for lunch, he grabbed a turkey sandwich on white bread with mayo and lettuce at the corner deli, with a bag of chips on the side. In Steve's mind, this was a great stride toward good health.

"Plus," he told me proudly when he first met me, "I don't smoke . . . and I go jogging every weekend."

Steve thought his efforts were good. But apparently they weren't good enough, for his physician informed him one day that his cholesterol was a high 249—the normal level being under 200. His triglycerides were also high. Steve was buckling under the burdens of his job, his diet, and his stress. Constantly haunting him as well was the specter of his father, who had died of coronary artery disease at the young age of forty-seven. Having just celebrated his forty-second birthday, Steve was ever aware—and frightened—of his faulty genes and his possible fate. Steve's doctor informed him that he would have to take cholesterol medication daily for the rest of his life in order to fend off heart disease. Refusing to surrender his whole life to a bottle of pills, Steve came to me seeking a more natural way to lower his high triglycerides and cholesterol—and to prevent coronary artery disease at all costs.

As I talked to Steve about his daily routine, I immediately understood its negative effect on his health. But his most serious problem was his diet, which lacked the important vitamins and nutrients that he needed to fight heart disease.

"What do you eat?" I asked him.

"I never have time to cook," he told me sheepishly. "And I don't like vegetables so much. But at least I eat low-fat foods. I mean, I never eat butter or red meat. I live on bagels, which are practically fat free. And I only put a pat of margarine on it."

I shook my head as Steve repeated this message of the masses. The turkey sandwich and bagels he faithfully ate every day contained practically none of the vitamins and nutrients he needed to stay healthy. People think that low fat is synonymous with "good for you," and it's not. Without fruits and vegetables, Steve was missing out on important vitamins and minerals, particularly vitamin B_{12} and folic acid. Carbohydrates were increasing his triglycerides. Not surprisingly, when I tested to see his homocysteine level, it was all the way up to 27. Excess homocysteine is an early marker for vitamin deficiency, and I knew Steve needed all the fortification he could handle. I recommended daily doses of B_{12} and folate, and I asked him to take dietary supplements of 10 milligrams of vitamin B_6 a day. Within three months, Steve's homocysteine levels had dropped to 7.

Steve was also eating too many refined carbohydrates, which was leading to his astronomically high triglyceride count of 500—the normal range lies under 150. Instead of white breads, whose nutritional value has been vastly decreased due to processing and milling, he should have been eating more fiber-rich carbohydrates, such as whole-wheat products. After three months of a diet that was more nutritionally sound, including more leafy greens, citrus fruits, and whole grains,

Steve's triglycerides dropped to 290. Although this was a huge improvement, it was still far from the normal, healthy range. But not all health victories can be won at one time; we had to be satisfied with the dramatic decrease in his homocysteine levels and with the healthy, heart-smart diet he had begun. Had we not looked into protecting him from possible arteriosclerosis, he would remain at far greater risk of disease.

In the end, there are no miracle cures, and only time will tell whether Steve's vitamin fortification regimen will be enough to ward off heart disease. In any case, however, limiting carbohydrate intake and getting enough B vitamins can only have a positive effect on his health. We owe it to ourselves to do whatever is in our power to fight impending disease.

Love Your Vitamins

Steve was not alone in neglecting to pack his diet with the proper nutrients. In fact, the United States as a whole is guilty of consuming insufficient amounts of B vitamins. While the optimal dose of folic acid is 650-1,000 micrograms a day, for example, most of us only get about 200. Getting enough folate is important because it plays such a key role in keeping us healthy. A deficiency of this vitamin is suspected to assist in the initiation and development of cancer. Even slight deficiencies of folate can damage white blood cells, eventually leading to anemia. Luckily, there are many places to find folic acid. Good sources include broccoli, spinach, turnip greens, legumes, green vegetables in general, and cooked lima beans. Unfortunately, 50 to 90 percent of the folates in most cooked foods are lost, so it's necessary to eat as much as we can get our hands on. This is safe, since there are reportedly little to no known side effects from taking high doses.

One of the few downsides of folic acid is that high levels mask a vitamin B_{12} deficiency, so you should make sure to consume lots of this nutrient, too. Getting enough B_{12} into the body is actually quite difficult, since it absorbs slowly, and peak levels may not show up for eight to twelve hours after ingestion. What's worse, absorption rates decrease with increased intake, so the more you eat, the slower your body is at storing it. This is why it can be especially hard to recover from a B_{12} deficiency; no matter how much you eat, your body cannot get enough. Inadequate absorption of B_{12} is actually responsible for 95 percent of the vitamin deficiency in the United States. Getting enough of the cagey vitamin is worth it, though, because it keeps our nerves myelinated and protected, as well as warding off anemia. Both B_{12} and folic acid deficiencies have been shown to cause psychiatric illness, such as dementia. B_{12} can be found in products like chicken, fish, eggs, and legumes.

Last but not least is vitamin B_6. Severe deficiencies of B_6 can produce some scarey physical responses: glossitis (a swollen tongue), seizures, and debilitating fatigue. Bioavailability of the vitamin depends on how much your food has been processed, since much of it can be lost through heating, cooking, and canning. Its absorption rate, however, is a fairly high 71 to 82 percent. Like its B_{12} relative, B_6 can be found in foods like salmon and chicken, as well as nuts and bananas.

B vitamin deficiency is not very difficult to remedy. Just by eating the right foods, or taking daily supplements, you can protect your heart from a prolific killer. One study found that taking a combination of all three vitamins reduced homocysteine concentrations in the blood by 49.8 percent. Fortifying yourself with vitamins is a win-win situation. You not only eliminate the risk of heart disease, you eliminate the risk of being vulnerable to illness at all.

Generally, I recommend 5-10 milligrams of B_6, 50-100 micrograms of B_{12}, and 400 micrograms of folic acid daily. However, this may vary from individual to individual based on their weight, health history, and needs. I may reduce this amount by half for people with normal homocysteine levels and no risk factors for heart disease. In other patients, I may increase the dose.

Feel Better with B Vitamins

Helen Smythe was alarmed when, at sixty-two, she awoke one morning without feeling in her lower extremities. A housewife and mother of three grown children, Helen had settled down to a quiet life of watching TV with her husband, Frank, throwing Tupperware parties, and volunteering for Mothers Against Drunk Driving. One morning, however, when she tried to get out of bed, she literally fell to the floor because she could not stand on her feet. It was as if, she told me later, her legs could not support her body. Her lower half was completely numb and tingly from that point on, and she could only move around by hobbling and shuffling, since she could barely feel where her feet were and where they were stepping.

I suspected that she had adult-onset diabetes, because it ran in her family, and one common symptom of the disease is peripheral neuropathy, which would explain her numb legs. After a number of tests, I saw that, indeed, her blood glucose was a moderately high 132. Her homocysteine levels were high at 20. High homocysteine may be a marker of heart disease, but it has also been found in diabetics with neuropathy. Vitamin B_{12} has been shown to reduce homocysteine levels in diabetic patients experiencing neuropathies.

The clear answer for treatment, I knew, was a heavy dose of the B vitamins. I prescribed 25 milligrams of B_6; 1,000 micrograms of B_{12}; and 800 micrograms of folic acid. I added garlic pills—garlic has been shown to lower cholesterol and blood sugar—and I suggested a low carbohydrate diet to help keep her diabetes under control. I also gave her a substance called chromium picolinate, which helps reduce insulin resistance. Finally, I added phosphatidyl serine and acetyl L-carnitine to the mix, since both not only improve alertness and mental clarity but also may alleviate peripheral neuropathies (see chapter 19). An exercise regimen of daily walking and stretching would also stimulate Helen's circulation and help decrease her blood sugar levels.

Six months later, Helen walked back into my office with firm strides and a big smile on her face.

"I can get around most days. My legs still feel a little tingly, like pins and needles, but at least I know they're there."

It was true; while Helen's legs were still numb at times and never as capable as they had once been, she did feel much more energetic, and her nerve weaknesses were much less crippling after treatment began. Her homocysteine levels dropped to 12, leading me to believe that this amino acid must have played a great role in her neuropathy.

Homocysteine and Stroke: The Hidden Connection

Joseph Conley had always loved to eat, but even more, he had loved to cook. When he was a young boy, he would help his mother peel potatoes; when he was in high school, he persuaded the principal to let him take home economics instead of auto shop. It was only fitting that he eventually became a successful chef. Whipping up delicacies at an upscale New York brasserie, Joseph was surrounded with mouthwatering roast beef, tender salmon filets, and creamy cheesecake all day. He had long known, however, that eating everything he cooked would make him fatter than the hams he carved up, not to mention a walking heart attack candidate. As a result, he was very careful about "just tasting" the savory entrees and rich sauces he concocted. He also checked his cholesterol and triglyceride levels frequently. Unfortunately, despite Joseph's dietary diligence, he discovered that his triglyceride levels were extremely high. He was worried and confused. He stayed away from fatty foods, yet over the next few years several relatives of his died of strokes, and as the years went on, Joseph worried that he would be next.

In frustration, and fearful of heart disease, Joseph tried every method advertised to help prevent the condition and experimented with every diet he could find. He went to health spas that fed him rabbit food and infinitely tiny portions of grilled chicken. But it was not enough, for at the age of forty-four, Joseph had a stroke, which left him helpless for a time. Although he recovered quite quickly, Joseph emerged from the experience even more scared and angry because of what had happened. Hadn't he taken all the proper health precautions? How could he prevent this from happening again? Was there something that his doctors hadn't seen, something they could have easily repaired that they all missed? Joseph came to me for a fresh opinion, and an answer. As he recounted his ordeal for me, one simple word came to mind: homocysteine. Exercise and healthful food are good steps to take to prevent heart disease, or any disease for that matter, but his blood tests did show high levels of homocysteine. I immediately instructed him to supplement his already nutritious diet with B_{12}, B_6, and folic acid. Within weeks, his homocysteine levels had begun to fall. Granted, we cannot be sure if this precaution will rule out any possibility of his having another stroke in the future—but vitamins may be the key to keeping his heart beating.

LIFE-SAVING NUMBERS TO KNOW

- Normal homocysteine range: around 12 micromoles a liter, although the lower your homocysteine count, the better

- Normal cholesterol range: between 160 and 220 milligrams per deciliter

- RDA for folic acid: at least 400 micrograms for premenopausal women, 180 micrograms for postmenopausal women, 200 micrograms for men. (Reference point: 1 cup cooked spinach has 260 micrograms.) The RDA for vitamins and minerals does not currently take into account the latest findings on homocysteine.

- RDA for vitamin B_6: 1.6 milligrams for women, 2 milligrams for men. (Reference point: 1 banana has 0.7 milligrams.)

- RDA for vitamin B_{12}: 2 micrograms for men and women. (Reference point: 1 cup milk has 0.9 micrograms.)

Remember One Word

You may not realize it, but an exciting new era of medical discovery is unfolding as you read this book. We are truly in the midst of not only a nutraceutical revolution, but a health care revolution in general. For years, the cholesterol theory of heart disease has reigned. So, however, has heart disease itself, which has killed more people in America than any other medical condition. Clearly, there was a key to the puzzle that even the experts were overlooking. Homocysteine seems to be one of the keys, and, as I've said, it's a key that keeps showing up in a wide range of other debilitating illnesses, from cancer to arthritis to diabetes. And while homocysteine may not be the last word in heart disease, it is an important part of an emerging story.

Even more novel is the finding that three simple nutrients—B_{12}, B_6, and folic acid—can directly lower your levels of this harmful substance, and maybe save not just your heart but your life.

HOW MUCH SHOULD I TAKE?

For General Health
50-100 mcg of B_{12}, 400 mcg of folic acid, 5-10 mg of B_6
After Meals
Special Conditions

Elevated homocysteine levels (above 12), heart disease/ arteriosclerosis, diseases of the nervous system (including depression, schizophrenia, multiple sclerosis, Parkinson's, Alzheimer's, cognitive decline), diabetes, arthritis, alcohol ingestion, osteoporosis, cancer, birth defects, elevated cholesterol/triglycerides.	500-1,000 mcg of B12, 400-800 mcg of folic acid, 50-100 mg of B_6

12

Vitamin E and Tocotrienols: Antioxidants for the Entire Body

Angioplasty. Open heart surgery. Coronary bypass. These painful procedures, where arteries are forced open like balloons or the ribs are literally sawed in half, are the cornerstone of cardiovascular surgery. Meanwhile, EKGs, Doppler, echocardiograms, and angiography, where dye is injected into the heart so that every little artery can be viewed, are all the latest techniques available to cardiologists. One in every three American deaths each year is due to heart disease. Cardiology, as a result, is one of the most high-tech, sophisticated areas of medicine—a place for doctors with the spirit of warriors and the minds of scientists: high stakes, modern medicine at its most dramatic. That's why it amazes me that, in the last few years, cardiologists have openly conceded that one of the most potent protectors against heart disease is not a fancy new procedure but the simple nutrient vitamin E, and that many cardiologists pop the vitamin along with their morning coffee. A survey reported several years ago in the *Medical Tribune* found that nine out of ten physicians not only recommended vitamin E to their patients but enthusiastically used it themselves. And at a recent medical conference given by the American College of Cardiology, it was found that most attendees took vitamin E supplements! Not vitamin C. Not iron. But vitamin E.

Vitamin E is the "crossover" nutrient, the one brave voyager in nutritional medicine that has made it into the mainstream intact and has been embraced by the doctors themselves. And rightly so. For, as new research is showing us, vitamin E is one of the most important and powerful protectors we have. And it's not just a single vitamin. It turns out that vitamin E and its chemical cousins may actually be made of a whole range of related substances, all of which protect our hearts and our bodies in unprecedented ways. In fact, different types of vitamin E are helpful for different illnesses.

The existence of vitamin E was first uncovered in 1920, but Agnes Fay Morgan and her colleagues at the University of California at Berkeley are credited with the 1937 discovery of vitamin E's special role in the body. While myriad studies have shown the promise of other natural herbs and supplements, the case for vitamin E has been unusually and irrefutably strong. One after another, in study after study, the results consistently showed that taking alpha tocopherols, a special form of vitamin E, caused a clear improvement in the reduction of cardiovascular problems. And a recent astonishing series of three studies that used enormous numbers of health professionals themselves as the subjects have convinced mainstream doctors that vitamin E counts. It is, in a country where heart disease is ubiquitous, a treatment even the doctors could not do without.

- The vitamin reduced the risk of cardiovascular disease by an astonishing 47 percent, according to the most famous study of vitamin E, called "CHAOS" (Cambridge-Harvard Anti-Oxidant Study).

- Vitamin E was clearly linked to a reduced risk of heart disease, according to a study reported in the *New England Journal of Medicine* of thirty-nine thousand male health professionals.

- The higher your vitamin E intake, the lower your risk of coronary heart disease, according to a study of thirty-four thousand postmenopausal nurses.

The fact that a natural therapy has finally been embraced by physicians everywhere is a huge step for both nutritional and modern medicine. And, as it turns out, vitamin E may be the ideal heart protector—but that's not all. It also is a powerful antioxidant, and it may even be a kind of fountain of youth.

An All-Purpose Antioxidant

Vitamin E's claim to fame may be its heart-saving abilities, but it can be used to help prevent other significant health problems. Not only can it boost the immune system, inhibit cancer cell growth, and reduce the damage associated with diabetes, but new research suggests that vitamin E can be used to halt the brain deterioration caused by Alzheimer's disease. Some conditions vitamin E can help treat or reverse follow.

HEART: Vitamin E's most promising quality is in preserving or restoring the health of the heart. Not only does this vitamin ward off myocardial infarctions, coronary artery disease, and coronary heart disease, it can increase the survival rate of patients undergoing bypass surgery and is implicated in decreasing angina and coronary spasm.

DIABETES: Free radical damage can cause long-term chronic conditions such as diabetes. A study shows that vitamin E may be helpful in reducing this diabetic damage by reducing protein kinase C, which is activated by sugar and can form harmful oxidative by-products. In addition, retinal damage is common in people with diabetes, and vitamin E has been shown to alleviate this as well.

ALZHEIMER'S DISEASE: Exciting new research indicates that vitamin E may also be used to prevent the deterioration of neurons involved with Alzheimer's. A study sponsored by the National Institute on Aging showed that the progressive dementia associated with the disease can be slowed by at least six months with high doses of vitamin E.

CANCER: A Tokyo study found that tocotrienols, which are vitamin E-related compounds, inhibited tumor cell growth in vitro. Tocotrienols have also been shown to be particularly effective against breast cancer and are a recommended therapy adjunctive to tamoxifen, the most popular breast cancer drug, according to a 1997 study in the *Journal of Nutrition*. Tocotrienols may also protect against skin cancer; according to a study in *Experimental Biology* in 1996, these cousins of vitamin E tend to be stored in the skin and protect against ultraviolet radiation. Yet another study in the *International Journal of Cancer* found that gamma—and delta-tocotrienols strongly inhibited the growth of tumors.

CHOLESTEROL: Vitamin E has been shown to lower blood levels of this artery-clogging substance. When tocotrienols were taken together with tocopherols (vitamin E), "bad" LDL cholesterol, triglycerides, and total cholesterol decreased in the body. A 1997 study in the *Journal of Nutritional Biochemistry* found that twelve weeks of tocotrienols lowered blood cholesterol. And a 1995 study in *Lipids* reported similar results: changing to a diet recommended by the American Heart Association and taking 200 milligrams of gamma-tocotrienol for four weeks decreased cholesterol levels by 13 percent.

ORGAN REJECTION: A study on heart transplants in the journal *Transplant* showed that vitamin E significantly reduced the risk of organ rejection.

IMMUNE FUNCTION: Especially in the elderly, vitamin E can enhance immune response. A study in the *American Journal of Clinical Nutrition* showed that vitamin E boosted white blood cell counts and reduced lipid peroxide free radicals in thirty-two older patients.

VITAMIN E: YOUR HEART'S NATURAL PLUMBER

Vitamin E has won kudos from doctors as excellent prevention against high cholesterol and other hallmarks of cardiovascular disease. How does it work its magic? This nutrient is an antioxidant, or a scavenger that collects and eliminates harmful free radicals as well as toxins that we breathe in from the world around us. Containing just a lone electron spinning in a lopsided orbit, free radicals have the capability to destroy cells and reduce the power of enzymes that keep our bodily processes functioning properly. They have been identified as playing a deleterious role in at least fifty different diseases, from arthritis to cancer.

While millions of these oxidized particles streak through us daily, damaging whatever they touch, production of some free radicals is beneficial to us because it helps us fight disease. For example, the bursts of caustic free radicals spewed out from white blood cells are part of an immune system mechanism designed to kill viruses. Detoxification and normal metabolic processes also lead to free radical production.

What we need is a balance between free radicals and our ability to clean them up. Not surprisingly, our body is ready with a complex defense system to protect us from excess free radicals, and antioxidants are the major arsenal. They donate their electrons to these particles and neutralize them, rendering them harmless. For this reason, antioxidant supplements are particularly beneficial.

Vitamin E seems born to handle a particular kind of free radical above all: lipid (fat) peroxides. Have you ever smelled the rancid odor of milk or cheese that has gone bad in the refrigerator? That's oxidized fat. That can happen in your cells. Vitamin E is the most important lipid-soluble antioxidant we have—that is, it dissolves and is absorbed only in fat. The membrane that encases each cell in our bodies is made up of chains of fat molecules strung together to protect us from the environment. Oxidized fat in the form of cholesterol can ultimately destroy the heart and blood vessels by damaging cell membranes. Vitamin E, however, protects us from this potential danger by preventing oxidation of cholesterol.

In particular, vitamin E is heralded as the best antioxidant protection against cardiovascular diseases. It has an affinity for cell membranes, where cholesterol can cause damage. It can prevent the oxidation of LDL or bad cholesterol. That oxidation forms free radicals called lipid peroxides, which profoundly damage the walls of arteries and blood vessels. That may be why high cholesterol is a marker for blockage and damage of arteries.

Because the American diet is traditionally rich in fat and cholesterol, we are especially vulnerable to the oxidation of these fats, known as lipid peroxides. Numerous studies show that by blocking the oxidation of cholesterol, vitamin E keeps the heart beating a healthy rhythm.

Post-op Vitamin E

Max Firestone was sixty-seven years old and the father of five grown children when he made his first appointment with me a decade ago. A former vice president of Citibank, he was now retired and hoped to buy a condo in Florida with his wife.

On his first night of retirement, however, he woke with a stabbing pain in his chest. He was rushed to the local hospital and immediately underwent bypass surgery for severely clogged arteries. Even after the operation, Max's angina remained unstable, and his heart was only able to pump at a third of its normal level.

Max was determined to investigate alternative therapies for his condition. We agreed that the first step was the heart-healthy diet popularized by Dean Ornish, MD, a pioneer of the link between heart disease and diet. He made the revolutionary discovery that an extremely low-fat diet that allows just 10 percent dietary fat a day can actually reverse dangerous plaques that clog the arteries. Max agreed to go on a Dean Ornish-style diet.

I prescribed supplements of coenzyme Q_{10}, a powerful heart protector that boosts blood flow and circulation, plus 4 grams of fish oil to thin Max's fat-congested blood. Most important, however, I put him on a course of vitamin E. A 1993 study of forty-five physicians in the *New England Journal of Medicine* showed that men taking at least 100 units of vitamin E a day lowered their incidence of heart disease by 26 percent. Even more impressive, a study in the *Journal of Cardiothoracic Surgery* showed that in subjects who had undergone bypass surgery, vitamin E increased their postsurgery survival rates.

Ten years later, Max is healthy and much stronger. We still need to monitor his health carefully, since his bypass surgery and weakened heart were serious impairments. But even his cardiologist has given him a clean bill of health, despite his initial misgivings. Max walks a mile each day with his wife, and he is free to enjoy the time he has earned to relax and enjoy life.

The Many Faces of Vitamin E

Vitamin E seems to be more than just a single vitamin. Vitamin E actually includes eight different compounds. Four of these are tocopherol subtypes, called alpha, beta, delta, and gamma. Alpha and gamma are by far the most important. Alpha tocopherol, the best-studied form of vitamin E, is mostly found in dietary supplements, while we can get gamma tocopherol primarily from the food we eat. Studies of alpha tocopherol revealed that this tocopherol form is most effective at saving us from heart disease.

Scientists have theorized that other compounds must exist that act like vitamin E tocopherols and work similarly to keep us fit. And in searching for these vitamin E mimics, we discovered that what we currently know and accept about vitamin E is just the beginning. Tocopherols may be just a small part of the whole story. There are now substances in the vitamin E family that are being studied and show great promise. These compounds, called tocotrienols, are another powerful group of free radical quenchers. These two types of vitamin E, the tocopherols and tocotrienols, may work synergistically in the body, creating an exciting new way to improve our health.

Tocotrienols have the same four subtypes (alpha, delta, gamma, and beta). The tocotrienols that have been studied have usually been isolated from palm oil. Tocotrienols seem to specialize in treating cancer and in lowering cholesterol and perhaps preventing heart disease, as the studies I've mentioned earlier in this chapter indicate. There is still much research to be done in this area, since not all tocotrienols have the same effects. For instance, a recent study in the *International Journal of Cancer* found that gamma and delta tocotrienols powerfully inhibited cancer cells in vitro. They did this by inhibiting the activation of Epstein-Barr virus, a common virus that most of us have been exposed to but that seems implicated in cancer in some vulnerable individuals. What does this mean for the average individual who wants to protect him—or herself from the common ailments of our time—heart disease and cancer? Eating foods rich in vitamin E is one solution. Certainly all of us could benefit by taking a supplement of 400 units of vitamin E daily, as mixed tocopherols, so that we benefit from each one's abilities. For those who are already ill, higher doses of vitamin E, along with supplements of tocotrienols, may be indicated. Tocotrienols and tocopherols can both be found in the same foods, like wheat germ, bran, leafy green vegetables, and vegetable oils. Most supplements that you will find in your local health food store contain only the alpha tocopherol of vitamin E, though. Cutting-edge nutritional supplements include mixed tocopherols and tocotrienols.

For cardiovascular disease, from angina to coronary heart disease, tocopherols are your best bet. They are particularly vigilant against cholesterol's clogging effects. Tocopherols prevent the oxidation of LDL cholesterol and inhibit free radical damage to the heart. In fact, they may truly save us from heart disease. In particular, alpha tocopherols have been shown to be the most effective prevention of heart disease. Gamma tocopherols, which don't last as long in the body, may be the key for inflammation and immune boosting. One of their major benefits seems to be the quenching of a particular type of inflammation, involving our immune system's white blood cells. These cells, called phagocytes, attack bacteria during infections. They use lethal hydrogen peroxide to kill invaders, but this causes free radical damage, which gamma tocopherols are particularly good at cleaning up. If left unchecked, chronic phagocytic inflammation can be one of the triggers of cancer. In this way, gamma tocopherols provide an important tool against cancer. A 1996 study showed that patients with coronary heart disease had reduced gamma, but not alpha, tocopherols. One study also demonstrates that gamma tocopherols are better than their alpha siblings at limiting the oxidation of LDL cholesterol. Alphas may be best for the heart, while gammas may be particularly effective in inflammation and immune response.

Tocotrienols, as I've noted, are good for the heart, hormones, and immune system. They are effective in keeping cholesterol from clogging our arteries. In fact, alpha tocotrienols are more effective in neutralizing LDL cholesterol than alpha tocopherols. Tocotrienols are also cancer fighters. In one study, these nutrients inhibited the growth of melanomas, a virulent form of skin cancer.

Tocotrienols also shine as hormone helpers: they balance out excess levels of hormone by acting as estrogen inhibitors. Too much estrogen in the body can lead to breast cancer and ovarian cysts. A study in the *Journal of Endocrinology* showed that tocotrienols prevented the onset of polycystic ovary disease, which is often triggered by a hormone imbalance.

In sum, it's time to revisit vitamin E. The nutrient may have much more to offer our health than we ever dreamed.

Vitamin E: Cholesterol Cop

A slew of studies supports the old adage that we are what we eat. In countries with a lower incidence of coronary heart disease, like Italy and France, citizens also boast higher plasma levels of vitamin E, which is strongly associated with their eating habits.

Ed Robinson, forty-seven years old, was one to know about eating habits; he was an incredible chef. He had an enormous network of friends, many of whom he had made—and kept—through his fabulous cooking abilities. An Ed Robinson dinner party was an event not to be missed.

Unfortunately, Ed had a family history of heart disease. His father had suffered three heart attacks, and his grandfather had died from complications of stroke. Ed himself had high cholesterol and triglyceride levels—over 300—and he suffered severe migraine headaches. He also had experienced elevations in blood pressure of late, and his HDL, or "good," cholesterol was under 40, putting him at high risk for heart disease. His cardiologist had prescribed beta-blockers to lower his blood pressure, but Ed continued to feel sluggish. His sex drive was also reduced for the first time. Ed finally came to see me on the advice of a friend. He had already sensed that the answer to his blood pressure and high cholesterol lay within dietary change, and he turned to me to help him improve his condition. When Ed mentioned to his cardiologist that he was going to try a natural approach to saving his heart, the doctor scoffed, "Just take the medication. Beta-blockers are a proven blood pressure treatment."

After conducting blood glucose tests, I found that he had a condition known as insulin resistance, the inability to handle carbohydrates properly. Insulin resistance may be a precursor to full-blown diabetes. If caught early, a change in diet can usually prevent any complications or full-blown diabetes.

Ed was unique in his knowledge about food and his willingness to make changes in his diet. Next, he had great willpower and was incredibly motivated to start a heart-healthy program. Not everyone has the inner strength to stick with the health programs I prescribe, for they can be stringent. Ed stuck to a healthy, balanced low-fat diet with lots of vegetables and few carbohydrates. Studies have shown that essential fatty acids can improve insulin's effect on receptor sites, so we enhanced his treatment by giving him fatty acid supplements in the form of flaxseed oil. Feverfew, an herb proven to reduce migraines, was prescribed for his headaches, and ginkgo to improve circulation throughout his body. I also gave him antioxidants, of which vitamin E was one of the most important. Within a year, Ed's triglyceride levels dropped in half. He's only had one migraine since I first saw him, he's feeling rested, and he lost twenty-five pounds. Ed still throws soirees, now featuring low-fat fare. Apparently, his friends find his dinners as delicious as ever, a tribute to a truly talented—and heart-smart—chef.

Vitamin E: Cellular Fountain of Youth

There are some puzzles in life that medicine may never decode, some holy grails we may never capture. One of these is the possibility of eternal youth. The mystery of longevity intrigues me as much as most people. When I observe elderly patients who have defied statistics and are enthusiastically enjoying long lives, I have to wonder about the biochemical secret of their success. One of the best ways to protect your body for the long haul is including vitamin E supplements in your daily diet. Good heredity counts for a lot, but so does nutrition. The life of Claire Darwin, a patient of mine who is ninety-three years young and loving it, is a case in point. Claire was born into a very different world from ours, in South Carolina, the daughter of a carpenter and his homemaker wife. When Claire graduated from finishing school in the early 1920s, she traveled to New York to visit her older brother. There she met her husband, Todd Darwin, and she has resided in the Big Apple ever since, for seventy-odd years and counting. Claire taught school for a while and raised two boys, but what's most remarkable about the latter part of her life is that she has not fallen victim to a single ailment that most women her age suffer. While many of her friends had strokes, heart disease, osteoporosis, or cancer over the years, Claire remains in the best of health. She takes ballroom dancing lessons twice a week. When she came to consult with me about a minor backache, I had to shake my head in wonder at her otherwise vigorous good health.

She was a small woman, but sat regally in her chair. Ever the Southern debutante, she was beautifully dressed. "Actually, I've never felt better in my life than in my last twenty years," she confided.

Twenty years? Twenty years ago, Claire was seventy-three. But even today, she looked as if she were hardly a day over seventy-five. How could she look so great at ninety-three?

DO ANTIOXIDANTS EVER FAIL US?

Although free radicals usually cause damage to our tissues in cells, causing complications ranging from cataracts to asthma, there are some situations in which free radicals are beneficial. As I've noted, immune system cells often kill invaders with free radicals (such as hydrogen peroxide). And chemotherapy drugs actually promote free radical damage to assist the reduction of abnormal cell growth. The problem is when there is an excess of free radicals that the body cannot adequately mop up or neutralize.

Antioxidants are powerful healers, but they don't work across the board 100 percent. For instance, a Finnish study revealed that antioxidants, like vitamin E, may pose additional risk to certain individuals. In the study, smokers with lung cancer who took beta-carotene, an antioxidant, were more likely to die than nonantioxidant users. Unfortunately, the same is likely to be true for vitamin E. The researchers suggest that the excess smoke taken in by these patients may be powerful enough to oxidize the vitamin supplements, causing further free radical damage. We are still learning more about the effects and benefits of antioxidants. So far, their benefits do seem to far outweigh their risks. But an unhealthy lifestyle may actually accentuate the negative side of antioxidants such as vitamin E, rendering them useless for some and dangerous for others.

"Twenty years ago," she continued, "I started taking vitamin E 400 units a day." A huge fan of nutrition, Claire had long taken a complete vitamin supplement regimen including vitamin C, drunk fruit and vegetable juices daily, eaten a good balance of healthy foods, and made sure to consume lots of fiber. Then she heard that vitamin E can prevent heart disease. Claire is certain that her excellent health habits have given her a golden old age.

HOW MUCH SHOULD I TAKE?

For General Health
Foods rich in vitamin E, such as wheat germ, or 200 iu/day
After Meals
Special Conditions

Cardiovascular disease	400-800 iu/day (tocopherols)
	25-100 mg/day (tocotrienols)
Diabetes	200-800 iu/day (tocopherols)
	25-100 mg/day (tocotrienols)
Alzheimer's Disease	400-1,000 iu/day (tocopherols)
	25-100 mg/day (tocotrienols)
Cancer	400-800 iu/day (tocopherols)
	25-100 mg/day (tocotrienols)
Cholesterol	400-800 iu/day (tocopherols)
	25-100 mg/day (tocotrienols)
Hormone balance	400-800 iu/day (tocopherol
(polycystic ovary disease)	25-100 mg/day (tocotrienols)
Hypertension	200-800 iu/day (tocopherols)
	25-100 mg/day (tocotrienols)
Insulin resistance	200-800 iu/day (tocopherols)
	25-100 mg/day (tocotrienols)

Word of Caution

Antioxidants such as vitamin E should be taken in conjunction with other antioxidants such as vitamin C, a lipoic acid and selenium. Consider a multivitamin/antioxidant when deciding on a nutritional regimen and always consult a physician to determine your unique requirements.

13

Ginkgo: Circulation and Energy

My office is on the Upper East Side of Manhattan, a few blocks from one of the most beautiful islands of green in the world: Central Park, with its acres of hills and valleys, rock outcroppings, lakes and plazas, and flora and fauna from all over the world. Sometimes, during a busy day with patients, I duck out for a quick lunch and a walk around the park's reservoir. The skyline of New York City circles the park like a steel and glass crown of amazing size and scale; sunlight filters through the leaves of the trees, and I find myself slowing down and calming down. Still, it is always hard to believe that one of the most important remedies I can offer my patients is growing in Central Park. It's an extract of a leaf from a tree that has made the crucial difference in the conditions of patients suffering from a wide range of illnesses, from asthma to stroke to poor memory.

It's called *Ginkgo biloba*. When I first learned about ginkgo over a decade ago, I just didn't believe it could work. How could there be an herbal supplement that could actually be useful in the treatment of vascular problems or memory loss? It seemed too simple. There are dozens of research scientists at universities and laboratories around the world who've spent years trying to develop a drug that might sharpen the memory and benefit the millions suffering from Alzheimer's and other memory ...npairments. I also know that many researchers have been struggling to find a safe ... to improve circulation for people suffering from diseases like diabetes.

...en though I knew a lot about the power of herbs and nutrients, I just didn't ... early studies I read about this herb. I knew it had been used for thousands ... that very few herbs had such a long history. But most of that research ... However, as the years passed, I discovered that an amazing amount ...en done in Europe on this herb. Literally hundreds of studies ...go has powerful therapeutic effects. The European medical community holds the herb in high regard for its ability to enhance circulation, and ginkgo[1] has even been adopted as a leading herbal medication in Germany.

Then, in 1988, Harvard University actually isolated one of the most powerful substances in ginkgo, ginkgolide B, which has specific and potent pharmacological activity. It seems to increase circulation and help quench the clumping of platelets, cells involved in inflammation and clotting.

Patients kept coming to me and reporting its benefits. I began to silently thank the ginkgo tree in my walks in Central Park. It seemed to me like an old and patient friend that never forgets you, that is always ready to help when you call upon it. Usually, I found that higher doses (like the amounts used in studies) of ginkgo are necessary—up to 120 milligrams per day for about six weeks—before an obvious effect is seen. Lower doses are often ineffective.

Maryann Forbes was one patient who was helped simply by taking ginkgo. A thirty-one-year-old mother of three, she recounted how she'd left her new puppy in the car when she went to the mall and then couldn't remember where she'd parked. Other equally upsetting events were occurring. She lost her keys constantly, couldn't recall the names of her acquaintances, and would regularly misplace things. Because she had a three-month-old baby, she was extremely concerned that her memory loss might cause her to put the baby in peril. However, her doctor said her symptoms were due to the stress of recent childbirth and that eventually her memory would return. He had no particular solution. She felt helpless and anxious, and as a result, she was also having problems swallowing and digesting her food. Her stomach was often upset.

Pregnancy and childbirth are indeed stressful, and although they could have been contributing to Maryann's symptoms, there was no reason for her to live with constant digestive distress. I started her on a low dose of ginkgo, only 60 milligrams a day. If ginkgo is known for anything in particular, it is the herb's potent ability to improve memory.

I thought of prescribing ginkgo because of a few fascinating studies I had read about the herb's ability to help stomach and intestinal distress. One study in Scandinavia showed that the herb can protect the mucosal lining of the intestines and increase blood flow throughout the digestive system. Another study in 1989 had shown that the herb inhibits some of the substances in the body that help trigger stomach ulcers. If I had to pick one nutrient that might address all Maryann's symptoms, ginkgo seemed the winner. I planned to add other nutrients that might help digestion—such as aloe vera and acidophilus (a healthy bacteria, see chapter 8)—but first I wanted to see just how well ginkgo worked by itself.

Maryann came back two weeks after our first appointment; there had been no change at all, and she was becoming despondent. I increased the dose to 120 milligrams per day, and when she came back for her third appointment, she was smiling. There had been an improvement in all her symptoms, she said. Within three months, her memory had returned, and her stomach distress had diminished. Ginkgo gave Maryann Forbes her life back. I didn't even need to add other nutrients to her program. How did a mere herb accomplish so much, and without any side effects?

Ginkgo in Action

Blood flow is the essence of life, for every blood cell is a tiny powerhouse that distributes nutrition, vitality, and oxygen throughout the body. Like the rivers and oceans that vitalize earth, adequate circulation is essential for good health. And ginkgo is key in the treatment of poor blood flow.

Traditional Chinese medicine considers the ginkgo leaf one of its prized medicinal treasures. This tree dates back to the time of the dinosaurs and has been found among fossils over two hundred million years old. Its ancestry makes it a mix of a fern and a modern-day tree. Today, there is only one species remaining; it does not grow in the wild.

It is in the leaf of the ginkgo tree that the most prized medicinal properties are found. It was the 1988 Harvard University team that made this momentous discovery when they finally isolated the mysterious active ingredient that had eluded researchers for so long. They named this extract, which is distilled from plant chemicals called ginkgolides, ginkgolide B. Ginkgolide and a host of other substances in the leaf are part of classes of compounds known as terpenoids and flavonoids (also found in many fruits and vegetables, from oranges to raspberries), which allay free radical damage and potent inflammatory factors in the body.

Ginkgo has two primary properties: it is a potent anti-inflammatory herb and a platelet inhibitor. A platelet is a crucial part of the healing process because of its ability to promote clotting, repair damaged blood vessels, and seal leaks in those vessels. Without platelets, our wounds would not heal. Platelets adhere to blood vessels that are injured, and once they stick to a site, they send out chemical messengers that attach to other platelets, causing them to cluster and to secrete an inflammatory chemical. Inflammation signals the body to rush in its troops of white blood cells, which then kill any bacteria that may have entered the wound or leak. Clotting and inflammation are key steps in wound healing. However, when there are too many platelets, or the platelets are too active, blood clotting occurs more easily, predisposing the body to conditions such as heart attacks and stroke. Heart attacks can be triggered by long-term, chronic, excessive platelet buildup that blocks the crucial small coronary arteries.

Obviously, everyone needs platelets, but it's the proper balance that's most important. This is particularly true when we consider the role of platelets in inflammatory disease. As I said, platelets release substances that promote inflammation. Although some inflammation is necessary, for example, to protect areas of the body where blood vessels are being repaired, excessive or chronic inflammation can be extremely damaging. Every day our own inflammatory cells release chemicals that do more than just kill invaders—they damage our own tissues, and our body must repair the damage and expel the toxic waste by-products. Ginkgo can help regulate this process when it veers out of control.

Ginkgo also keeps one other trick up its herbal sleeve: it contains flavonoids, healing compounds found in many different plants. The human body cannot produce these. There are many different flavonoid compounds that are essential to our diet. Originally, flavonoids were thought to be useless plant pigments that simply gave the world of fauna their beautiful greens, reds, purples, and yellows. Recently, research has shown that these pigmented substances offer significant health benefits, because they are potent free radical quenchers.

Ginkgo helps improve circulation in other somewhat mysterious ways. It seems to directly stimulate the release of two important substances in the body, both of which relax blood vessels: an endothelium-derived factor and prostacyclin. This is yet another reason that ginkgo has great promise in the treatment of vascular disease.

It's this one-two-three-four-and-more punch that makes ginkgo such a star. By reducing inflammation and excessive platelet activity, the herb protects blood vessels, helps keep the blood thin and flowing easily, controls excessive inflammation, and offers the body potent free radical quenchers to help repair any damage done by illness or toxins.

Why Ginkgo Is Valuable

Ginkgo is surprisingly effective in a wide range of conditions. Here are a few examples of ginkgo's powerful effects:

Brain: Studies on brain tissue show that ginkgo can protect the neurons that conduct information through your brain and spinal cord from suffering stress due to free radical damage.

Heart: Studies have shown promising evidence that ginkgo has a protective effect on an oxygen-starved heart. In a study using rabbits with damaged hearts, ginkgo significantly reduced levels of lipid peroxide, substances associated with permanent heart damage following heart attack.

ASTHMA: Ginkgo has long been a treatment for asthma in Chinese medicine, and now that we are beginning to learn of its profound ability to inhibit platelet activity and therefore inflammation, we understand how it can help in inflammatory diseases like asthma. A study in Barcelona showed that ginkgo could not only reduce airway constriction, it even stopped the bronchial tubes from contracting when they were challenged by allergens.

CLAUDICATION: This is a condition in which poor circulation results in muscle pain. A study in Germany showed that ginkgo increased the ability of patients to walk without suffering claudication pain.

CEREBRAL INSUFFICIENCY: Many elderly patients suffer from a lack of oxygen to the brain. Some have suffered from strokes. They often show symptoms such as depression, forgetfulness, and distractability. A German study of fifty such patients found that ginkgo improved both mood and recall. Another study of nineteen patients evaluated the effect of ginkgo on the brain and found that the herb improved blood flow as well as sugar consumption in the brain. Since sugar is the brain's main fuel, this was remarkable news.

ALZHEIMER'S DISEASE: A study of fifty patients with Alzheimer's found that ginkgo improved their sociability and overall mood. In research on one hundred twelve patients with memory problems, elderly patients who received ginkgo showed significant improvements in short-term memory and alertness. The impact of ginkgo actually increased as time went on.

CIRCULATION: Ginkgo exhibits antioxidant abilities and inhibits the oxidation of the fatty acids in our cell membranes, which occurs when free radicals attack a cell's membrane and damage its fat content. Also, as discussed, ginkgo guards against heart disease.

IMPOTENCE: Blood flow is crucial in impotence, an increasingly common problem today, as prostate conditions are on the rise. Fifty patients with impotence were given ginkgo, and after six months, an astonishing half of them had regained potency. That's almost as high a success rate as some drugs on the market. My only caveat is that individuals taking ginkgo for this problem should be patient, since significant results may take several months.

Depression: In patients with depression, ginkgo showed a 50 percent reduction in symptoms after six to eight weeks. In a study of forty middle-aged patients with mild to moderate depression that did not respond to medication, patients were given either ginkgo or a placebo. In the ginkgo group, there was a 50 percent reduction in the severity of depression after four weeks and a 68 percent reduction after eight weeks. In the placebo group there was only a 10 percent reduction in four weeks.

Cellular Repair: Intriguing studies around the world have found other potential uses for ginkgo, including liver and blood repair, indicating that ginkgo's benefits may extend far beyond circulatory problems. Ginkgo may even be useful in radiation exposure, according to one study that looked at damage to the blood in Chernobyl victims. Excessive exposure to radiation can be traced as clastogenic factors, which damage chromosomes and are thought to be triggers for cancer. In another study done in China, eighty-six patients suffering from chronic hepatitis took ginkgo for three months. This condition, which is sometimes fatal and is notoriously hard to treat, improved simply through the use of this herb. After three months of treatment, the majority of patients were in remission.

Although these studies are only preliminary and were done on only a small number of patients, they provide intriguing evidence of further potential for this most useful herb.

Ginkgo and Blood Flow: Some Treatment Surprises

As noted, ginkgo can help with a variety of circulatory problems, from strokes and heart attacks to varicose veins and embolisms (blood clots in the lungs or arteries), and even in mystifying conditions like Raynaud's phenomena, where circulation to the hands drops so suddenly and acutely that the hands become cold, numb, and bluish.

The usefulness of ginkgo in combating chronic low blood flow in the brain has been documented in over forty clinical studies done around the world. When ginkgo was administered within six hours of a stroke, significant improvements were noted in the control subjects. In one recent study, 120 milligrams per day of ginkgo extract was given to eighteen patients with impaired memory and concentration. Although short-term memory did not improve immediately, ginkgo did restore it over time. In another study of ninety patients with cerebral insufficiency, ginkgo was more effective than a placebo in improving the condition. In a study of memory impairment, ginkgo improved memory at the end of the six-month trial period.

WARNING

Ginkgo may be so powerful that sometimes it can cause problems when taken with blood-thinning medications. Although ginkgo is considered to be nontoxic, a recent letter to the *New England Journal of Medicine* described a case in which ginkgo combined with aspirin caused bleeding to occur in a stroke patient. This situation will need to be monitored and studied further. If you are taking aspirin or Coumadin (a blood thinner), consult your physician about this if you are considering taking ginkgo.

HOW MUCH SHOULD I TAKE?

For General Health
30-60 mg/day (optional)
After Meals
Special Conditions

Memory	60-120 mg/day
Circulation	60-120 mg/day
Asthma	60-180 mg/day
Claudication	60-180 mg/day
Cerebral insufficiency	60-180 mg/day
Alzheimer's Disease	120-180 mg/day
Impotence	120-180 mg/day
Depression	60-180 mg/day
Cellular repair	60-180 mg/day
Tinnitus	120-180 mg/day
Peripheral neuropathy	60-120 mg/day
Diabetes	60-120 mg/day
Fatigue	60-180 mg/day

That's why I recommend ginkgo for such a wide range of conditions. It's a versatile and critical treatment that gets to the root cause of many problems and helps speed nutrients to a needy cell in any part of the body. Whether I use ginkgo to help other herbs and nutraceuticals get to where they need to go, or simply for its own ability to quench free radical and inflammation activity, this herb lives up to its ancient reputation.

14

NAC: Breathe Easy

Free radicals: when I was in medical school, I rarely heard a word about them. Only a small group of "kooks" would rave about the powers of vitamins and minerals. It wasn't until my own struggles with asthma in the late 1980s that I began to appreciate the benefits of antioxidants; only then did I appreciate the genius behind the discovery of free radicals, how important it is to combat free radical production, and how crucial antioxidants are in preventing disease. Vitamins C and E helped me escape the respiratory infections I'd had every year of my life.

As I explained in chapter 12, free radicals are highly charged molecules bearing an extra electron. That electron makes them extremely unstable. Imagine them as lightning bolts crashing into cells and causing damage.

How do these unimaginably tiny particles inflict their widespread damage on your body? Surprisingly, it's the very defense mechanisms that our bodies employ for safety that release free radicals into our systems. And it's the very air we breathe that fuels them.

Oxygen is essential for life. But oxygen can turn against us. That's because each cell produces both energy and free radicals. Two percent of the body's oxygen actually undergoes free radical reactions. Free radicals are unstable, and so they streak through us, searching everywhere for extra electrons to bond with to help them stabilize, and inevitably those electrons are snatched from our other cells. This path of destruction, like an atomic bomb, is a series of chain reactions in which free radicals steal electrons from each other, attacking cell membranes and creating even more hyperactive free radical molecules in the process. In their wake, they leave behind tissue and organ damage. In excess, this can lead to a shocking number of health problems, from cancer to liver disease, cataracts, and emphysema.

Why does our body generate free radicals in the first place? One reason is because they're such powerful warriors, and we need them to kill invading microbes. Our white blood cells release a caustic peroxide designed to kill whatever comes its way. This peroxide releases strong free radicals—it's actually the same substance found in products we use to clean our homes and kill germs.

The good news is that our bodies are designed to mop up these free radicals after they've done their job. But in today's world, that simply isn't enough. Close to 150 million tons of pollutants are released into the atmosphere each year in the United States, and most of these contaminants promote harmful free radicals. Every time you walk past a bus belching out a cloud of fumes, clean your floors with ammonia or chlorine bleach, spray your garden with pesticides, pump fuel into your tank at the gas station, or inhale ozone from smog; or as a by-product of computers and photocopiers, you are subjecting your lungs to free radicals. Even greasy foods like hamburgers, pizza, and french fries contains harmful fats that become oxidized, creating free radicals. Perhaps the absolute worst—and most ubiquitous—free radical damage stems from cigarette smoke, whether you puff it out or get it secondhand. In the face of this onslaught, our bodies need supplemental antioxidant assistance.

Antioxidants chase free radicals through the body, stabilizing and neutralizing them. Among the most powerful of antioxidants ranks an amino acid called NAC, N-acetyl cysteine. NAC protects us in many ways, but above all it's the lung's guardian, and since our lungs are so vulnerable to free radicals in this polluted world, I believe this is a nutrient crucial to general health—a nutraceutical many of us could benefit from.

Glutathione's Trusty Sidekick

The potent antioxidant NAC not only has powerful restorative effects of its own, it is a primary building block for glutathione, the preeminent antioxidant in the body. Glutathione is thought to strengthen the immune system, protect cells against heavy metals and free radicals, and aid in general cell metabolism. Together with NAC, glutathione is extremely effective in repairing damage done to the lungs. The delicate airways and lining of the lungs are extremely vulnerable to free radical damage, because of the many poisonous environmental toxins that assault them, leading to defensive inflammatory and immune reactions. NAC soothes the lungs both alone and in concert with glutathione and is particularly helpful in combating respiratory illnesses like bronchitis, asthma, or emphysema. If gluthathione is the superhero antioxidant, then I like to think of NAC as its trusty sidekick.

So why not just take glutathione, instead of its trusty backup? Because glutathione has an incredibly short half-life. We can take it in supplement form and even absorb it into our blood, but it will quickly dissipate in a few minutes. To keep levels of glutathione up for long-term protection, we should take NAC.

How NAC Can Work for You

NAC may be especially helpful in keeping our lungs healthy, but that's only one of the roles it plays in helping prevent and ameliorate common illnesses. Some examples follow.

Cancer: Promising research indicates that glutathione can lower the risk of cancer. A study of one thousand eight hundred participants in the *American Journal of Epidemiology* showed that glutathione reduced cancer risk substantially. NAC also seems to reduce the side effects of adriamycin, a potent drug used in chemotherapy.

Heart Attack: Nitroglycerin is used by doctors to help dilate blood vessels and relieve heart problems. However, heart patients rapidly develop a tolerance to it and must increase their dosage of the drug over time. A study in the *American Journal of Cardiology* in 1997 showed that NAC reduced nitroglycerin intolerance in patients with angina over a forty-eight-hour period. While fourteen out of fifteen patients in a control group stopped responding to nitroglycerin, only five out of sixteen patients on NAC developed a tolerance to the drug. A combination of NAC and nitroglycerin may improve heart health when nitroglycerin alone just isn't enough.

Muscle Fatigue: In a study in the *Journal of Clinical Investigation*, NAC was shown to inhibit muscle fatigue in humans.

Bacterial Infection: NAC has been shown to fight staphyloccocus bacteria; it may actually protect your immune cells while they kill microbes.

Viral Infection: Modern science offers very few drugs to combat viruses, but NAC may offer hope in this area. A study in *Anti-Viral Research* reported that NAC inhibited replication of the hepatitis B virus, reducing viral DNA fiftyfold. Exciting new research also indicates that NAC may protect the body against HIV.

Aging: High levels of glutathione are linked to increased life span. Indeed, a report from the University of Nebraska's journal *Drugs and Aging* states that life expectancy can be increased by five years with a healthy diet and antioxidant supplements.

BRONCHITIS: A 1997 study in the *European Respiratory Journal* showed that NAC reduced bronchitis infections: in sixteen smokers taking 1,200 milligrams of NAC daily, only three succumbed to bronchitis, compared to fifteen out of twenty-one smokers not taking NAC.

CHRONIC OBSTRUCTIV PULMONARY DISEASE (COPD): A study in the journal *Chest* showed that in patients with COPD, a debilitating and chronic lung disease, NAC significantly enhanced the antifungal activity of the immune system, as well as increasing the destructive activity of white blood cells fighting invading bacteria. Another study in the *American Journal of Respiratory and Critical Care Medicine* found that NAC improved breathing capacity in eighteen patients who suffered from fibrosing alveolitis, a condition where lung tissue becomes scarred and fibrous. The patients took 600 milligrams of NAC three times daily for twelve weeks, along with their usual medication. Their lung fluid was analyzed and showed increased glutathione levels.

AIDS: Dr. Leonard Herzenberg and other researchers at Stanford University reported they had used NAC to bolster immunity in 204 AIDS patients. The results, published in the *Proceedings of the National Academy of Sciences*, found that AIDS patients taking 600-1,200 milligrams a day were twice as likely to live two years longer than patients who chose not to receive long-term treatment. Herzenberg theorized that NAC was restoring normal blood levels of glutathione.

REAL-LIFE ADVENTURES WITH NAC

Stacy Shaw, a twenty-five-year-old with chronic bronchitis, was always taking cough medications, and her throat was so sore and raspy that her friends actually told her they were jealous of her "sexy growl."

Stacy loved her gig as a bartender at a jazz club, but the smoky air was proving to be a problem. Her bronchitis kept her up at night, and although she took melatonin, a hormone used as a natural sleeping pill, it didn't help. It was her cough, not insomnia, that was keeping her up at night.

As Stacy ran down her list of problems, it became clear that her work environment was a major culprit. A study from 1983 stated that secondhand smoke can be even more toxic than smoke directly inhaled from a cigarette. I suggested to Stacy that she try to avoid smoke as much as possible.

"I can't. There's no way I can get away from smoke—it's always right in my face. I'd have to avoid every single person I work with. Even my manager smokes."

Not only was Stacy continually inhaling secondhand smoke, she had no access to fresh air because the club was in a basement.

Everything Stacy told me convinced me that her job was seriously compromising her health, allowing free radicals and carcinogens from cigarette smoke to devastate her lungs. I couldn't force her to find a new job, but I could try to improve her situation to the best of my ability. I told her to get a portable air purifier and place it at the far end of the bar countertop. I myself probably wouldn't be able to live in the chemical paradise that is New York City without air purifiers at home and in the office. I also prescribed 1,000 milligrams of NAC daily, along with a complete vitamin and mineral program.

When Stacy came back for a follow-up visit one month later, she was breathing more easily. She also informed me that she was looking for a new job.

"Working the bar was such a blast," she told me, wistfully. "But after we talked, I realized this job was ruining my health." She had made the right decision. Nutrients can help us tremendously, but they can't change the world we live in.

NAC Helps Cleanse You from the Inside Out

Gail Kantor was a sixty-four-year-old retired widow who lived alone. Fiercely independent, even stubborn, Gail only came to see me when her asthma actually interfered with her daily schedule.

"How long have you had asthma?" I asked Gail on her first visit to my office.

"About seven years," she told me.

"And why did you suddenly decide to see me after seven years? Your symptoms must have gotten much worse."

"Oh yes," she agreed, nodding her head vigorously. "At my age, keeping fit is very important. I don't want anyone's help, and I'm not about to depend on the kindness of strangers. But lately it's been so much harder to walk on my treadmill. I become short of breath and my throat fills with mucus."

"Have you been doing anything different lately that might cause these changes?"

"Everything's exactly the same as it was seven years ago . . ." she trailed off, playing with the hem of her shirt.

"Gail," I said firmly, "I want to help you as much as possible. But I can only do that if you're honest with me about the changes in your life."

"OK," she admitted, eyes flashing at me. "I got a cat a year ago, and every time I'm with her, my symptoms get worse. But I love Betsy. She's my companion, now that my husband is gone. There's no way I'm giving her up."

That was the key to her asthma. She was allergic to Betsy. Well, I thought, she won't give Betsy away, but maybe the cat isn't the only cause of her asthma.

"Where do you exercise?"

"My treadmill is in the basement."

"Is your basement damp?" She must have thought my questions were strange. But indoor air can become polluted by mold spores, and a large percentage of my asthma patients are sensitive to molds and fungus. I explained this to Gail.

"Yes, it's damp and chilly. I exercise down there because it's the only place the treadmill will fit."

"Are you taking any medications?" I asked.

"I was, but they stopped working years ago. And . . . I know you're going to hate this . . . I smoke," she admitted.

I told Gail that there were many things we could do to improve her situation. Smoking is one of the worst ways to damage your lungs. Smoke contains particles that embed themselves deep within the lungs and carcinogens processed through the liver. The first step was getting her to quit smoking.

Second, I told Gail if she could not move her treadmill, she should consider biking outdoors or at a gym. I asked her to remove carpeting, rugs, and drapery from her home, since cat hair and allergens tend to accumulate in these places. Wooden floors and miniblinds, frequently washed and cleaned, would help eliminate excess cat dander. Finally, I put Gail on a program of NAC, plus other supportive nutrients like magnesium, zinc, and vitamin C. Gail agreed to try to give up cigarettes, perhaps relieved that I hadn't insisted she give up Betsy instead. She called me a few weeks after she quit smoking, complaining, "I've been coughing more than ever in my entire life, and I haven't touched a single cigarette! I've even stopped exercising in the basement. Are you sure this is going to work?"

I reassured her that, with time, the treatment would come through for her. Paradoxically, smoking can often act as a cough suppressant. In ancient Sicily, asthmatics often traveled to a volcano to inhale its smoke and diminish their cough. In the long run, quitting smoking would save her lungs. Sure enough, a few months later, Gail's symptoms were improved, even with her cat by her side. She still had occasional asthma attacks, but her immune system was better equipped to handle them, thanks to NAC.

NAC Fights Lung Disease

A simple vacation can become a living nightmare for people who have lung disorders. Tiffany Zane, a forty-seven-year-old saleswoman for an international trading company, had lived with COPD since she was just seven years old. Two of the most common forms of COPD are emphysema and bronchitis. Emphysema's hallmark is the destruction of alveoli, the small air pockets in our lungs where oxygen is absorbed. Bronchitis, on the other hand, is defined as inflammation of the mucous membrane in the lung. Both incarnations of COPD are widely prevalent among us: autopsies reveal that 60 percent of men and 15 percent of women are found to have emphysema, and at least 15-20 percent of adults are believed to have bronchitis.

Tiffany had been receiving allergy shots for most of her life, but she felt that they were useless against her illness. Despite her breathing problems and phlegm-filled lungs, Tiffany refused to let COPD diminish her passion for life and adventure. She loved to travel as part of her job, and she had returned from Thailand just three weeks before seeing me for the first time. Unfortunately, Tiffany's curiosity about foreign cultures had nearly ended her trip. After sampling all the Thai delicacies she could get her hands on, including a piece of meat from a roadside stand in Bangkok, she suffered from alternating spells of diarrhea and constipation. She was also allergic to monosodium glutamate (MSG), an ingredient used in Asian cooking. As a result, a weary Tiffany made it back to the United States dehydrated and seriously ill with a respiratory infection. Tiffany finally sought my help because she wanted to cleanse her system and return it to a natural state. Only then, she believed, could she feel healthy again.

My first concern with Tiffany was her dehydration. Her bouts of diarrhea were still ongoing and debilitating. I immediately put her on a course of glutamine, zinc, and acidophilus to repair her intestinal tract and replace the healthy bacteria she'd lost. In about a month, results of a stool test showed that Tiffany had no excess pathogenic bacteria in her system. However, bacterial infections continued to plague her, and she developed bronchitis. To purge her lungs of allergens and phlegm, I had her take 1,000 milligrams of NAC and 3 grams of vitamin C daily. Within three weeks, Tiffany's lungs felt stronger, and she could breathe much more easily. She still had mucus, but she did not show any signs of the infection that mucus often promotes.

"This is the first time in recent history that I've had mucus in my lungs that didn't lead to infection," she informed me. The excitement she felt was almost overwhelming enough to make her sign up for a safari to Africa—but not quite.

NAC Protects the Liver

The free radicals spewed out by an inflamed lung are similar to those emitted during liver detoxification. In chapter 7, I explained how milk thistle helps the liver to remove chemicals and harmful particles from the blood. I often use milk thistle in conjunction with NAC, since both help the liver.

Joanna Huang benefited immensely from this potent combination. A public relations manager with a sunny smile, Joanna had a number of allergies, and she had been diagnosed two years earlier with hepatitis A. At a recent business dinner, she had ordered the most expensive item on the menu: lobster. Unfortunately, the seafood triggered an acute allergic reaction that caused every part of her body from her lips to her feet to itch uncontrollably.

By the time one of her friends referred her to me, Joanna had been itching for a whole month.

"I kept thinking it would go away," she confided. "At work, people walk by my cubicle, and I'm scratching my legs with pencils, doing anything I can to relieve this itch."

Joanna also had frequent urinary tract infections. I don't often use antibiotics in my practice, but it was clear she was harboring bacteria that kept flaring up into an infection. A week of antibiotics, along with a daily glass of unsweetened cranberry juice, cleared her infection right up. Her itching, however, would take more work. Knowing her history of hepatitis, it was clear that her liver was having problems with detoxification. To give Joanna the powerful antioxidant defense abilities she was lacking, I put her on a healthier diet along with both silymarin and NAC. Within a month, Joanna's itching was gone. She continues to eat more healthily—and watches what she orders on business dinners—and is back to being her exuberant self.

Defend Your Life with NAC

The chemical interactions between our body and the environment are part of a grand but precarious balance. Free radicals belong in this category. Think of these electron radicals darting through our bodies like quasars or comets. In a finely tuned system, free radicals are necessary intermediaries of the our body's defense system, created from the very air we breathe and used to power the enormous undertaking of life itself. Rebalancing the body's free radical scavengers with natural antioxidants like NAC allows us to harness the willful energy of free radicals for our own healthy advantage.

Dosages are generally from 500 to 2,000 milligrams daily for conditions such as asthma or bronchitis. Patients with serious liver disease or HIV infection take between 1,000 and 2,000 milligrams per day. For maintenance doses in healthy individuals, 50 to 100 milligrams should be adequate. Since NAC is a powerful antioxidant, it works synergistically with other vitamins, such as vitamin C, selenium, and lipoic acid.

HOW MUCH SHOULD I TAKE?

For General Health
100 mg/day (optional)
Before Meals Divided Doses
Special Conditions

Bronchitis	500-2,000 mg/day
Asthma	500-2,000 mg/day
Emphysema	500-2,000 mg/day
Cancer	1,000-2,000 mg/day
Heart attacks	1,000-2,000 mg/day

15

Tyrosine: Stress Buster

What if I told you there was a nutrient so important to energy and stamina that the United States military was conducting studies on its benefits, as if concocting some secret strategy for their troops? The day may soon come when troops are sent into battle with weapons, K-rations, and a little vial of tyrosine.

With bullets flying, bombs exploding, and death and destruction all around them, soldiers are expected to keep their cool. It's no wonder that the government takes interest in any measure that will improve performance under pressure, and the amino acid tyrosine has been shown to do just that, decreasing battle fatigue and increasing the ability to handle a trigger under stress.

But, you say, I'm not a gun-toting army cadet. I'm a peacekeeping parent of two whose main concerns are impressing the boss at work, managing the household, and getting the kids to bed on time without having a nervous breakdown. Or maybe you're an athlete or a student who has to be "on" all the time, leaping hurdles or making the grade. Or perhaps you find yourself hopelessly lethargic, wanting to go out and conquer life but constantly lacking the energy. If you are chronically fatigued, must consistently perform well under high-pressure circumstances, or find that stress is severely handicapping your ability to get the simplest tasks accomplished, then tyrosine may help. Tyrosine could be the natural antidote to today's fast-paced lifestyle.

Of all the supplements I study and prescribe in my practice, tyrosine is one of my absolute favorites. Under its guidance, I've seen people emerge from the fog of depression, handle stress better, and generally improve their energy.

Tyrosine: Nature's Antidepressant

Tyrosine is an amino acid—a building block for protein—that we encounter every day in dairy products such as cheese and milk, and meats such as chicken and turkey. While all of the twenty-odd amino acids that form our bodily proteins serve as building blocks for the brain, tyrosine plays an especially important role in keeping our nervous system alive and running. Just like two other amino acids, tryptophan and phenylalanine (which is found in the sugar substitute aspartame), tyrosine is known as an "aromatic" amino acid and has a special ring structure shaped like a hexagon. Unlike nonaromatic amino acids, any dietary tyrosine we consume is readily absorbed into our brains. This quality allows tyrosine the heady power to tinker with our moods, feelings, emotions, and cognitive abilities.

You may have never heard of tyrosine, but this nutrient is the proud precursor of three of the most crucial neurotransmitters used as chemical messengers by the neuronal cells that wire our brains: dopamine, norepinephrine, and epinephrine (otherwise known as adrenaline). The life-changing power of antidepressant drugs is often due to their ability to increase both dopamine and norepinephrine. Though the role of norepinephrine is subtle; it is absolutely necessary for preparing our bodies for the fight-or-flight reaction. It conserves energy and stimulates adrenaline release. A 1989 study in *Military Medical Journal* shows that intensely stressful situations, like fighting in a war, can deplete our stores of norepinephrine. Tyrosine not only restores low levels of norepinephrine but also improves performance and cognitive functioning during times of extreme pressure.

Studies of human subjects at high altitudes and freezing temperatures show that tyrosine supplements prevent the learning, motor, and memory difficulties that usually arise in stressful environments. Second, tyrosine is a source of energy. A study on lab animals showed that tyrosine renewed the enthusiasm and motivation normally eliminated by stressful surroundings. Similar research has shown that tyrosine can restore significant amounts of energy to sufferers of chronic fatigue syndrome and dysthymia—depression that is not as severe as full-blown clinical depression—by acting as a natural stimulant. This brain-boosting nutrient can also be useful as an analgesic and as a potential treatment for disorders like narcolepsy, and it may even help ameliorate PMS.

Anna Darvington, a forty-six-year-old medical assistant who was suffering from chronic stress, came to me seeking solace from PMS symptoms like hot flashes and irritability. As it turned out, PMS was the least of her problems. After being diagnosed with breast cancer in 1990, Anna was told that she would need a mastectomy. She'd been quite worried about how her husband would react. In addition, frequent urinary tract infections, yeast infections, and colitis continued to plague Anna. Meanwhile, she was finding it increasingly difficult to maintain her concentration at work. As an emergency-room nurse, she was expected to perform numerous repetitive tasks like administering injections and putting in IVs quickly and efficiently in chaotic surroundings. But Anna was having trouble focusing on the day-to-day problems that the emergency room posed. She often had problems getting the vein right for her IVs, to the distress of her patients. She was always tired and easily distracted from her job of saving lives.

"I feel like a space cadet," she told me. "As if I'm floating around in my own little world. Today in the hospital, I was poking some poor kid's arm for ten minutes trying to insert a simple IV."

In cases like Anna's, I know that tyrosine is important for treatment. People who are having trouble completing repetitive tasks or are buckling under the pressure of illness or career demands are excellent candidates for tyrosine's energy-boosting powers.

I prescribed the herb St. John's wort for Anna's depression, coenzyme Q_{10} to increase her energy (it helps the energy powerhouses in our cells, the mitochondria, function more efficiently, see chapter 6), and 1 gram of tyrosine before each meal. When she came back for a follow-up visit two months later, she was happy to report a significant change.

"I haven't missed an IV in months," she said, visibly livelier. "I am so much more productive at work—I can concentrate so much better."

The Brain: Our Own Grand Central Station

How can a single amino acid affect memory, mood, concentration, and energy? It all begins in the brain. Our bodies are wired with a complex network of hundreds of billions of interconnecting cells called neurons, which take information from the outside world and relay it to our central command center, the brain. The brain is responsible for integrating and making sense of all the sounds, sights, smells, and data rushing in from the world and translating them into the movements we make and the emotions we feel.

Neurons, like living telegraphs, send messages through our nervous system in two forms: electrical impulses, which shoot signals down the length of a neuron, and chemical messengers, which carry these signals between cells. These chemical messengers are known as neurotransmitters, and the trillions of notes they send through the brain every second make them amazingly fast purveyors of information.

Our brain's instantaneous coordination of the over fifty known or suspected neurotransmitters is crucial. Each neurotransmitter has its own unique character and can pass news on only to neurons that have receptors fitting its chemical shape. Some excite the brain while others calm it and diminish the impact of their chemical counterparts.

A lot of what we know about the importance of these chemicals, unfortunately, comes from what happens to people who are lacking these important messengers. Dopamine, for example, helps regulate movement and is also a profound pleasure chemical that helps us fall in love, savor a chocolate fudge sundae, and set and achieve goals. But it can also trigger addictive behavior. The degeneration of dopamine-using neurons in the brain can lead to Parkinson's disease, a terrifying illness that inhibits the conscious ability to initiate, sustain, or terminate movement. Too little dopamine in certain centers of the brain may lead to attention deficit disorder or depression.

For people who are stressed, norepinephrine is a crucial neurotransmitter. When you are walking alone down a dark alley and hear footsteps close behind you, your heart begins to pound, you breathe rapidly and shallowly, and you feel suddenly alert. Your body has just released a flood of stress hormones, including norepinephrine. This response to stress shuts off normal processes like digestion and immune response in order to save energy for fighting off—or fleeing—the alley prowler.

Unfortunately, constant stress can deplete necessary norepinephrine levels. That's where tyrosine, as a building block for norepinephrine, is so valuable.

How Stress Can Hurt You

You can see how important neurotransmitters are in maintaining our psychological and physiological well-being, even in times of stress. The fascinating association between stress and illness is still not accepted enough today, even though it has long been researched. In 1936, Hans Selye, known as the founding father of stress studies, published a groundbreaking paper on the long-term consequences of stress in the renowned British journal *Nature*. Selye was the first to conceive—and brilliantly so—that stress can wreak havoc with our health and that it's our response to stress that makes all the difference to our bodies. In fact, it is our response to stress that actually is the stress. If we can keep stress from affecting our lives, he believed, then it ceases to be a problem.

The evidence of stress-induced chemical cascades that Selye proposed so long ago in his paper holds up, even today. He suggested that when we're stressed, neurotransmitters caused a part of the brain known as the hypothalamus to produce a substance called corticotropin-releasing factor (CRF). This stress substance travels to our hormone factory, the pituitary gland, and signals the release of adrenocorticotropic hormone, another chemical that warns our bodies about life's pressures. Finally, this hormone cues the adrenal glands to secrete cortisol and adrenaline. The result? Increased blood sugar, faster heart rate, and higher blood pressure.

Many people reach a saturation point, where they can no longer tolerate stress and its effects on the body. Eventually, norepinephrine becomes depleted, and the immune system is suppressed. A study in the *New England Journal of Medicine* found that psychological stress increases the risk of acute infectious respiratory illness. There is even evidence that stress hurts us at the most basic cellular level. Each of our cells contains a powerhouse called the mitochondrion, which regulates energy production all through the body. In rats, acute stress was found to cause severe mitochondrial damage, illustrating the far-reaching powers of sustained pressure.

Even the stress of exercise can have an impact on health, depending on your genetic legacy. A study in one neurology journal showed that hard physical activity can lead to a decrease in the synthesis of norepinephrine.

Neurotransmitters like norepinephrine can become depleted if our stress levels are excessive. One extreme example of this is chronic fatigue syndrome (CFS). An epidemic that has reached its highest levels this decade, chronic fatigue syndrome has gone by many names, from chronic fatigue immune dysfunction syndrome (CFIDS) to “the yuppie flu.” Part of the mystery of CFS stems from the fact that we still don't know what virus causes the syndrome. Epstein-Barr virus, or HHV-6, another member of the herpes family, has been implicated. There is even some speculation that it is triggered by what are thought to be “stealth” viruses, which may actually evade the immune system's powerful surveillance.

Whatever the cause, one thing is certain: CFS is not just fatigue. While most of us have been exceedingly tired at some point in our lives, sleep eventually restores our energy and vitality. For sufferers of CFS, however, there is no such thing as a good night's sleep. They are constantly plagued with a deep, unrelenting exhaustion that sleep cannot remedy. They have the will and the desire to live a normal life, but their fatigue wears them down. This fatigue interferes with a normal life, normal relationships, and normal day-to-day functioning. CFS has been defined by the Centers for Disease Control as a set of major and minor criteria, one hallmark being a debilitating fatigue lasting at least six months that reduces average daily activity to below 50 percent. One group of criteria for CFS suggests that hypotension, or abnormally low blood pressure, may be associated with CFS in some people.

Many patients suffering from CFS report that stress exacerbates their condition. Clearly, stress is not just a mental dysfunction; it can dismantle the health of the whole body. Because tyrosine can replenish norepinephrine, it is a great way to restore that neurotransmitter in times of excess stress. And because high levels of norepinephrine can raise blood pressure, it makes a great energy source for chronic fatigue victims. Although the connection between low blood pressure and CFS has not yet been proven, studies irrefutably show—and I have seen in my practice—that tyrosine has been extremely effective in this regard.

In 1970, the *New England Journal of Medicine* suggested that the job of a clinician is not just to treat disease but to alleviate distress. In fact, alleviating distress may be key in treating disease. Many people come to see me with a variety of medical conditions for which there may be no known antecedent, such as severe lower back pain or an acute onset of chronic conditions like asthma, heart disease, or arthritis. Inevitably, a specific stressor—or several—clearly predated the illness. Sometimes the stressor is a treatment offered by another doctor. For instance, many medications can actually worsen depression, like antihistamines, hypertensive medications, and stimulating drugs like over-the-counter decongestants, theophylline (an asthma drug), and even caffeine. Physical symptoms as different as nausea, blurred vision, and muscle weakness are all common signals of internalized stress. So are debilitating conditions like irritable bowel syndrome, high blood pressure, migraines, sexual dysfunction, and fatigue, just to name a few.

EFFECTIVE WAYS TO COPE WITH STRESS

Tyrosine can be a great energy boost and stress reliever. It works best, however, when norepinephrine levels are low in the body. If you prefer not to resort to supplements to give you energy, tyrosine is certainly not the only answer to distress. All of the following techniques have been proven to eliminate fatigue from a hectic schedule. In addition to techniques I mention in my book *Reversing Asthma*, such as meditation and yoga, the following also have been found to be helpful.

Biofeedback: Biofeedback has recently become a popular, accepted method for improving health. Biofeedback machines allow you to tune in to the subtle state of internal, involuntary processes like heart rate, brain wave activity, and blood pressure that you might not otherwise perceive. Using this feedback, you can consciously alter these processes to improve their functioning. Most machines use devices like bells or lights that sound or flash when your blood pressure rises, for example, or when your muscles tense. By learning to control the speed of the sound or flashes coming from the biofeedback machine, you control the precision of your biological processes. In many cases, biofeedback is a great way to will yourself well. It can allow you to monitor and control your stress level and improve it using the power of the mind.

Sleep: Getting enough sleep is one simple but often overlooked way to reduce frustration and anxiety. Even if you don't have enough time to sleep in every morning, napping for twenty to thirty minutes in the middle of the day fits in with your natural circadian rhythms and can temporarily restore energy.

Along with other nutrients, tyrosine shores up your inborn coping defenses. Of course, it will not reverse longstanding psychological problems, nor will it miraculously transform patients. But the nutrient does seem to improve sustained concentration and replenish a sense of energy so that individuals can resume their everyday lives.

Relationships: Being alone, it seems, can only contribute to your stress. Studies show that social ties improve immune function and lower mortality rates. A study of ten thousand men at Tel Aviv University found that love and support were the biggest predictors of health, and elderly people have been shown to thrive when visited regularly. Learning to spend time with friends and relatives can relax you mentally and protect your body physically.

Eliminate Smoking, Coffee, and Alcohol: All three of these are no-nos for the pressured person. Drinking more than two ounces of alcohol a day has been shown to raise blood pressure and increase stress, while caffeine can leave you anxious and jittery. Smoking carries such high risks of lung cancer and heart disease that quitting can improve your body's health immensely; within just three days, quitters notice enhanced lung function. Within three years, risk of cancer diminishes.

Exercise: Regular exercise, be it walking or running marathons, not only improves health but is essential for reducing stress, boosting self-esteem, and lowering anxiety.

Time Management: Making lists of "things to do" and planning carefully what needs to be accomplished each day can save us the panic of trying to remember everything and trying to do too much in one day. Just the act of writing down essential events and errands can relieve stress and reassure us that we are prepared for what comes our way. Remember, though, to make time in your daily planner for relaxation; taking a few minutes to breathe in fresh air and meditate not only reduces anxiety but lowers blood pressure and the risk of heart disease.

And You Thought Your Stress Was Bad
True Tyrosine Tales

Tammy Griffith was a sixty-five-year-old woman who could easily benefit from a little help focusing in life. A retired housewife, she was also a partner in the family automotive repair business. Yet you'd often have to call Tammy's name two or three times before she realized you were addressing her. Her own family thought she was senile, that she was losing touch with reality as part of the normal aging process. Her family physician even told her that she might be showing early signs of Alzheimer's disease.

As it turned out, Tammy's distraction was coming not from a neurodegenerative illness but from her own family—or their workplace, anyway. Knowing that auto repair shops are usually swimming in toxic gases and fumes and that exposure to these toxins could have stressed her liver to the point where it could not rid the body of the chemicals (see chapter 7), I asked her how often she visited her relatives at work.

"I'm actually working there, so I'm there all day in a little room in the back," she said. "They need me to do the books."

"Tammy," I said, "toxins are constantly being released into the air where you work, and in a small back room you aren't getting any fresh, clean air. That alone could be stressing your body, burdening your liver, and causing your symptoms."

"I know," she said, "but they need me there, and I have so much free time on my hands now that I'm retired."

I convinced Tammy to stop working at the auto shop, and her mind grew clearer within weeks. She continued to keep the books, but now she did her work at home. Not only did this allow her to watch her grandson during the day, but it saved her from the autoshop's chemicals. She was much more attentive and felt more in tune with her surroundings. Still, some of her symptoms persisted. Her memory and concentration remained faulty. I put her on 1 gram of tyrosine, taken in two divided doses before meals, as well as ginseng to help reduce her blood sugar. Tests revealed that she was mildly diabetic with a slightly elevated blood sugar, which can usually be controlled by diet. Eliminating sugar and adding ginseng would, I felt, balance her blood sugar.

Her blood sugar did stabilize quickly, but her concentration still flagged. She noticed no difference in her ability to get things done under the pressures she faced at home. I increased her dosage of tyrosine to 3 grams, and in a few weeks Tammy was noticeably more productive. I knew the tyrosine had taken effect when her brother called my office.

"I used to think my sister was going crazy—or maybe just lazy. Now she's like a whole new person."

"Don't thank me," I told him. "Thank tyrosine."

Tammy was not alone in being called crazy because she was perpetually listless or tired. Murray Heffner, a fifty-five-year-old TV executive under enormous pressure to make ratings and close deals, suffered from chronic fatigue syndrome (CFS), weakness, and insomnia. His wife complained that he was never home, and that when he was, he was completely inattentive to her needs. One particular point of contention was his recent inability to perform sexually.

His coworkers warned that he was increasingly unreliable. When he took clients to dinner, hoping to wine and dine them into giving him their accounts, he inevitably woke up the next morning with an excruciating hangover. When I first met him, he looked haggard and worn as he sunk into a chair in front of me.

"My doctor tells me to see a shrink," he told me. "But I don't think the problem is in my head. There's got to be some way to make me more alert and more efficient at work besides going into therapy."

I tested for causes of severe fatigue such as low thyroid function, chronic allergies, low blood sugar, and Lyme disease and found them all negative. Since Murray wanted a natural approach, I started him on mood-boosting herbs like St. John's wort and strengthening supplements such as ginseng. None of these, however, seemed to alleviate his depression and fatigue. I finally asked him to visit the hospital for a tilt test, which would detect any problems with his blood pressure. This is a test where the patient is strapped to a table and moved from a reclining to vertical position to test whether they become faint or dizzy as a result. Researchers at Johns Hopkins University examined subjects with CFS in a tilt table test, where patients were monitored as they were moved from a reclining to an upright position. Those who suffered from low blood pressure became dizzy when tested. Murray's test came up positive, and the hospital specialists recommended that he begin taking a cortisone drug called Florinef to increase his blood pressure. However, I was convinced that natural supplements could restore Murray's vitality back in a safer, gentler way.

After examining his case, I thought tyrosine might help Murray. I had just seen a study of lab rats that were placed in water, an immensely stressful situation. Usually, when faced with this threat, rats strike an immobile posture, unable to deal with the problem at hand. Rats administered tyrosine, however, retained mobility and showed actions similar to those stimulated by caffeine and amphetamines. Despite the obvious differences between television executives and rats, Murray was not unlike a rat sunk in water, paralyzed by the pressures he faced at work every day and the negative feedback he received from his wife and colleagues.

Murray also had several of the markers I determine to monitor chronic fatigue syndrome. Tests showed that he had low levels of natural killer cells, which usually roam the body looking to obliterate cancer or viruses wherever they lurk. This is a common finding in chronic fatigue syndrome. Tyrosine is an excellent way to energize and revitalize anyone suffering this exhausting disorder. I put Murray on 3 grams of tyrosine daily, plus coenzyme Q_{10} to improve his energy and ginkgo to enhance circulation to the brain. I also gave him licorice extract, which has been shown to help in chronic fatigue syndrome patients. It raises blood pressure and seems to function much as the body's natural cortisone does. Finally, I prescribed a calming herb, valerian root, for insomnia. Now Murray's state of health is much improved. Of course, the stressors that led to his chronic fatigue and depression are still present in his life, and he is still resisting psychotherapy. We are talking instead about biofeedback and meditation techniques to help him deal with his stress.

Concentration Improves with Tyrosine

A pharmacist's job may seem fairly simple: take someone's prescription and give the customer their medicine. But in truth, pharmacists need to constantly monitor prescriptions and customers and inform them of potentially dangerous side effects and interactions. Robert Enrico, a forty-four-year-old pharmacist, used to be able to remember a customer's medication as soon as he or she walked in the door. He was well-known and loved in his neighborhood for his diligence and care. Yet lately his mind had been wandering as he stood at the counter filling bottle after bottle with pink, blue, and white pills. On several occasions he caught himself filling a few prescriptions incorrectly, leading to irate customers and physicians, and one near overdose. He began to double- and triple-check himself, and his resulting slowness drove customers away.

"These are friends, family, people I've known for ages," he told me sadly. "But now they want to take their business elsewhere."

Robert also noticed that he was increasingly fatigued throughout the day and having trouble sleeping at night. When I conducted tests for any underlying medical problems, such as thyroid disease or diabetes, I found out that he had elevated triglycerides, which are dangerous fats associated with high cholesterol. When I confronted Robert with these results, he confessed that his diet was unhealthy—every lunch hour he ordered a greasy burger and doughnut from the diner next door, and every night he ate ice cream while he watched *The Late Show*. We eliminated all junk food from his daily routine, substituting healthy snacks like dried fruit for the honey-dipped doughnuts he loved so much, whole grain carbohydrates in place of pasta and white bread, and leafy green and colorful vegetables at least twice a day. He switched to tuna sandwiches instead of hamburgers and fresh fruit salads with low-fat frozen yogurt instead of ice cream.

Finally, I gave him 1 gram of tyrosine three times a day to improve his concentration. At first, Robert was skeptical of this natural remedy. He did lose twelve pounds from his dietary changes in about four months, and his acne began to clear up. I noted that his triglyceride levels had improved, but he was still forgetful and distractible. After moving his dosage of tyrosine up to 2 grams before each meal, however, Robert began to see clear changes in his mental capacities. He informed me that he was sleeping better, but, most important, he was able to be very attentive and focused in the tasks he needed to perform quickly at work.

WHAT YOU SHOULD KNOW BEFORE USING TYROSINE

Although tyrosine can be a great way to promote concentration under stress, it should not be used as a permanent part of your diet. This is especially true if you have any kind of kidney disease or reduced kidney function, since concentrated amino acids can be stressful to the kidneys. In addition, tyrosine, as the precursor to norepinephrine, can boost levels of this neurotransmitter when they are low due to stress. Once your levels return to normal, however, excess norepinephrine may elevate your blood pressure. Use the nutrient as support for times in life when you feel like you're truly buckling under pressure, but only as a personal 911 number to be used only when necessary. If you have been diagnosed with chronic fatigue syndrome, chances are that your blood pressure is consequently low, and tyrosine use for lengthier periods is safe. Tyrosine should be used cautiously in patients suffering anxiety. It is best taken before meals and should not be taken before bedtime.

A 1992 study on tyrosine showed that sustained work periods involving the loss of sleep led to stress, mood deterioration, and performance deficits. Norepinephrine also decreased in periods of extended wakefulness and sleep. A follow-up study found that individuals on tyrosine significantly improved their performance and reduced something called lapse probability. Lapse probability indicates the amount of time between repeated tasks, such as loading shells in the military. This landmark study shows that in times of stress, which often leads to insomnia or less available sleep time, tyrosine improves our reasoning as well as the ability to complete tedious tasks quickly and efficiently. I told Debra to take 500 milligrams of tyrosine three times daily, before meals. Not only was Debra able to concentrate better on her track drills, she could read her science textbooks for chapters at a time without getting distracted by the phone or her friends. She enters medical school in the fall.

Resilience Is the Key to Health

Any number of situations have the ability to create stress: bereavement, a new job, unemployment, a new relationship, a rocky relationship, illness, withdrawal from drugs, school, work. Our health depends on our return to a calm, steady state of "normal," so that we can recover and cope normally with any pressures that come our way. As stresses increase in life, it is crucial to learn to adapt to these situations. Ultimately, as Hans Selye so brilliantly put it, it's our resilience in the face of stress that determines whether we will be strong enough to live—and thrive—through these pressures. That resilience is both mental and physical, and what is unique about tyrosine is that it boosts both energy and mood. It works on both levels at once. The mind and the body are profoundly connected, and where stress is concerned, tyrosine sits at the crossroads between the two, sending help in both directions.

Considering the incredible popularity of antidepressants like Prozac, which help many people face life's challenges with greater equanimity, I'm surprised tyrosine is not more widely known. I believe it's a safe alternative to drugs in many cases. It's when stress leads to fatigue rather than anxiety that tyrosine works best.

HOW MUCH SHOULD I TAKE?

For General Health
500 mg/day (optional) twenty minutes before meals

Special Conditions

Depression	500-2,000 mg/day
Stress/Cognitive functioning	500-1,000 mg/day
Fatigue (including CFS)	500-2,000 mg/day
Memory, mood, poor concentration	500-3,000 mg/day

Note of Caution
If you are currently taking an antidepressant, do not take tyrosine unless your physician specifically instructs you to do so.

16

Lutein: Sight for Sore Eyes (and Zeaxanthin) Vision and Eye Health

Virginia Hartman was sixty-seven years old when the world began closing in on her. Like most people, Virginia took the clarity of her good vision for granted. Over the past two or three years, however, she had begun to notice that the TV reception wasn't as sharp as it once was and that in the noonday sun, objects in her kitchen looked a little fuzzy around the edges. She understood the problem was not the TV or the sun but her own eyes. Virginia wondered, "Am I going blind?"

According to the National Institutes of Health, eye problems are the most feared medical diagnosis. Macular degeneration, a process that obstructs vision by initially damaging fragile capillaries in the eyes, is the leading cause of irreversible central (though not total) blindness among Americans over age fifty. Over 13 million adults currently suffer from age-related macular degeneration (AMD); up to 37 percent of people over the age of seventy-five have some form of AMD, and by the age of eighty, 25 percent of all Americans will have lost eyesight due to this disease. One type of AMD occurs when the tiny vessels in the back of eye are weakened, allowing blood to seep out and leaving the eye defenseless to damage from the sun's powerful rays. This can cause a dark spot that blocks—or blurry lines that distort—anything in your field of vision. Legal blindness from AMD can sometimes take its toll in mere weeks. And AMD isn't the only threat to aging eyes. Glaucoma, which is the most common cause of blindness in all age groups, affects the optic nerve and usually remains undetected until a significant amount of vision has been lost. Cataracts, too, are quite common, afflicting two-thirds of individuals over age seventy with the inability to focus. Although vision problems are pervasive in the elderly, over one-third of the 10 million diabetic Americans also suffer from some form of eye disease.

Unfortunately, even in this age of medical progress, there are no cures for eye disease and resulting blindness. Cataract operations and laser surgery, for example, benefit only a minority of patients, and although they can delay vision loss, they cannot prevent it. Indeed, there was little hope for aging eyes—until now. Luckily, we now know that risk of eye disease can be reduced by controlling one simple factor in our lives: nutrition. New medical research indicates that specific antioxidants can lower the risk of eye disease and prevent macular degeneration, cataracts, and glaucoma from occurring. These antioxidants include vitamin E, vitamin C, and an amino acid called taurine. But the most important defenders of the eye are a class of compounds called the carotenoids, which include beta-carotene and most notably a versatile and potent nutrient known as lutein.

Concentrated in the retina as well as present in fruits and vegetables, lutein appears to prevent the risk of macular degeneration and other eye illnesses by protecting the fragile back of the eye from harmful blue light. Lutein, as it turned out, was Virginia Hartman's savior. She was diagnosed with macular degeneration, and her doctor said that at some point it might be necessary to use laser surgery. Virginia was afraid of such a painful-sounding procedure and worried that it might destroy her eyes rather than heal them. After reading about lutein and its protective powers, Virginia called my office to make an appointment and find out more about this carotenoid. As I listened to her story, it became clear that she was a prime candidate for lutein, as she was in the early stages of macular degeneration—but we'd have to act quickly, before she lost more of her vision. Although lutein has been shown to reverse mild blurriness and overall eyesight (not to mention its preventive effects), there is currently no way to cure complete blindness. Because Virginia's eyes were already showing signs of disease—the blurriness—I put her on a comprehensive program of eye-friendly antioxidants. I prescribed 200 milligrams of another antioxidant, zeaxanthin (lutein's buddy, also found in the retina) once a day. But the cornerstone of her anti-AMD regimen was lutein, at a healthy dose of 20 mgs gram per day, to be taken as an oral supplement.

At first, Virginia was frustrated. A few weeks passed, and she noticed no difference in her eyesight. When she woke each morning, she kept her eyes tightly shut for a moment, hoping that when she opened her lids, she would see a clear, sharply defined world. But the objects around her continued to blur. After a few months, however, Virginia began to accept her fate—and that's when things changed. She opened her eyes one morning, looked into her husband's face, and the ever-present dark smudge in the center of her visual field was smaller. Even better, her sight was much clearer than it had been in months. Virginia decided to stay on her antioxidant program, and although the blurring never completely disappeared from her line of vision, and her eyesight was never as sharp as when she was young, there was no doubt in my mind—or in hers—that her condition had not only stabilized but gotten considerably better. Lutein reopened the world for Virginia by restoring the gift of sight.

The Quiet Carotenoid

Virginia's condition improved with her course of nutrients; however, had she begun taking lutein years earlier, she might not have lost any vision at all. Lutein isn't just for the old and ill; in the youngest and healthiest individuals, it can prevent life-altering blindness and keep the eyes strong and clear. A growing body of research suggests that regular consumption of nutrients called carotenoids can boost your overall vision, slow the deterioration caused by AMD, and, most important, prevent the onset of disease.

Carotenoids are a group of antioxidants found in concentrated quantities in fruits and vegetables; in fact, they provide the pigments that color our produce. There are two major classes of carotenoids: the carotenes, including beta-carotene, and the xanthophiles, which include lutein and a similar compound called zeaxanthin. While beta-carotene, responsible for the yellow and orange of foods like squash and carrots, is the most famed carotenoid, it is virtually absent in the eye. This is where lutein and zeaxanthin enter the picture.

Age-related macular degeneration occurs when cells break down in the macula, a yellow spot at the center of the retina that is responsible for our clear, central, or focused vision. This breakdown process slowly and progressively destroys sight in the center of the field of vision, although it does not affect peripheral vision. Lutein and zeaxanthin work by accumulating in the macula and screening out harmful blue light that can damage the back of the eye (unlike ultraviolet light, which can also damage the eye, blue light is part of the visible spectrum, known as the short wave). They accomplish this by giving the macula its yellow pigment. Although xanthophiles are found primarily in leafy and green vegetables, especially kale, spinach, peas, lettuce, and broccoli, they are actually yellow and orange in color, a fact hidden behind the chlorophyll that gives these veggies their rich, dark hue. By pigmenting the macula, lutein and zeaxanthin act like sunglasses, filtering out destructive rays from the daily onslaught of light waves. They also fight free radicals that threaten to impair our vision.

It may seem too simple that eye diseases with no known scientific cure could be prevented so easily, but it turns out Mom was right: you should eat your vegetables. Research indicates that eating leafy greens packed with lutein and zeaxanthin can ensure clear sight for most of us as long as we live. A groundbreaking 1994 study in the *Journal of the American Medical Association* analyzed the dietary patterns of 356 case subjects aged fifty-five to eighty who had been diagnosed with advanced AMD during the year prior to enrollment in the study and 520 control subjects. They concluded that those with the highest dietary intake of carotenoids had a 43 percent lower risk for AMD compared with those who had the lowest intake. Lutein and zeaxanthin, which are primarily obtained from dark green, leafy vegetables, were most strongly associated with a reduced risk for AMD. In particular, a higher frequency of intake of spinach or collard greens was associated with a substantially lower risk for AMD.

Although these carotenoids are best known for their effectiveness in combating AMD, they are also devoted disease fighters in other parts of the body.

- A study by researchers at the University of Michigan showed that there was a correlation between high lutein levels and a high number of estrogen receptors (ER) in the female breast. ER-positive breast cancer is associated with improved survival since more treatment sites are available to treat this disease.

- In the Fiji Islands, lung cancer is considerably lower than in the United States despite a comparable rate of smoking; a 1995 study found that lutein consumption in these islands—where residents ingest 18-23 milligrams a day—was strongly correlated with lower lung cancer rates.

- Finally, research shows that antioxidant carotenoids, especially lutein, may prevent coronary heart disease. A study from Cambridge University, comparing carotenoid intake in Toulouse, France, and Belfast, Ireland, showed that the French subjects had twice the level of lutein as the Irish, and the French subjects had less plaque clogging their arteries than the Irish. Nutritional supplements allow us to prevent disease before it has a chance to start. Consuming lutein in both supplements and produce can help us see our way to a healthy old age.

Lutein should be part of an eye-healthy antioxidant program. We can increase our daily intake by eating foods such as kale, spinach, broccoli, and brussels sprouts. A portion of kale or spinach will supply you with your daily requirement; otherwise, a lutein supplement of at least 5 milligrams a day will help you protect your eyes.

MURIEL'S EYES

Scientists and doctors alike will tell you that there is no cure for AMD. Muriel Ganz knew nothing about medicine, but she can now tell you that while there's no definitive cure for AMD, there's at least a way to slow it down. A seventy-five-year-old widow, Muriel was a popular debutante and Southern belle who had once ruled the state of Georgia as Magnolia Queen a record three years in a row. Blonde and brainy, Muriel enjoyed her hometown fame but was far more concerned with photography. Forced to study it as a high school elective, she became smitten with the art, clutching a box camera wherever she went. This love affair developed into a lifelong career. Muriel was one of the few successful female photojournalists of her time, and the evidence of her talent was framed on the walls of her cozy home in Connecticut.

But over time, as Muriel married, raised children, survived the death of her husband, and grew increasingly fragile, picture-taking became less an active pursuit than a fond memory. Now she was content to stitch needlepoint and play with her grandchildren. Still, because vision—both physical and mental—had been the fuel for her artistic passion, Muriel was perhaps more anxious than most when she noticed one day that her sight was not what it used to be.

Muriel's complaints of blurry vision led to a diagnosis of macular degeneration. She refused to accept the diagnosis or the doctor's grim prognosis. Muriel made an appointment at my office to see if any other course of treatment would be helpful. Ophthalmologists use an Amsler grid, an effective way to check for AMD. The grid is black with horizontal and vertical white lines across it, like graph paper. To test for AMD, you close one eye and stare at the grid with the other. The lines on the paper are continuous, but if they appear wavy, then there's a good chance that you have macular degeneration. Another hallmark of the disease is having holes in your vision; if pieces of the grid are missing when you look at it, AMD might be causing it. Sure enough, Muriel saw three lines on the grid as wavy where they should have been straight, which convinced me that she did have AMD. However, since Muriel still viewed the entire grid intact, I knew that her condition was not terribly advanced. While Muriel was facing other major age-related problems such as osteoporosis and elevated cholesterol, her biggest worry was the loss of her sight. In order to halt the free radical damage to her macula and prevent further degeneration, I prescribed her supplements of B vitamins, taurine, and essential fatty acids. The crux of her anti-AMD program, however, was a daily dose of both lutein and zeaxanthin.

Eager to restore her sight, Muriel consented to my provision regimen. Initially, however, she was extremely upset because the treatment didn't seem to be working.

When it comes to an area as complex as the eye, I told her, healing takes time; we couldn't expect to undo years of damage in a few days. Worried, but knowing she had little other recourse, she continued to submit to treatment. One day, while walking up the stairs of her home, gazing at the black-and-white photos hanging there and lamenting the loss of her sight, Muriel realized that the pictures looked sharper than they had in years. She went to her eye doctor to confirm that her vision was truly improving after months of natural treatment.

"You aren't just seeing things," he told her, amazed. "There's a definite improvement in your vision. Whatever you've been doing, keep doing it."

What she'd been doing, of course, was taking lutein and zeaxanthin to shield her eyes from harmful light rays. Not only did the carotenoids seem to protect her from further macular damage, they appeared to reverse degeneration. That finding was remarkable enough, but two months later, Muriel noticed even further improvement. Details of objects popped out like never before; edges were more defined than ever. Inspired by her renewed sight and the almost forgotten clarity of life around her, Muriel dusted off her camera and set out to capture her new vision on film once more.

The conventional wisdom is that macular degeneration is irreversible, but Muriel's case shows that this simply is not true. With the aid of lutein and zeaxanthin, the body can help heal and even reverse age-related vision loss.

The Miraculous Eye

The human eye is a marvel of structure and function. Inside its tiny orb lie numerous complex layers that allow us to perceive the vast world around us in incredible focus and detail. Our eyeballs are protected by a tough outer casing called the sclera, which covers the inner structures and maintains the rigid form of the eye. As the sclera approaches the front surface of the eye, it becomes thinner and transparent and is called the cornea, which allows light to enter the eye. Behind the cornea sits the lens, a clear ball held in place by flexible ligaments that focus light to the back of the eye, and the iris, which dictates eye color and uses muscles to control the amount of light let into the eye by constricting or dilating the opening called the pupil.

Lying just inside the sclera is the choroid, a sheet containing blood vessels that nourish the other structures of the eye. The choroid is filled with black pigment to absorb excess light entering the eye. Lining the posterior two-thirds of the choroid is the retina. All light that enters the eye is directed back to the retina, which is composed of neural tissue containing light-sensitive receptor cells. Light passes through the cornea and lens, which is then refracted back to the retina where it forms an image. The retina is divided into two types of photoreceptor cells, both named for their shape: rods, which handle general light detection and motion, and cones, which allow us to see color and have high visual acuity. The human eye contains an estimated 125 million rods, most of which are concentrated at the corners of the eye. Cones, on the other hand, are most abundant in the fovea, a small indentation in the middle of the macula that is the area of sharpest vision in the eye. The approximately 6.5 million cones in each of our eyes have red, blue, and yellow pigment, which allow us to see the world in glorious technicolor. Incoming light is perceived by rods and cones as either present or absent, and the pattern of light that is picked up by these receptors is sent to the brain by neurons that, together, unite to form the optic nerve. The area at the back of the eye where the optic nerve passes out of the eyeball to the visual areas of the brain's cerebral cortex forms our "blind spot," where there are no rods and cones to pick up images.

Sitting in the center of the retina, the macula is about the size of a pencil eraser and is one hundred times more sensitive to small-scale images than the rest of the retina. This tiny structure is responsible for our acute vision. The depression in the center of the macula called the fovea contains only cones and lacks blood vessels. Without this, we could not differentiate between a friend's face and that of a stranger; we could not negotiate the distance needed to climb a simple flight of stairs; and although we could get a general sense of what was happening around us, we would miss the objects right in front of our noses. People with macular degeneration don't become completely blind, since their peripheral vision remains unaffected. Still, the disease unarguably compromises one's quality of life. As macular damage builds and central vision fades, the world before our eyes begins to dissolve into an indistinct blur.

Tax-time Blues

Arthur Shipley, a sixty-year-old bachelor, knew how incomprehensible everyday life could become when macular degeneration took hold. Unfortunately, other people depended on him to simplify their lives. He was an accountant, and his clients expected him to decipher the bewildering financial jargon of decimal points and bank account balances for them so they could sleep easy at night. Around tax time, in particular, Arthur became a veritable patron saint of number crunching. Usually, maintaining people's finances and tax returns were no problem for this math whiz. This year, though, tax time was giving Arthur a big headache. The myriad forms that he normally handled with ease seemed harder to read than usual; the words and numbers on each page were blurry. At first, Arthur thought he needed new glasses. His ophthalmologist confirmed that he needed new lenses, so he picked out some snazzy new frames to go with his new prescription. Much to his dismay, Arthur realized that the glasses did nothing to improve his foggy vision. Perplexed, he wondered whether the monotony of repeatedly calculating figures on forms all day might not be causing eye fatigue. Once again, he visited his ophthalmologist, who finally realized that the problem at hand might be macular degeneration. An Amsler grid test further confirmed this diagnosis.

Understandably, Arthur was extremely concerned about the effects that macular degeneration might have on his life. His job meant everything to him, and he was still in the prime of a very successful career. Skeptical of his ophthalmologist, who had failed to initially diagnose his condition, he also felt helpless in the face of an untreatable disease. Arthur heard my radio show one Friday morning and decided to call in, in the hopes that my natural approach to medicine had something to offer him.

"What have I done to deserve this?" he groaned over the phone. "No eyesight, and my work goes down the tubes."

"Well," I asked, "how old are you? Do you smoke? Do you have some form of heart disease?"

"I'm in my sixties, but I've never had a problem with my ticker in my whole life," he boasted. "I'm as healthy as a fellow half my age. As for smoking, I do smoke two packs a day, which I admit isn't the healthiest move. But it's my only vice."

"That vice could be the downfall of your eyes," I told Arthur.

While age is the main risk factor for AMD—and Arthur was getting up there in years—smoking is another major risk factor. A 1996 study in the *Journal of the American Medical Association* showed that people who smoke more than one pack of cigarettes a day have an incidence of AMD more than twice that of nonsmokers, and this risk remains high even up to fifteen years after quitting the habit. Smoking tends to deplete the protective antioxidants in the eye, while creating dangerous free radicals.

"What can I do to get rid of this disease? Or is it too late?" he asked.

I suggested that Arthur visit my office so that we could discuss treatment options. He came in that very afternoon. First, I told him, he would have to quit smoking to reduce the free radicals that cigarettes were spewing into him. Most important, though, he'd have to take 1 gram each of lutein and zeaxanthin supplements daily, along with vitamin C, selenium, and zinc, to boost the level of antioxidants in his eyes. Arthur vowed that he would try to stop smoking. Within six months, his vision was less blurry, and he was better able to concentrate on his accounting duties. He visited his ophthalmologist who urged him to continue whatever treatment had caused such an improvement. True, Arthur's sight never completely returned to normal. He was unable to quit smoking, and the damage that his eyes had suffered over the years was too great to completely overcome. Overall, however, his eyesight became notably better due to consistent nutritional therapy. He is now happily back to work, ready to tackle tax time with a vengeance.

How Macular Degeneration Affects You

There are two types of age-related macular degeneration: dry and wet. Dry AMD is the less severe of the two and accounts for 90 percent of all cases. In dry AMD, yellowish spots called drusen begin to accumulate below the macula, breaking down its light-sensing cells and causing distorted vision. If dry AMD advances far enough, it can become wet AMD, so named because it arises when tiny abnormal vessels begin to grow behind the retina toward the macula. These vessels can leak blood and fluid that damage the macula, not to mention the scar tissue from burst vessels or vision blockage from new vessels that may occur. Seeping fluid leads to rapid and severe vision loss. Wet AMD almost always takes place in people who have already suffered dry AMD and usually results in legal blindness. Legal blindness is defined as visual acuity less than 20/200 or visual field restriction to 20 percent or less.

Macular degeneration is probably caused by oxidative damage and poor circulation in the macula. Studies in animals demonstrate that the visible light entering our eyes each day, especially ultraviolet light, can lead to extreme free radical damage. Light, of course, is essential to the health of the eye. Without it, not only would we see nothing, but our retinas would shrink. Light also stimulates the production of certain hormones (although its absence does the same to other hormones; melatonin, a sleep hormone, is secreted only when we're in the dark). Unfortunately, the ultraviolet component of all visible light coming from the sun can also hurt us with free radical damage, producing cataracts, macular degeneration, and even cancer with its free radicals. The fatty outer layer of the macula is particularly vulnerable to oxidative damage from the sun, which is why this area is the most common locus of degeneration. Although the retina and the macula are packed with carotenoids, especially lutein and zeaxanthin, to fend off harmful free radicals, the outer edge of the macula is less protected by these antioxidants than the rest of the eye. In sum, the more we shield our eyes from excess sunlight and the more we boost our intake of sight-saving carotenoids like lutein and zeaxanthin, the better we'll be able to preserve the macula—and our vision—for a lifetime.

When Eye Problems Strike the Young

The last person you'd expect to fall victim to blindness was a hip, healthy young man in his early thirties. Simon James, at age thirty-one, was already the executive editor of an upstart political magazine. The son of two influential parents, both editors, Simon was witty and urbane and was riding an early wave of success that surprised nobody who knew him. His sheer satisfaction in his life and luck was clearly evident. He had the respect and envy of his publishing peers.

Only one part of his life worried him: his eyes. Simon had worn glasses as a child and then later switched to contacts as an appearance-conscious teen, but his eyesight had never been a cause of concern. Soon after he'd been named head of his magazine, however, he noticed a blurring of his vision. At first, Simon hoped that this fuzziness was merely the result of long days before the computer screen and late nights partying. But as the days passed and his eyesight grew worse, Simon felt afraid for the first time in his life. The master wit, who'd always been praised for his sharp mind and biting humor, faced his first serious problem. Now he lay awake at night wondering what would happen if he went blind. He couldn't imagine any other life but that of an editor.

Simon soon consulted one of the best ophthalmologists in Manhattan, who confirmed that the young man's eyes were ailing. Simon was suffering from a rare condition of the macula involving a thick rapid overgrowth of blood vessels obscuring the eye. Eventually, said the doctor, his vision would progressively deteriorate until the blood vessels would completely obliterate his central eyesight—a process that would occur over the next twelve to twenty-four months. There was no scientific cure for this disease, and the only therapeutic option, laser surgery, would zap the blinding blood vessels but in the process would nearly obliterate his sight.

Simon was absolutely devastated. He took time off work. When he came back to the office, he paced aimlessly. Finally, a colleague, hearing his tale, recommended me as a possible source of information and treatment. He immediately called me, hailed a taxi, and came up to my office an hour later.

This was clearly a devastating blow to someone so young. I knew that I would have to work quickly, and I began with a two-pronged approach. First, in order to reduce the free radical damage to his delicate eyes, I knew that lutein would be crucial to protect the macula as well as possible, and I prescribed him 1 gram of this carotenoid twice a day. I also advised him to pack his diet with fruits and vegetables high in lutein, like spinach, kale, and other leafy greens. Second, I asked him to take a slew of star antioxidants, including taurine, zinc, and vitamins C and E, as well as shark cartilage, which can slow angiogenesis (growth of blood vessels). Simon went home with a care package of nutrients, but without much hope. He truly believed the grim prognosis and was trying to prepare himself emotionally for surgery and loss of his sight.

I hoped that Simon's sight would improve, or that the process might at least be slowed and even halted. I never expected that it would completely reverse itself.

Simon continued to see his original ophthalmologist, who could most accurately detect progress. After two months, the doctor noted clear signs of improvement, though Simon could barely detect any difference in his eyesight. But over the next few months, his vision started to improve rapidly, and his eyes simply healed themselves.

When we are young, the body, given the right chance and nutrients, can actually heal itself completely. Simon continues to take his natural treatments, and, miraculous as it may seem, his eyesight is back—for good.

Foresight for Future Sight

Lutein can heal other eye problems as well. Cataracts, which can cause severe visual distortion and blindness, can also be prevented with these power carotenoids. Alice Winters was smart enough to use this knowledge, plus an understanding of her family's health history, to her advantage. Alice was a divorced mother of three boys and a high school English teacher. She loved to travel, and on her summer vacations she would pack up the family van and drive all over the country with her sons, stopping to see the sights and learn the history of cities from Bangor, Maine, to Sedona, Arizona. Although raising three children and teaching a rigorous schedule on a small salary was stressful and demanding, Alice was in excellent health. She was worried, however, that her luck would soon run out. The Winters family had a strong history of cataracts, and practically every member had developed the eye condition by the age of sixty. At the age of fifty-five, Alice was concerned about the fate of her eyes.

Cataracts involve the clouding of the lens and are believed to be caused by excess sun exposure, poor nutrition, and free radical damage. The cells in our lenses are built for life; they cannot be regenerated and therefore must last a lifetime. As the lens faces the onslaught of light and oxidation, it thickens, causing foggy vision and the inability to focus on objects, making life very difficult for sufferers.

Alice was particularly fearful of cataracts because of the experience her mother had had with the condition and her subsequent cataract surgery. Although this procedure is extremely common and usually goes without a hitch, Alice's mother experienced a complication in which her lens was not placed in her eye properly, leaving it blurry for life. Alice's fear of losing her vision either from cataracts or from surgery to treat cataracts was so great that she was inspired to try to prevent the disease any way she could. Diabetes also ran in Alice's family, putting her at particular risk for cataracts. Because she knew that the cornerstone of a nutritional approach like mine is prevention of future illness, she came to me for a program designed to ward off her family's cataract curse.

In order to maintain the health of her lenses, I knew that a diverse but comprehensive program of foods and supplements would be the best course of action. I prescribed nutrients such as cranberry and bilberry, which were given to British pilots in World War II to sharpen their night vision. Selenium is another supplement that would be instrumental in keeping cataracts away. Selenium prevents the binding of sugar to proteins in the eye, which produces lens-clouding protein disulfides. But the most important part of Alice's preventive program were carotenoids and antioxidants taken both in supplements and in food. In 1991 the *American Journal of Clinical Nutrition* reported a study of seventy-seven people showing that those who took vitamin C, vitamin E, and carotenoids displayed a lower incidence of cataracts. Another study tracked a group of fifty thousand nurses for eight years and discovered that total carotenoid intake was inversely associated with risk of cataracts. Therefore, not only did I suggest that Alice take 20 mg of lutein and zeaxanthin a day, but I told her to pack her diet with antioxidant- and carotenoid-rich fruits and vegetables like spinach, kale, peas, broccoli, green beans, and corn. (I prefer this, in most cases, to carotene supplements, because we are not certain of the impact of an isolated carotene such as beta-carotene on health. There are over five hundred carotenoids in fruits and vegetables, and it's best we get a sampling of them all.)

In the five years since Alice first visited my office, she has developed adult-onset diabetes, but she has not as yet displayed any sign of cataracts. Certainly, it's true that she may yet get cataracts, or that she may never have been destined to get them, despite her family history. But research does indicate that certain supplements and foods can protect the eyes from free radical damage, making it entirely possible that her prevention regimen kept her eyes free and clear of danger. We will continue to monitor her eyes as the years go by. For now, her diabetes is under control. She is watching her diet and taking her supplements.

Keeping Your Eyes Open to Good Health

Longevity is a primary concern in my practice. The best way to maximize the benefits that nutritional therapies and dietary supplements have to offer is by using them to prevent the diseases that attack as our bodies decline with age. I found it extremely wise that Alice Winters came to me to maintain her good health instead of trying to find a quick fix for her ailing health in the future, especially when she knew her family history put her in danger of cataracts. Many people overlook the importance of stopping disease before it starts, and any illness that impedes eyesight puts us in extreme jeopardy as we get older. With age, it becomes more and more difficult for us to maneuver our bodies and maintain our balance, and eyesight becomes an increasingly important tool for helping us make it through the world. What strikes me about eye problems like cataracts, glaucoma, and macular degeneration is that while all are genetically linked, the common denominators are free radical damage due to excess sunlight and poor nutrition that leaves us defenseless against free radical oxidation. If you spend a great deal of time outdoors, sunglasses that filter ultraviolet light can be helpful.

ARE YOU AT RISK FOR AGE-RELATED MACULAR DEGENERATION?

If you meet any of the following risk factors for AMD, you should look into preventive treatment to protect your eyes.

Age: The main risk factor for AMD. In the United States, an estimated 14 percent of people between the ages of fifty-five and sixty-four have this disease, increasing as we get older.

Diet: Because the fragile cells of the macula are extremely vulnerable to free radical damage, it is important to stay away from saturated fats and cholesterol, which are particularly instrumental in facilitating free radical reactions. Alcohol can deprive the body of protective antioxidants. By eating a varied diet of fruits and vegetables, you can ensure that your eyes have the antioxidants they need to counteract the threat of free radical damage.

Sunlight: The very light that allows us to see can also take that ability away. The ultraviolet component of light is especially harmful to the macula, causing excessive free radical damage. Wearing sunglasses or taking care to shield your eyes from constant sunlight will reduce the deterioration of the macula.

Smoking: Smoking reduces the amount of free radical-fighting antioxidants in the eye, more than doubling the risk of AMD.

Heredity: Several studies show that AMD may be inherited. If any of your immediate relatives have the disease, it might be in your best interests to focus on preventing it in your own eyes.

Gender and Race: Caucasians are much more likely than African Americans to lose vision from AMD. Women over seventy-five have twice the risk of developing AMD as men the same age.

Eye Color: Individuals with light-colored eyes (blue or green, for example) have much higher risk for AMD than those with darker eyes.

Heart Disease: Good eyesight depends in part on proper blood flow through the eyes. High blood pressure or other forms of heart disease can increase your likelihood of getting AMD because they usually mean poor circulation to the eyes.

But remember, the eye, like the rest of the body, does need some sunlight to remain healthy.

By taking a full complement of supplements including vitamins C, E, and A, selenium, zinc, taurine, and antioxidants like lutein and zeaxanthin, not to mention eating a healthful diet filled with leafy greens and juicy fruits, you can keep your eyes alert and strong enough to see you into a beautiful old age. I recommend 5 to 20 milligrams a day of lutein.

HOW MUCH SHOULD I TAKE?

For General Health
Through leafy green vegetables, or 1 mg/day
After meals divided doses
Special Conditions

AMD	20 mg/day
Cataracts/Glaucoma	5-20 mg/day

17

Quercetin: The End of Allergies

The sun bathes the world in golden warmth, the flowers bloom in vibrant reds and violets, the birds sing a sweet song—and you're too busy sneezing and rubbing your itchy eyes to enjoy it. Sound familiar? These are the rites of spring for the over 20 million Americans who suffer allergic rhinitis. Nine percent of all visits to the doctor stem from these sinus, ear, nose, and throat irritations. In my practice, that ratio is even higher. Thankfully, natural remedies are remarkably helpful in banishing allergies for good. Unlike many drugs, which suppress symptoms, natural treatments bring the body into balance as they quench allergic reactions.

If you're under forty, you're especially prone to runny noses and scratchy throats, since the risk of allergy is even higher for this age group (20-25 percent) than for the total population (7 percent). Women are more likely to get allergies than men. Allergies carry a strong genetic link, so your chances of developing them is even greater if your parents have them—30 percent if one parent has allergies; 50 percent if both. If you're prone to asthma or eczema, you probably have allergies.

Allergies can be as wide-ranging as the world itself. Perhaps the most common form is allergic rhinitis, the technical name for the sneezing, coughing, runny nose, watery eyes, and itchiness that many of us experience yearly. The seasonal pollination of trees, grass, and weeds distributing airborne allergens varies little from year to year, causing the predictable return of symptoms at the same time and place annually. While spring, with its freshly mown lawns and free-floating pollen, is usually associated with allergy onset, the early fall is also prime time for allergies, since hay fever season (also known as ragweed season) lasts from August to October. But many allergies aren't seasonal at all, and you don't have to be in the great outdoors to fall victim. Sensitivities to cockroaches, mold, dust, pets, household chemicals, and wood mean that you could stay indoors your whole life and still develop the itchy, scratchy symptoms of allergic rhinitis.

True, there are a panoply of pills and capsules lining drugstore shelves that claim to relieve your allergies. Many of these medications, however, have irksome and often dangerous side effects. Benadryl, for example, can lead to severe drowsiness. Nasal decongestants and cough suppressants can also cause mental and physical impairment (hence, the warnings on the box against "engaging in use of heavy machinery" while under the influence of these drugs). Recently a commonly used antihistamine, Seldane, was pulled off the market after causing 127 cardiovascular "incidents."

Would you rather relieve your allergies with a natural antihistamine and anti-inflammatory agent guaranteed to help you breathe in the fresh springtime air without sneezing—or fall into a drugged stupor? Look no further than the strange-sounding nutraceutical called quercetin, a seemingly innocuous plant pigment proved to clear up your sinuses without clouding your head.

Allergy-Quelling Quercetin

Quercetin belongs to a class of nutrients known as bioflavonoids, compounds better known for the blue and red color they give to plants than for the antioxidant benefits they provide the body. Once merely considered useless plant pigments, flavonoids were originally unearthed by Albert Szent-Gyorgyi, Ph.D., the Nobel Laureate who discovered vitamin C in the 1930s. Szent-Gyorgyi found that flavonoids were able to strengthen capillary walls in a way that the common cold comfort vitamin C could not. Over four thousand flavonoids have since been identified, and they are increasingly being recognized as a crucial key to health and longevity. One of the most frequently discussed flavonoids is a pigment known as proanthocyanidin, found in red wine, and hypothesized to retard heart disease. This substance is thought to be one reason that wine-swilling French citizens manage to eat four times as much butter and lard as we do with significantly less heart disease. Other flavonoids, such as the catechins found in green tea, are not only heart smart but are believed to prevent cancer. Other nutraceuticals mentioned in this book, such as garlic, bilberry, ginkgo, and silymarin, also exert their healthy powers through flavonoids.

Of the many bioflavonoids known to us, quercetin appears to be the one with the highest degree of antiallergy activity, according to a study in the *Journal of Allergy and Clinical Immunology*. Quercetin stops allergies in their tracks via two routes. First, it is a powerful anti-inflammatory, keeping the lungs, nasal passages, and eyes from swelling as they normally do when allergens like pollen come into contact with the body. For this reason, quercetin may also be useful in treating inflammatory conditions such as arthritis and asthma. Second, quercetin is a potent antihistamine that prevents the release of itchy chemicals that make our nose run and our eyes water. Best of all, this natural one-two punch of allergy defense is achieved without the drowsiness or jitters that medication can cause; it is extremely rare for quercetin to cause side effects.

Not only does quercetin provide sweet allergy relief, but it also has been shown to protect the stomach from ulcer disease and gastric distress. Nonsteroidal anti-inflammatory drugs (NSAIDS) such as Advil or Motrinare commonly used to stop headaches, cramping, and fever; but they are actually the current leading cause of gastric bleeding in the United States. A study in the journal *Pharmacology* showed that quercetin protected the gastric mucosa from damage after being exposed to NSAIDS. Quercetin also has been shown to inhibit cell cancer lines and oral tumors and to boost the benefits of chemotherapy treatment for ovarian cancer, as described in the *Journal of Anti-Cancer Drugs*. Yet another study suggests that quercetin might halt the cell proliferation in bone marrow, which could be helpful in treating leukemia. Most people, however, are drawn to quercetin's amazing ability to alleviate allergies, which is its forte, especially when combined with other natural antihistamines and anti-inflammatories like vitamin C, vitamin B_{12}, bromelain (an enzyme), and nettle (a plant).

I recommend using quercetin whenever you would reach for an antihistamine, or when you are about to enter a season that is particularly difficult for you, such as hay fever or pollen season. The initial dose is 300 milligrams twice a day, although I may recommend doses as high as 1 or 2 grams in some severely allergic patients. Short-term use of one to two months is recommended. I generally don't suggest long-term use unless there is a chronic allergy, such as one related to dust mites.

Anatomy of an Allergic Reaction

Many of us have sneezed, scratched, and blown our noses in allergic agony without considering the irritating causes of our distress. There are many symptoms that signal allergy onset: a sore throat, postnasal drip in the back of the throat, swollen nasal passages and membranes, and nasal polyps. Normally, the nose increases the temperature and moisture content of inhaled air and filters out incoming dust particles. A potent system of enzymes and trapping mechanisms removes most airborne allergens, dust, and pollen from the nostrils, but when the mucous membranes of the nose become swollen, allergens have a better chance of penetrating the barrier lining and enhancing nasal hypersensitivity.

An allergic reaction begins when a stimulus, known as an allergen, binds to an immunoglobulin created by our immune system called IgE that is located on mast cells. Allergens can be anything from the seasonal pollen that is disseminated by trees, weeds, and grasses to the dander spread by beloved pets around the house. In response to allergens, the mast cells rapidly release histamines, the pesky compounds that cause the familiar nasal congestion, watery eyes, rash, itchy throat, sneezing, swelling, and inflammation associated with allergies. Depending on where the IgE antigens bind to mast cells, that's where you'll get your symptoms: allergic rhinitis if the cells are in your nose, asthma if they're in your lungs, or hives if they're in your skin. Histamines can also be released from white blood cells called basophils. Mast cells reside in the skin and organs, whereas basophils circulate through the bloodstream. Other substances released by cells in response to this allergen trigger are called leukotrienes, which lead to symptoms similar to those caused by histamines. All contribute to create allergic reactions.

Quercetin is an especially effective allergy fighter because it works in two ways. Unlike drugstore antihistamines, which prevent the binding of IgE and antigens to mast cells, quercetin blocks histamines at the site of release by stabilizing mast cells and basophils and—more important—by inhibiting inflammatory enzymes and decreasing the number of leukotrienes coursing through the body. It also inhibits enzymes like lipooxygenase, which are found in the inflammatory pathways that cause allergy symptoms. Studies in journals like *Progressive Clinical Biology Research* and the *Journal of Allergy and Clinical Immunology* confirm the dual action of quercetin in stopping allergies at the source of the problem.

Onscreen Sniffles

For a TV anchorperson like Kelly Levin, a clear speaking voice and clean breathing are professional necessities. Kelly rarely contracted colds, but she feared her allergies would eventually get her fired. Ever since she was a grade-school student pretending to be Jane Pauley in her bedroom mirror, Kelly had suffered from allergies. This thirty-two-year-old blonde spitfire had always hacked and blown her nose till her throat was raw and several boxes of Kleenex were depleted. Through the years, Kelly had sampled every antihistamine and allergy medication on the market, and had relied on her favorite orange Sudafed liquid-filled capsules to help her through a communications degree, broadcasting internships, and finally a job anchoring the nightly news. Although Kelly's composure, personality, and clear locution on the air helped her to rise through the ranks, behind the scenes there was another story. Every night, before taping the news, Kelly would have sneezing attacks, and during breaks, she would always have tissues nearby, dabbing and blowing her nose before going back onscreen. Somehow, she managed to pull herself together before each news segment, but she was tired of trying to suppress nasal congestion and coughs while on camera. She was also tired of depending on Sudafed and didn't like the light-headed feeling it gave her.

Kelly, who listened to all kinds of news and newscasters to hone her craft, heard my Friday-morning show on a talk radio station on the way to work one morning and immediately called me from her cell phone.

"Allergies," she virtually barked at me when I answered her call. "I've had allergies my whole life and am sick of the runny nose and sneezing and raw nostrils and tissues and drugs. Is there some natural way I can get rid of this once and for all?"

I scheduled her for an appointment the very next day. Although Kelly was vivacious and warm, I could see the toll that allergies were taking on her usual charm and cheer. Allergies may seem a minor annoyance if you've never had them, but over a lifetime they can be bothersome and persistent enough to drag you to the pits of despair.

I performed a laryngoscopy, where a flexible tube is used to peer inside the body, showed that Kelly had polyps, which are clumps of tissue dense with allergen-binding mast cells, lining her nostrils. In order to shrink these, I prescribed her 1 to 2 grams of quercetin daily, plus nettle to boost its antihistamine, anti-inflammatory effects. I also advised that she use a nasal steroid spray called cromolyn. Many people are surprised when I prescribe synthetic medications. "Aren't you the natural health guy?" they ask. "Don't you hate drugs?" The truth is, many drugs can be more harmful than helpful. But there are medications out there that are greatly beneficial in treating medical conditions, and when I find these, I like to use them in conjunction with nutraceuticals to provide the best route to good health. Cromolyn is one example of an exemplary drug. It is synthetic, but it's derived from an ancient Egyptian plant used to treat asthma. Similar to quercetin in structure and function, it blocks histamines from being released and displays few side effects. Using cromolyn and quercetin together further ensures allergy relief.

Like many of my patients, Kelly was anxious to try natural compounds, plants, and vitamins but was skeptical of using a nasal spray, no matter how safe; after all, she had come to see me for an alternative approach. Finally, though, she took my recommendations and went back to work.

A month later, Kelly bounded back into my office with a sparkling smile on her face—the very smile, no doubt, that had landed her promotion after promotion. "I feel great," she enthused. "No more sneezing between takes, no more stuffy nose."

Since she had shown such dramatic progress on a combination of medications and nutrients, I told her that we'd begin to wean her off the medication so that she could maintain her allergy-free state solely with natural supplements. Taking drugs for an extended period of time, no matter how beneficial they are, can be detrimental to the body.

"What drugs?" she asked innocently, avoiding my eyes.

"The nasal spray I asked you to use," I reminded her.

"Well . . . I never took it," she admitted, with a guilty look on her face. "I really didn't want to use drugs. So I thought I'd give the supplements a chance first, and they worked so well!"

I was stunned. As confident as I am in the power of nutritional supplements, even I didn't believe that she could see such results in such a short time without the boost of a steroid. But Kelly took her health into her own hands, willing to wait and see what the effects of natural compounds would be, and she had a terrific response. Kelly is now more confident and lively—on and off screen—than ever before, and she attributes it all to quercetin. Every so often, when she is visiting her summer home—a tree-lined, grassy haven that she rarely frequented when allergens were her nemesis—she sends me a postcard to remind me how allergy-free quercetin has allowed her to be.

Shock Treatment

Bob Maxwell, thirty-eight, desperately needed an effective alternative to the traditional antihistamines, nasal sprays, and allergy shots normally offered to allergy sufferers. A graphic designer, Bob was a victim of chronic sinusitis and rhinitis, and he found that his symptoms would peak in the late summer, when ragweed season terrorizes many with stuffy noses, itchy eyes, and scratchy throats.

Much to his relief, I had an arsenal of allergy-fighting nutrients and techniques at my disposal; as the first part of my allergy control program, however, we'd have to test Bob for any and all allergies that he might have. First, we found that he had spring fever, meaning an allergy related to grasses. He also showed an allergy to wheat, which sometimes cross-reacts with grass and was confirmed by food-tolerance tests. Much to Bob's dismay, we advised him to cut all wheat out of his diet. We also detected allergies to dust mites, as well as ragweed, which would explain his late-summer symptoms. Finally, a laryngoscopy used to evaluate the nasal passages found polyps.

One of the first—and easiest—ways to rid yourself of allergies is to remove or replace anything in your home or office that might exacerbate them. For example, HEPA air filters can control the amount of pollen and pollutants floating around you; new hypoallergenic mattress and pillow covers can minimize exposure to dust mites in the sleeping environment. I also gave Bob an anti-inflammatory aloe wash to flush his nasal passages out every night before bedtime. This treatment shrinks polyps, which can grow during the day in response to environmental allergens. Finally, I prescribed him 1.2 grams of quercetin daily, accompanied by a healthy dose of the herb nettle. While the air filter and aloe wash did wonders for Bob's allergies, he noticed the most startling difference in his health after taking quercetin. Not only did his symptoms lessen within several weeks, but within three months he was able to wean himself off all the numerous nasal inhalers that he had previously used to clear up his nose. Lastly we started him on weekly allergy shots, using extracts of the same substances he was allergic to. This technique is called desentization and is an effective adjunctive therapy. He just kept improving over time. Now, three years later, Bob is breathing freely and is medication free.

The Antiallergy Program

From home to office and in between, allergens are everywhere. Say someone works in an environment with a poor ventilation system. This office may harbor allergenic compounds, rodent or insect hairs, and dust. The workplace may also contain environmental pollutants like formaldehyde. At home, pests and pets might pose a problem. And in the great outdoors, pollutants from cars, buses, and factories saturate our air. This often makes it difficult for me to decipher the root of allergies. There are even some cases where there is no distinguishable cause for allergic symptoms, just a particular combination of irritants in the environment. Foods can also cause the sneezing, runny nose, and watery eyes that seem like allergic rhinitis, though not as commonly. And there are many foods that share similar compounds with common allergens. For instance, wheat and grass can both cause a kind of cross-reaction. So can, oddly enough, bananas and latex.

Because of the large number of allergens surrounding us at every turn, one of the best allergy treatments that I can recommend—in addition to supplements—is avoidance. In a word, simply avoid any animal, object, or area that you think might be causing or instigating your allergies. If you're allergic to pets, for example, giving away your cat or refraining from adopting that adorable dog at the pound will relieve your symptoms. However, what pet owner finds that easy—or even possible? In such cases, HEPA air filters are a great way to purify both the work and home environments. A good HEPA air filter can run $300-400 with smaller units units running about half, but it's well worth the expense in most cases. There are also special shampoos for cats and dogs to control dander. Molds can grow insidiously in dark, wet areas in the home, and you should seek to eliminate them whenever possible. Your physician can test for them with mold plates to place in your home. Allergy-proofing your home with cotton blankets, sheets, and pillow cases as well as perfume-free detergents can also reduce your symptoms. Carpets can hide dust, mites, and dander that can instigate allergy symptoms. Removing carpets, if at all possible, can make a big difference. (For more information on allergies and allergy-proofing your home environment see my book *Reversing Asthma*.)

As part of an overall approach to treating allergies, I try to eliminate the unhealthy habits that many of my patients initially come with, such as high alcohol intake, smoking, poor diet, and lack of exercise. I also encourage them to seek stress reduction by taking up yoga or meditation. An unhealthy lifestyle can make almost anyone vulnerable to allergies and is a particular burden for people who are physically prone to them. Avoiding foods containing MSG, additives, preservatives, dyes, sulfites, stabilizers, guar gum, and colorings will also help you relieve your allergy symptoms. Switching from a meat-heavy diet to one chock full of vegetables and fruits for cleansing the liver will also help, as will increasing your consumption of omega-3 fatty acids through fish and flaxseed oil to control inflammation. The more pure your diet, the better you'll feel.

Smoke Gets in Your Eyes

As the manager of her family's raucous Irish pub in midtown Manhattan, twenty-eight-year-old Molly Tracey was as far removed from a pure diet and environment as she could get. Although smoking is strictly prohibited in restaurants, the patrons of O'Shaughnessy's couldn't have cared less; to them, a pub wasn't a pub without Guinness and clouds of smoke, and Molly's family was happy to oblige. Peddling ale and waitressing, surrounded by cigarette fumes and snacking on greasy Buffalo wings and nachos all day and night, Molly would arrive home at one o'clock in the morning, ready for bed. The next day, however, she'd feel completely awful. Her throat would be sore, her nose congested, her eyes tearing.

When Molly's mother, Rose, who was a faithful patient of mine, described her daughter's symptoms to me, I figured that the carcinogenic smoke and fatty foods at work were her main health concerns. But it turned out that her home was no allergy haven, either. Rose informed me that Molly's home was filled with magazines and books, not to mention a fluffy fat cat named Princess. I realized that even when Molly came home from her polluted work environment, she was being assaulted by two potent allergens—dust and pet dander.

Upon administering allergy and skin tests, I found that Molly was allergic to her cat, her dusty home library, and the bar's ubiquitous cigarette smoke.

"But what can I do?" she asked, shrugging her tiny shoulders. "I can't let my family down by quitting my job at the pub. Plus, I enjoy it. And there's no way I'm giving up Princess. Isn't there some other way to get rid of my allergies?"

Molly wouldn't change her mind about her job or her cat; it was her life and her prerogative, so it was up to me to improve her stuffy nose and itchy eyes despite these allergenic factors. First, I instructed her—and her mother—to install a HEPA air filtration system in her home, plus new allergy-controlling mattress, pillow, and comforter covers to protect her from dust mites as she sleeps. (It is actually the feces of these microscopic bugs that cause allergies, as they shack up in carpets, pillows, mattresses, and blankets.)

After purifying her home, my next step was to desensitize Molly to her allergies by giving her extracts of allergens in shots. Resistant as she was to quitting her smoke-filled job and giving up her furry cat, she was extremely compliant when it came to her allergy shots and even administered them to herself at home. Finally, I asked that she begin taking nettle, vitamin C, and other antioxidants to protect her from free radical damage in her nose, eyes, and lungs. The cornerstone of her antiallergy program, however, was quercetin.

After a month of living in a clean house and faithfully taking her nutrients, Molly's condition had barely improved. I doubled the amount of quercetin to 2 grams a day. A month later, Molly's symptoms were so much better that she woke up most mornings feeling energized and breathing easy. Since she insists on waitressing at the pub and keeping her cat, her allergies and congestion have not completely disappeared, but they're markedly better.

NETTLES

Anyone who has ever brushed up against the plant called stinging nettle regrets it: the juice of the dark green leaves instantly irritates the skin, causing it to burn and prickle painfully. Internally, however, the juice is truly healing to the body and has almost the opposite effect. It soothes allergies.

The Latin term for this herb is *Urtica dioica*, derived from a word meaning "to burn." The leaf has been shown to be anti-inflammatory and works by preventing the body from making inflammatory prostaglandins. It is used in Europe as a spring tonic and a detoxifying remedy. Containing more than twenty-four different chemical components, from vitamins to proteins to flavonoids, the herb has the following effects:

- It's a diuretic, increasing urine flow, and soothing inflammation in the bladder and prostate.

- Freeze-dried nettle helps sinusitis and allergic rhinitis. In one study, sixty-nine hay fever sufferers took nettle, and 57 percent had remarkable improvement in their symptoms.

- Nettle is a great companion nutrient to quercetin. I generally recommend one or two 400-milligram capsules every four hours. Symptoms should start to clear up almost immediately. Nettles can be taken whenever allergies flare up.

Say Good-bye to Allergies

Research over a forty-year period has consistently proved that bioflavonoids like quercetin have antiallergy benefits. Only recently have we begun to appreciate the role they play in keeping us from sneezing, coughing, and scratching our way to misery. When you compare the available drugstore and over-the-counter medications and their drowsy, fuzzy-headed side effects to quercetin's problem-free, natural solution to springtime distress, the answer to allergies is clear. With the help of quercetin, many people can now enjoy the beauty of the seasons, the comfort of their homes, the familiarity of their offices, and the love of their pets symptom free.

HOW MUCH SHOULD I TAKE?

For General Health
See special conditions below, as needed
Divided doses after meals
Special Conditions

Allergies	300-600 mg/day
Peptic ulcer disease	300-600 mg/day
Chronic sinusitis/rhinitis	300-600 mg/day

When considering any treatment for allergies, first consider any underlying causes in your environment, foods you eat, or exposures at work or home. Then embark on a program to eliminate them.

18

Valerian and St. John's Wort: The Key to Calm

More people suffer from anxiety than any other health problem. An estimated 23 million Americans suffer from severely debilitating anxiety disorders that require serious medication. But an even greater number—an astonishing 65 million—experience a milder form of anxiety that can still tug at their days like a strong undertow in seemingly calm waters.

Virginia Curry, a forty-five-year-old hairstylist, lived with constant low-level anxiety daily. Her customers were the glitterati of the New York social scene who would visit her before galas, film premieres, balls, private parties, and benefit dinners.

Ten years earlier, Virginia had gone through a very difficult divorce. Her husband sued for custody of their daughter, Trina, and Virginia countersued, using up her entire savings. Though Virginia won custody, Trina had been angry and resentful since the divorce; after her boyfriend broke up with her, she became especially uncommunicative.

Virginia's family physician had listened sympathetically when she was going through her divorce and had prescribed Valium. At first, it seemed a godsend, but Virginia soon found herself hooked. Studies show that the addictive properties of Valium can take hold within just five days of consumption. With a half-life of seventy-two hours, the drug stays in the bloodstream for several days and can cause memory lapses and severe drowsiness. Doctors now recognize its dangers and prescribe it much more carefully as a result; New York has actually passed laws to prevent the overuse of such medications. In the 1980s, however, these drugs were in vogue and much prescribed. It took Virginia five years to kick her habit. Now she was again in need of an anxiety reliever, but she was understandably reluctant to use Valium or a similar medication again.

Drugs for anxiety and depression are among the top sellers in the country. Newer benzodiazepines, the class of drugs to which Valium belongs, have shorter-lasting effects, but they still have the same side effects and can also be addictive. Prozac and other selective serotonin reuptake inhibitors (SSRIs) are given for depression along with anxiety (the two often go together) and may indeed prove calming. They also are not as addictive as tranquilizers or benzodiazepines, but a common side effect is a diminished libido. Virginia had tried Prozac and found herself losing interest in sex. As she said, "I'd rather be anxious than live like a monk."

Fortunately, there were answers for Virginia, and for the millions of others suffering from constant anxiety. They are called valerian and St. John's wort.

The Root of Anxiety

Anxiety is a normal part of our lives. The jitters that come before your first day at a new job and the stress you experience when you feel you have too many responsibilities to juggle are actually signals from our brain that it's time to slow down, to take care, to focus. Becoming frightened in dangerous situations can prevent and protect us from harm. So fear is not necessarily our enemy: it may be an essential part of our survival skills, stimulating our senses and keeping us alert.

It's when anxiety becomes constant that we stress our bodies and souls. Symptoms like rapid heartbeat, jumpiness, shortness of breath, insomnia, headache, fatigue, nausea, abdominal discomfort, sweatiness, chest pain, numbness, loss of appetite, or voracious appetite can result from chronic anxiety.

According to Harold Bloomfield, author of *Healing Anxiety with Herbs*, even low-level anxiety over the long term can cause genuine medical problems. Stress and anxiety suppress the immune system, leaving you more vulnerable to illness.

Whether you take an herb or a synthetic drug, it's crucial that you understand the root of your anxiety before beginning any kind of treatment. Otherwise, you cannot truly relieve your tension. This is especially important if you are facing major life issues, job stress, or family problems. I've noticed my own tendency to put myself in stressful situations: as a doctor who grew up with childhood asthma, I often had to face health challenges and to push myself twice as hard to succeed at activities like sports. I grew accustomed to seeing myself as someone who could come from behind, who could overcome challenges, and in my adult life I often unwittingly placed myself in situations where I had to do just that. Whether it was my tennis game or a business venture, I seemed drawn to high-stress, high-reward situations. Lately, I've begun to change that approach, and my own anxiety has markedly diminished.

The sweaty palms, fluttery heartbeat, and churning stomach that warn of anxiety seem to be rooted in a small almond-shaped part of the brain known as the amygdala. In an anxiety-producing situation, such as before an exam, your amygdala processes your fear before it even has time to be processed by the neocortical areas of the brain responsible for higher thought. In other words, our bodies feel fear before our brain has had a chance to understand it.

Without an amygdala, we would have no fear. Without fear and anxiety, we would be unable to avoid dangerous situations. However, when the amygdala is frequently alerted in response to situations that scare us, chronic stress disorders can result. Overstimulation of the amygdala may deplete our brain levels of the neurotransmitter serotonin; such depletion has been implicated in certain impulse and anxiety disorders. I find that anxiety and depression are closely linked in my patients, and the fact that depression also seems to stem from a lack of serotonin supports this observation.

Stress itself is not an event; it's a reaction to an event. I recommend to my patients that they look carefully at their own life patterns and try to stop stress internally, as well as with herbal aids such as kava. That is truly what we call an integrated mind-body approach—and it works.

Stop Job Jitters

Given the right combination of events and situations, even the most laidback and relaxed among us are susceptible to anxiety. Thirty-five-year-old Tim Anderson was facing such a scenario when he came to see me. A management consultant, Tim had feared public speaking since the third grade.

SLEEP SOUNDLY WITH VALERIAN

Valerian has been utilized to manage nervousness and sleeplessness for thousands of years in Chinese and Ayurvedic medicines. It's a large perennial plant native to South Asia and North America.

Valerian is a natural cure for insomnia. Indeed, valerian may work like Valium, by stimulating GABA receptors in the brain—without the side effects. Probably the only downside of taking valerian root is its distinctive smell of old socks.

Of the two hundred species of valerian, the most common is *Valeriana officinalis*, which flourishes all over Europe. Prescribed by the Greek physician Galen as a treatment for insomnia, by the eighteenth century, it was also established as a digestive aid, and today it is still heralded as a sedative. Studies show that valerian is the perfect supplement for the third of the adult population suffering sleep disturbances; two 1992 studies reveal that the plant seems to decrease sleep onset time and

So when he was promoted to group leader of his firm, requiring him to give talks and head meetings on a daily basis, he came down with a good case of the jitters. His new position also entailed flying all over the country to meet with company presidents and attend conferences, and Tim absolutely hated to fly. Needless to say, after just a few weeks as group leader, Tim was so anxious about going to work each morning that he soon became exhausted with worry, especially because he was having trouble sleeping at night.

"I just lie in bed, stressing out because I have speeches to make in the morning," he told me.

He was even more worried about afternoons, when, for some reason, his anxieties were even worse.

Management consulting is a lucrative but grueling field, especially at Tim's firm, and many of his colleagues recommended taking Xanax.

continue increase deeper, more restful sleep. Valerian also seems to reduce nighttime awakenings. One double-blind study found that 89 percent of subjects treated with valerian reported improved sleep.

In 1989, Drs. J. Holzl and P. Godau of the Institute of Pharmaceutical Biology in Marburg, Germany, discovered that valerian binds to the exact same brain receptors as benzodiazepines but works more gently. This milder action is the key to its efficacy, however, since it improves sleep in the same way without the same potential for addiction, withdrawal, or side effects. Valerian can also be quite beneficial in managing anxiety, especially since treatments that improve sleep tend to alleviate anxiety.

The German Commission E reports no side effects or contraindications to valerian. I have not found it to be useful as an adjunctive treatment for acute cases of insomnia; however, with persistent use, benefits seem to accumulate. Particularly potent when combined with other calming herbs like kava, St. John's wort, or passionflower, valerian proves that good health can return when you get a good night's sleep.

He was not convinced that these high-powered drugs would provide a quick fix to his problems.

"Those drugs can work," I said, "but they can knock you out, and that won't help you at work. If you'll give me just a few weeks, I'll bet you can get the same results without the side effects."

Tim decided he was game, and we made a deal: I'd give him natural treatments for a month, and if his anxiety wasn't relieved, I'd start him on benzodiazepines. I recommended that he take chamomile tea and St John's wort to three times a day. In order to treat his insomnia, I also asked him to take a supplement called valerian, a calming root particularly prized for its sedative effects (see box on page 247).

When I tested Tim's blood sugar and diet, I realized that his intensified afternoon anxiety stemmed from blood sugar fluctuations throughout the day. Blood sugar problems are an oft-ignored cause of anxiety symptoms and should always be investigated in these cases. In order to regulate his glucose levels, I suggested that he eat smaller, more frequent meals and more protein throughout the day.

After the first week of treatment, I received a message from Tim, who joked, "Get the Xanax ready!" But after three more weeks, I hadn't heard any more from him. I knew that he'd flown to the Midwest for a week during that time, and I was expecting complaints of stress and nerves. After a month, I finally called him to make sure he was faring well on his treatment.

"I didn't want to jinx myself by calling, but I'm feeling so much better," he exclaimed when I asked about his anxiety. "I slept right through my flight and made it through my speeches in the Midwest without the normal butterflies in my stomach or sweaty palms. Guess I won't be needing those drugs."

After two months, Tim returned to my office for a follow-up consultation. Not only were his anxiety symptoms reduced, but he was much better able to cope with the pressures of his job. Both Tim and I believe that this was due mostly to the calming combination of kava and valerian.

Environmental Anxiety

Kate Vogel, thirty-four, suffered from irritable bowel syndrome, characterized by gas, bloating, diarrhea, and food sensitivities, as well as shortness of breath. She had also been losing weight rapidly, shedding fifteen pounds in the last two months. Her job as a freelance computer analyst required her to hop from office to office, offering her expertise for a few weeks and then moving to the next job. She was beginning to crack under the stress of constantly starting over in new places, meeting new people, getting used to new systems, and then leaving again. Kate felt that her work was suffering as a result.

When I tested her vitamin levels, I found that she was extremely low in vitamin B_{12}, which was probably contributing to her fatigue and malaise. Giving her weekly injections of the vitamin slowly increased her appetite. Still, her stress continued.

Kate noticed that whenever she had a day off work and stayed home, she felt much better and she could breathe more easily. She attributed this to the rare opportunity to relax, but I felt that there must be some other factors causing her problems.

Upon questioning her about her home and work environments, as I always do with my patients, I found that her studio was well ventilated, thanks to many open windows and a little humidifier she kept going at all times. Her work environments, however, were a different story. Although she roved from office to office, most workplaces had poorly ventilated interiors and polluted surroundings. I call these sick buildings, and Kate was catching their illness. Sick buildings can aggravate the respiratory system, not only making it difficult to breathe but also leading to anxiety. Mental triggers aren't the only causes of anxiety and depression; your physical surroundings may sometimes play as much of a role.

I advised Kate to sit in areas in her office that weren't so cluttered with dusty papers and away from photocopiers and areas where mold might be growing. Many companies, I've found, will make provisions for workers who truly are sensitive to environmental factors.

Finally, to treat Kate's anxiety and stress, I prescribed valerian each night before bedtime. Ultimately, Kate decided that what she really needed was a permanent full-time steady job; trying to find freelance work was a stressor she didn't need. Even at her new permanent workplace, however, Kate continued to take small doses of valerian when necessary to make sure she slept well and worked at her highest capacity.

Anxiety and Depression

Lila Ross first came to see me because of her frequent burning urination. Embarrassed but frustrated by her condition, Lila hoped that I could recommend some medicine or technique to curb her numerous trips to the bathroom. As I took her history, however, I began to realize that there was much more to the problem.

For Lila was under a lot of stress at home. Her mother had just been diagnosed with Alzheimer's disease, and Lila wasn't sure how to talk to her or deal with the situation. At age fifty-one and unmarried, Lila began to worry that she would be alone for the rest of her life. Even worse, she was beginning to go through menopause, which not only gave her hot flashes but reminded her that she had lost her opportunity to give birth.

Exhausted, nervous, and depressed, Lila displayed symptoms of both severe anxiety and depression. As I've mentioned before, these two conditions are linked in many people. Lila found herself unable to sleep at night, unable to wake up in the morning, and unable to relax during the day. This was a multifaceted problem.

Luckily, I knew of two supplements that, together, could alleviate most of her ailments. Valerian was the first for anxiety. In order to lift her depression, I prescribed St. John's wort, a plant that has been heralded as a mild answer to Prozac. I also recommended that she fill her diet with soy-based products like tofu and soy protein, since the gentle plant estrogens in soy foods can alleviate the symptoms of menopause.

When Lila first came to my office, she was brooding, quiet, and withdrawn. But as the weeks passed, I began to notice a gradual change in her demeanor.

LISTENING TO ST. JOHN'S WORT

One of the first nutraceuticals that made me recognize the power of herbal medicine was St. John's wort. It was among the first nutraceuticals to break through from alternative medicine to the mainstream world. I began to prescribe it on the basis of research indicating that the plant was an excellent natural alternative to antidepressants like Prozac without the side effects or addiction potential. A 1994 controlled, randomized study reported in the journal *Phytomedicine*, for example, found that taking St. John's wort elevated the moods of 67 percent of subjects with mild to moderate depression, while only 20 percent of subjects taking a placebo showed any mood difference. Furthermore, a study in the *Journal of Geriatric Psychiatry and Neurology* found no difference between the effects of St. John's wort and imipramine, a synthetic antidepressant; in fact, many subjects felt better on the herb than on the drug. The patients I treated with it convinced me of its worth in combating depression.

The active ingredient in St. John's wort is hypericin, which is also believed to have antiviral properties. The recommended dose is 300 milligrams three times daily. There are a few known side effects: the herb can make you light sensitive, so beware of excessive exposure to the sun; it can also, in theory, cause sensitivities to foods like wine, cheese, and yeast, all of which contain a compound called tyramine. St. John's wort seems to work like Prozac, which is an SSRI. Keeping serotonin coursing through the brain can fend off depression, which is characterized by a lack of this neurotransmitter. St. John's wort may also function as a monoamine oxidase (MAO) inhibitor; MAO is an enzyme responsible for the breakdown of serotonin in the brain.

Ancient folklore had it that the flower of St. John's wort could banish witches or protect you from their evil eye. The herb may not exert such supernatural powers, but it does seem to have an ability to diminish the depths of depression. I recommend this as a natural treatment for anyone engaging in the battle against mild depression.

The first sign that her natural medications were working was the news that her urination was back to normal. I spoke with her on the phone about twice a month, and each time I noticed a bit more cheer and life in her voice. The biggest breakthrough, however, came when Lila excitedly told me that she felt well enough to buy a dog. Strange as it may seem, this dog changed her life. Until she rescued Boomer from the pound, Lila told me, she was beginning to feel like she could never love or even connect to anyone again. But Boomer made her realize that life wasn't as difficult—or as lonely—as it seemed. Walking down the street with her new pooch, Lila was surrounded with strangers kneeling to pet the dog and compliment him, and she found herself enjoying the conversation. She also found the courage to face her mother and support her in her time of need. All of this, Lila felt, was due simply to the combination of nutrients I had given her. She couldn't explain her vast improvement any other way.

It may seem strange that mere dietary supplements could affect such profound change in someone's life, but we tend to overlook the power and potency of the plants around us. I truly believe that kava and St. John's wort, in particular, may have eased Lila's mental distress.

Conquer Anxiety

In today's world, none of us can entirely escape anxiety. And we may not want to: consider the fluttering, anxious thrill of falling in love, of performing onstage to an appreciative audience, of doing a challenging job well. Nonetheless, you can certainly take charge of your anxiety if it's hampering your ability to make it through life. Valerian or St John's wort or even chamomile tea has a long history as an effective traditional treatment for anyone looking to relax .

HOW MUCH SHOULD I TAKE?

For General Health
See special conditions below, as needed
Divided doses or bedtime
Special Conditions

Anxiety/stress (symptoms may include the following: rapid heartbeat, jumpiness, shortness of breath, insomnia, headache, fatigue, nausea, abdominal discomfort, sweatiness, chest pain, numbness, loss of appetite or voracious appetite)	*Valerian* Doses 125 mg 4:1 extract daily *St. John's wort* *Doses 300mg* daily .3% Hypericin
Soothe intestinal discomfort	800-1,600 mg/day

May cause drowsiness

Word of Caution

Anxiety and depression need to be treated by a physician. If you believe you suffer from the above, consult your physician before starting any treatment plan. Supplements should never be used as a substitute for medical treatment.

19

Phosphatidyl Serine and Acetyl-L-Carnitine: The Nervous System and the Mind

The brain is the body's crowning glory, a three-pound organ that is master conductor of all the daily functions we take for granted, from walking down the street to recognizing a friend's face. Some would say it is the seat of our soul, where our very identity resides. The thrills of falling in love, enjoying music, and recalling fond memories are all gifts given us by the brain. But the brain is vulnerable as well. Depression, Alzheimer's disease, schizophrenia, and many other conditions rob us—and our families—of life's joys and freedoms.

When the brain fails, the simple abilities of thinking, moving, and remembering can vanish. In certain types of brain damage, all capacity to store long-term memory is utterly destroyed, and the patient is caught in a permanent present, unable to remember a new face for more than a few minutes. Relatives of stroke victims often comment that their loved one is "no longer himself." And in Alzheimer's disease, perhaps the most devastating consequence is not the memory loss, but the personality change. Victims become irrational, irritable, even demented. One writer described her mother's early onset of Alzheimer's disease "a different kind of madness" that first became apparent when she had all her cats killed. The depths of the brain's mysteries and miracles are truly enigmatic, but one thing is clear: the brain is what makes us human.

Neuroscience is now making groundbreaking genetic discoveries that may predict devastating brain illnesses like Alzheimer's disease and offer hope of finding a treatment. New imaging techniques like PET scans and MRIs actually allow us to watch the brain in action as its circuits fire and direct our bodies into order.

Perhaps the most exciting new finding about the brain is that it has the remarkable ability to heal itself. In this chapter, I will introduce you to two of my favorite brain foods: a nutrient called phosphatidyl serine (PS), which is one of the five phospholipids essential to the functioning of all cells, and another called acetyl-L-carnitine (ALC), which is a form of a common amino acid, l-carnitine. Both occur naturally in the healthy brain and have the profound ability to protect nerve cells, keep them flexible and active, and even enhance their functioning. Over our lifetime, we lose half of our mental capacity. Unless we combat that decline with super nutrition—and with nutrients that work together synergistically, such as PS and ALC—we may be at risk of losing our truest, most vital selves.

Anatomy of a Thought

The brain is amazingly adaptable. Although nerve cells cannot regenerate, at least according to current research, they are flexible, or “plastic.” Consider the stunning example of severely epileptic children whose devastating seizures could not be controlled by drugs. Eventually some of these children had to undergo extensive surgery to halt their violent seizures. Although all the children lost nearly half their brains in the procedure, in all cases the remaining half assumed *all* the mental functions served by the severed nerve connections. These children were able to return to school and to live nearly normal lives.

The brain is also the absolutely mysterious home to a constant cascade of thoughts. How does it create a thought? What *is* a thought? A fireworks of neurons shooting their electrochemical signals to each other. And what is a neuron? A nerve cell that looks rather like a flower, with the dendrites as petals, the axon as the graceful thin stem, and the synapse as the chunky bulb at the tail end. One neuron connects to another by attaching its synapse to a dendrite on a neighboring neuron, and voilà! The flow of information begins.

The more dendrites and dendritic connections you have, the better your brain works. Unfortunately, as we get older, our dendrites begin to die off, which leaves less potential for synaptic connections and compromises our logic and memory.

Not only does aging cause our dendrites to wither away, it can also lead to the depletion of neurotransmitters. Stress is absolutely toxic to the brain. That’s because high amounts of cortisol, released during times of great stress, can seriously damage neurons. Stress impairs cognition, and since older individuals find it harder to calm themselves down in pressure-filled situations, they are particularly susceptible to such damage.

If these warnings sound bleak and pessimistic, their aim is only to encourage you to take hold of your own brain health and do what you can to preserve your mind. First of all, dendrites can be stimulated to grow. By keeping your brain active—by reading, engaging in interesting conversation, learning a new language or skill, or taking up hobbies—you can keep your synapses buzzing until you're well into your second century. Do what you can to avoid stressful situations that can poison the brain. If you take time to relax, you will not only keep your body healthy but preserve your mental powers for the long haul. Finally, using powerful nutrients like PS and ALC can protect your gray matter and keep you mentally fit well into a vital old age.

Jim's Story

Jim Weston was seventy-one years old when he first faced bypass surgery, back in 1994. Although he had had attacks of angina prior to surgery, causing frequent discomfort, Jim's mind had always been razor sharp. He was a retired army drill sergeant, as strong as he was smart.

After his surgery, however, Jim soon noticed that he was perpetually groggy and confused. He would forget where he'd put his reading glasses and turn the house upside down in their pursuit, only to realize that they were in his shirt pocket. Or he'd run into old acquaintances at the supermarket, knowing that he'd met them before but unable to remember their names. This was frustrating, to say the least. Jim, who in his prime had devised complex military strategies and maneuvers, felt he was losing his mental faculties.

"This is not just about forgetting to pick up milk at the grocery store," he told me. "I feel like a prisoner of my own failing mind."

Forgetting familiar faces, misplacing objects—these are signs of age-related cognitive decline, which tends to set in around the age of fifty. Other factors, like fatigue, nutritional deficiencies, hypoxia (lack of oxygen), medication, stress, and life traumas can also contribute to this decline.

Memory is the bedrock of the self. And one of the biggest concerns my patients voice is the fear of losing their brain fitness, particularly their memory. No wonder Jim was upset.

To return Jim's mind to its missile accuracy, I started him on a program of gentle aerobic exercise and natural supplements, including ginkgo to improve his circulation and help bring more oxygen to his brain and magnesium to help his heart function more efficiently. The most important supplement, though, was PS. A groundbreaking 1991 study by Dr. Thomas Crook showed that in 57 subjects with age-related memory decline whose average age was sixty-four, PS was able to turn back the mental clock by roughly twelve years.

Within three or four months, Jim was able to concentrate more on daily events, recall the names of acquaintances, and follow through on tasks like grocery shopping without forgetting what he was doing.

Brain Food

It may seem incredible that you can safely boost mental clarity by consuming a little-known nutrient with a long-winded moniker. Phosphatidyl serine, however, has rapidly been gaining notice and credibility over the past ten years. More clinical trials have been run on PS than on any other nutrient targeting the brain. Over fifty human trials demonstrate that, when used as a dietary supplement in a wide range of doses, phosphatidyl serine is incredibly effective at conserving stores of brainpower. Here's what Dr. Parris Kidd, a well-known proponent of PS, has to say about this nutrient: "PS is the first—and only—memory nutrient of promise. I have seen elderly patients with severe memory lapses recall previously forgotten names within minutes after being on a supplement program of PS."

PS is a building block of all your brain cells. It's one of four molecules known as the phospholipids, large fatty substances that hold together cell membranes. All cells depend on their protective membranes for survival, but nerve cells in the brain especially depend on this outermost layer in order to receive and conduct the impulses that allow us to think and move. Without PS, our neurons could not manufacture, package, or send out the neurotransmitters that travel from nerve cell to nerve cell, relaying messages throughout the brain. This is the secret to the heady success of PS.

I like to think of PS as the brain's personal bodyguard, loyally protecting each and every neuron around the clock, monitoring the comings and goings of substances through the membrane and, most important, guarding the priceless intelligence within.

By recovering synaptic and electrical activity within neurons, PS actually heals the brain, which encourages the restoration of mental function. Many studies show that PS, when administered to elderly subjects in various states of cognitive deterioration, significantly improves attention, concentration, recall of numbers and words, verbal ability, and short-term memory. Dr. Thomas Crook, founder of two memory assessment clinics in Bethesda, Maryland, has used tests of basic, daily tasks to demonstrate that PS can facilitate recall of telephone numbers and misplaced objects, improve sight recognition, sharpen short-term memory, and help the mind focus on reading and conversation. Most studies on the benefits indicate that 300 milligrams of PS per day is an optimal dose for treating the mental malfunctioning caused by age-related cognitive decline.

PS not only preserves the skills we need to get through the day but enhances mood; it has been shown to increase sociability and decrease depression and apathy among subjects. Most important, PS improves quality of life. And even younger people can use it, with a healthy diet and exercise, as prevention against future memory loss.

PS I Love You

Following are just some of the ways in which PS has been found to boost brainpower.

Memory: The largest study on PS to date, conducted by B. Cenacchi and colleagues in the *Journal of Aging*, monitored the effects of PS on 425 subjects with moderate to severe age-related cognitive decline. The researchers discovered that the nutrient benefited subjects in long-term memory storage, long-term memory retrieval, and total recall of past events.

Behavior: When mental functioning deteriorates, quality of life and self-sufficiency often fall by the wayside. A study by G. Palmieri and colleagues in the *Clinical Trials Journal* found that PS improved the ability of elderly subjects with moderate cognitive decline to complete activities required for independent daily living. PS also lessened the apathy and social withdrawal caused by cognitive deterioration.

Stress:Phosphatidyl serine can be beneficial in younger individuals by preventing later brain deterioration and reducing the harmful effects of stress on the body. In the *European Journal of Clinical Pharmacology,* P. Monteleone and fellow researchers studied young, healthy men subjected to exercise-induced stress by bicycling to near exhaustion. Men who took PS for ten days prior to the exercise session had reduced production of cortisol, which is usually released during stressful periods and can damage muscle as well as impair brain function.

Mood: Not only does PS improve cognitive functioning in the elderly, it can also repair associated mood problems. A study of elderly women on PS showed that the nutrient reduced anxiety and alleviated vertigo and depression. A 1995 trial, this time on elderly men, suggested that PS can similarly boost mood. As far back as 1981, researchers found lowered PS levels in the red blood cells of subjects with clinical depression.

Brain Physiology: New technologies, like PET (positron emission tomography) scans and EEGs that monitor the brain in action provide further proof of the strength of PS. The EEG rhythms measured in the brain reflect the activity of acetylcholine, a neurotransmitter that is often depleted with age, resulting in cognitive deterioration. A 1991 study showed that PS boosted the EEG rhythm in healthy young males by an average of 15 to 20 percent. PET scans, on the other hand, track glucose metabolism in the brain: the more glucose is being consumed, the better the mind is working. This study indicated that subjects taking PS demonstrated higher brain activity on PET scans.

Brain Geography, Briefly

Ever wonder just what your gray matter is composed of, and exactly what it does? The brain is comprised of three major regions: the brain stem, cerebellum, and cerebrum. The brain stem is the first part of the brain to be formed in the womb. Here, nerves run from the brain to the spinal cord, coordinating and relaying motor information. The brain stem also controls unconscious functions like breathing and heartbeat but has no capacity for memories, thoughts, or feelings. The first animals roaming the earth were believed to have only brain stems, which is why it is often called the "reptilian" or "lizard" brain. It's a powerful seat of instincts, drives, and perhaps our most primitive and irrevocable passions.

The cerebellum is the part of our brain that allows us to maintain our balance and move in synchronized patterns, like walking. This so-called little brain resides in the back of the skull and coordinates movement. Athletes have well-developed cerebellums, while those of babies are very undeveloped. Birds, as a percentage of their brains, actually have the largest cerebellums of all, due to the complex integration of information needed to take flight.

Now we get to the most interesting part. The outer layer of the brain, called the cerebrum, made its first appearance in the skull 80 million years ago with the evolution of mammals, making it the newest member of the brain family. Also known as the mammalian brain, the cerebrum is what we tend to think of when we picture the brain: a wrinkled, rounded mass with bulging hills and deep valleys running over its surface. The cerebrum is covered with a 2-millimeter-thick layer of brain tissue called the neocortex (or cerebral cortex), which is the location of all our higher thoughts and functions. The neocortex covers about 2.5 square feet, though much of it is hidden in grooves and fissures. The more grooves and fissures a brain has, the smarter the body attached to that brain. Birds, for example, have almost no neocortex at all, hence the insult "bird brain." The neocortex is our real-life thinking cap, where our abstract thoughts, deepest emotions, sensory skills, and cherished memories are born.

Memory for people or events requires every part of the brain, every sense we have. Try to remember, for instance, your grandmother. Your memory of her comprises many different elements, from her smiling face to her signature perfume, the sound of her voice, and the warmth of her hugs. Out of the vast net of neurons that span the brain, there are groups of nerve cells that must all fire together in a unique pattern across the brain in order to summon the memory of your grandmother. If a single group of neurons in this pattern degenerates, this memory weakens. This is why the degeneration of nerves that occurs with age, disease, drug use, and other conditions wreaks havoc with the mind.

The Dual Action of PS and ALC

Although PS is considered by many to be the most effective brain booster, it is well complemented by ALC, which has a different mechanism of action. ALC easily commutes across the protective blood-brain barrier to work within neurons. ALC, by enhancing fatty metabolism in the cell, ensures efficient function of the mitochondria, the little energy factories that reside within every type of cell we have, except red blood cells. ALC promotes efficient energy use in the brain and improves its supply of the neurotransmitter acetylcholine, which is crucial for memory function. Many studies document the use of ALC to repair the degeneration of neuronal tissue that can trigger the age-related deterioration of mental function. A 1994 study in the journal *Brain Research*, for example, showed that rats taking the nutrient as they grew older displayed a partial reversal in the expected breakdown of neurons with age. In humans, too, ALC can impact neurological function for the better. In a 1989 study, elderly subjects taking 3 grams of ALC daily for forty days showed vast improvements in judgment, depression, memory, self-sufficiency, and sociability.

While ALC directly enhances function of the brain's mitochondria, it also prevents the toxic accumulation of fatty acids in the mitochondria. PS regulates membrane function, which allows cells to communicate more efficiently. By enhancing membrane function and mitochondrial function, these deliver a powerful synergistic effect. I generally prescribe both nutrients together, particularly in case of memory loss or neuropathies. However, I might prescribe PS alone, initially, in memory loss, and add ALC as a backup when I need to give a patient an extra boost.

To quote a wise television commercial, a mind is a terrible thing to waste, and using PS and ALC together is one surefire way to restore the brain to its sharpest abilities.

Painful Memories

Melissa Raven, fifty-four, was a mystery to every chiropractor and physician whose help she sought. Just over ten years ago, Melissa underwent a laminectomy to remove several of the disks in her lower back. A decade later, Melissa was still experiencing severe back pain. Doctors and specialists prescribed painkillers and anti-inflammatory drugs, none of which seemed to work. Melissa's constant distress was taking a toll on her mental health as well, so she was put on antidepressants. As time went on, Melissa's problems began to multiply. Beyond depression and pain, she began to lose her memory. She grew confused and disoriented and consequently had problems sustaining social relationships. One doctor suggested that she might have early-onset Alzheimer's disease. Desperate and alone, Melissa came to me for yet another opinion on her condition.

Melissa's back was slumped in defeat. Although she was withdrawn and subdued, she was still alert when I spoke with her and even showed flashes of humor at times. Before mental cloudiness forced her to quit her job, Melissa had been a high school teacher with a master's degree; she also had been very active in championing women's rights. I could see that she had once been a vital and enthusiastic member of society.

Between her back surgery, her depression, and her cognitive decline, Melissa had a whole cauldron of problems brewing. I sensed that she was stuck in a rut, so enmeshed in her pain that it was depleting her nervous system and preventing her memory from functioning optimally.

In addition to a special program designed to alleviate her pain, I put Melissa on 300 milligrams of PS and 1,000 milligrams of ALC per day, plus ginkgo and tyrosine, all designed to restore her mood and memory.

Part of Melissa's mental confusion was probably due to her anxiety and stress over her back condition; her back surgery also may have caused the degeneration of neurons that run along the spinal cord. Several recent studies demonstrate that ALC can exert neuroprotective effects on peripheral nerve lesions.

Within a few months, Melissa found she was better able to focus on daily tasks like grocery shopping and reading the newspaper, which prior to her treatment had proved challenging. Her mind became sharp enough that she was able to return to the public school system as a substitute teacher, which allowed her to work with students while avoiding the strain of working full-time.

Still, Melissa was not completely herself. Despite my best efforts, her pain persisted, and several years later, she tested positive for rheumatoid arthritis. Sometimes the body takes its own time to declare the existence of a full-blown medical condition. Now that we knew the probable root of Melissa's pain, I prescribed anti-inflammatory nutrients for her such as glucosamine and fish oils, while her other doctors treated her with standard arthritic medications. Slowly, Melissa is shedding some of the pain that she has carried for years. Melissa's case teaches a valuable lesson about the body, however. When evaluating a patient, it is important to review every possible cause of illness. What if Melissa had gone through life awaiting the onset of full-blown Alzheimer's disease? Luckily, PS and ALC were able to repair the damage and convince Melissa that she was not losing her mind.

Alzheimer's Disease: Unraveling the Mind

While memory decline is a natural signal that aging is taking its toll on the mind, one of the greatest fears associated with old age is Alzheimer's disease, a nonreversible deterioration of mental functioning that affects millions of elderly people each year.

Alzheimer's disease has been diagnosed in over four million Americans. The threat of this disease clearly advances with age: less than 5 percent of people under the age of seventy-five have been diagnosed with Alzheimer's, but it affects about 20 percent of the population between ages seventy-five and eighty-four and around 40 percent of individuals over age eighty-five. These statistics are expected to worsen into the middle of the next century, when there will be as many Americans over the age of eighty as there are now over the age of sixty-five. While only 4 percent of the U.S. population in 1900 was over sixty-five, by 2020 that figure will increase to 20 percent. And although Alzheimer's disease tends to appear as we get older, there is no boundary for its onset. The youngest patient known to show signs of Alzheimer's is twenty-eight years old.

First brought to the national attention by its namesake, Alois Alzheimer, in 1907, Alzheimer's disease is the leading cause of dementia known in the United States. Dementia consists of cognitive disturbances that impair memory, motor activity, and thinking. While most elderly individuals experience the frustrating inability to remember where they've put objects or when they have appointments, Alzheimer's is a much more limiting, distressing kind of mental disturbance. The first sign is not memory loss but the difficulty carrying out complex and abstract thought and proper judgment. Later, memory, personality, and freedom of movement all suffer. By the end of a victim's lifetime, he or she will have suffered abnormal neuronal growths in the hippocampus known as neurofibrillary tangles. Also, the accumulation of dead material called plaques will have formed around a protein known as amyloid. Finally, there is a notable depletion in the neurotransmitter acetylcholine, which is one of the primary memory chemicals in the brain.

People with a genetic family history of Alzheimer's are at a greater risk for this disease, although many afflicted individuals have no genetic history of the disease. There is as yet no concrete way to diagnose this life-stealing disease; the only certain way to validate its insidious existence is by examining postmortem brain tissue.

Alzheimer's is a medical condition of the gravest concern, which incapacitates vital individuals without warning or cause. Unfortunately, PS and ALC have not been as useful for fighting Alzheimer's, once it has progressed, as many researchers had hoped. Perhaps they work in higher doses than have been tested or are more effective as a preventive measure; this will become apparent through research. For now, our best weapon against the mind-numbing forces of age is a healthy diet, exercise, careful monitoring of chemical substances like medications or alcohol, and natural brain builders like PS and ALC.

PS, ALC, and the Case of the Numb Limbs

The tightly woven net of neurons that makes up the brain also extends down the spinal cord, where it sends and receives messages from different parts of the body. When these peripheral neurons are damaged, they may not compromise memory or reasoning ability, but they can be very painful, as Francine Sutherland discovered. A fifty-five-year-old Avon saleswoman, Francine was the busy and contented mother of two twenty-somethings and a teenager—all boys. With her blinding smile and flawless makeup, Francine was a natural at her job. In 1988, she was diagnosed with adult-onset diabetes, which her mother had also suffered. Soon thereafter, she developed an alarming numbness in her feet that worsened over a period of months. Because Francine's job required her to walk door-to-door, this condition was especially incapacitating.

"I can't feel my feet well enough to know when they are planted firmly on the ground," she explained, when I asked her about the severity of her numbness. She looked at her practically useless legs. "I just stumble down the street."

I evaluated Francine for Lyme disease, and the test came up negative. I knew that a deficiency of vitamin B_{12} can result in peripheral neuropathies, which could have been causing Francine's loss of sensation, and, sure enough, a test indicated that she had low levels of that vitamin in her system.

Before Francine was referred to my office by a concerned coworker, her neurologist had prescribed her amitriptylline, which is normally used for depression but has been found to be helpful in patients with chronic pain or nerve problems. She did not respond well to this drug at all. When I constructed my own treatment plan for her, I was determined to use more natural approaches to her discomfort. The first step was to address the sugar-related problems I had detected. I thought that her numbness could stem from her diabetes, and I put her on a low-carbohydrate diet. Next, I put her on supplements of vitamin B_{12}, ginkgo to improve her circulation, resveratrol for antioxidant defense, and coQ_{10} to enhance mitochondrial function and produce more energy. Most important, I prescribed 300 milligrams of PS to promote the health and strength of her nerve cells as well as 1,000 milligrams of ALC. ALC is especially good at treating peripheral neuropathies, or the dangerous deterioration that can occur in nerves extending from the spinal cord into various parts of the body, like the legs. According to a study in *Diabetalogica*, peripheral neuropathy associated with diabetes is extremely common; there is as high as a 28 percent chance that the two will be paired. This suggests that Francine's numbness was coming from her diabetes. A 1995 study showed that sixty-three diabetics with painful neuropathies experienced significant improvement in movement and pain relief after taking ALC for fifteen days.

For almost two weeks after putting Francine on this nutritional program, I heard nothing from her. Then, one night, my beeper went off around midnight. It was Francine.

"Are you okay, Francine?" I asked when I returned the call.

"Doctor," she said, "I'm really worried. I couldn't fall asleep tonight because I'm feeling a painful sensation in my legs."

"What does it feel like? Can you describe it?"

"It feels like pins and needles, as if I'd been sitting cross-legged for too long and cut my circulation off."

I smiled in relief. "Francine," I told her, "that's exactly what you want to feel. You're getting the feeling back in your legs."

Certainly, diabetes and a B_{12} deficiency could cause this loss of sensation. Whatever the precise cause, PS and ALC have done a wonderful job of getting Francine back on her feet, as even her neurologist concedes. For a year after she started treatment, Francine continued to improve. Although she still has some discomfort in her legs, they feel much stronger than before, and she is back on her Avon route.

Improve Sleep with PS and ALC

Julian Van Beuren, forty-six, was far from the depths of mental decline and deterioration that Francine or Melissa had experienced. He was an ingenious computer specialist working long hours on his own startup software company.

Because new advances in computer technology are constantly being developed, Julian felt an enormous pressure to put out novel products as quickly as possible. But every time he came up with a brilliant new idea, a competitor would beat him to it. The stress and pressure of long hours at work began to exhaust him. On weekends, Julian had plenty of time to relax and catch up on lost sleep, but, alas, it was not to be. Five days a week of sleep deprivation had thrown his normal circadian rhythms out of whack so that he couldn't fall asleep until late in the night.

When I first saw Julian's haggard face, I knew that he needed to sleep as soon as possible. I started him on melatonin, which is used for the short-term treatment of sleep disorders. On Julian, however, the popular hormone had little effect. It seemed he needed some extra help. Taking tyrosine in the morning, I decided, would keep him alert during the day, when he needed to work with customers and beat the competition. In the evening, I told Julian to take PS and ALC to boost the sleep effects of melatonin. I had never tried the combination of PS and ALC with melatonin, so I was as curious to monitor the effects of this trio as Julian. However, I knew that PS would strengthen his neurons to give his brain the extra healing help it needed, and ALC has been shown to increase melatonin levels in rats by improving nerve transmission. Researchers theorized that, since both ALC and melatonin are free radical scavengers, these nutrients could reverse the aging process by increasing melatonin levels in the brain.

Happily for both of us, the nutritional hat trick worked—within three days of starting his supplements, Julian was sleeping well again.

Brain Ambition

You've seen the benefits of PS and ALC on the elderly, but why should anyone else heed its powers? The truth is, these brain-boosting nutrients may work even faster and more effectively in younger individuals than in their older peers. One of my patients, a twenty-nine-year-old named Tim Brinker, recently decided to attend law school. This was an incredibly ambitious decision, as Tim worked as a stockbroker by day to pay his bills and burned the midnight oil studying and taking classes. As one of the older students in his class at a top law school, Tim felt enormous pressure to ace his exams and pass the bar as soon as possible. Although he wasn't suffering any noticeable memory deficits, he wanted to stay at the top of his game and be as sharp as he could. I told him about the results of PS and ALC in my older patients with memory problems, and I wondered aloud what they could do for him.

"Give 'em to me, Doctor," he said fearlessly. "I'll try it."

Because these supplements have few—if any—side effects, I put him on the kind of rigorous memory-boosting nutraceutical program on which I put the elderly: 1,000 milligrams of ALC, 300 milligrams of PS, 120 milligrams of ginkgo, and 1,000 milligrams of tyrosine every day. To my surprise, the nutrients worked much faster in Tim than in my older patients. I have noticed in older individuals that PS and ALC can work wonders, but often after a sometimes frustrating period of months. In a matter of weeks, however, Tim began to handle his workload and juggle his home and school lives more effectively. Perhaps I shouldn't have been surprised: studies show that choline, which is related to PS, may concentrate more potently in younger people. Tim's results lead me to believe that one of the biggest benefits of mind-sharpening supplements like PS and ALC may occur in the young. Further research on the early use of nutrients to enhance academic performance may well bear this out.

Keep Your Mind Forever Young

Every day, over two hundred people celebrate their one hundredth birthday. Baby boomers are turning fifty. The magazine *Modern Maturity* now has the largest advertising base—25 million people—in the business. Aging is fast becoming a concern for the rapidly growing segment of our population entering their later years. But perhaps it's never too early to worry about the quality of life we'll have when we get older.

The exciting feeling prevails that, under the right circumstances, longevity can be ours. But longevity alone is not the only goal. We want advanced years with no diminution of the quality of life. New research shows that there are many things we can do to prevent the age-related loss of memory and mind. Exercise—both mental and physical—has been shown to improve memory. Stimulating the brain through social contact, pursuing interests, and learning new information also can boost memory.

One of the most important foundations of nutritional medicine is the mind-body connection, and studying the mysterious depths of the brain illustrates the strength of this inextricable link. Our thoughts and feelings work to produce physiological responses via hormones seeping out of the pituitary gland. Meanwhile, our behavior and reactions to the environment also can feed back to the brain, changing and fine-tuning the mind. In this "decade of the brain," many of us are learning to take control of our physical health—but what about our mental health? Ultimately, the two are joined, with one always

NO MAD COWS HERE

In the past, PS was extracted from bovine brains to be sold in supplement form. With the recent outbreak of mad cow disease in Britain, it is important to know that bovine PS is now rarely to be found in stores—if it can be found at all. Instead, a soy version of PS is currently on the market, which is not only safer than the bovine derivative but also just as effective in protecting neurons and preserving memory function.

affecting the other. The remarkable ability to remember someone's face, to reason through a difficult situation, and to simply take note of all the wonderful things life has to offer all depends on the continued strength of your mental faculties. By using PS and ALC, you can ensure that your brain keeps running smoothly and working efficiently, and that your mind can work its wonders for a lifetime.

HOW MUCH SHOULD I TAKE?

For General Health

Age 50 and over: 50-100 mg (PS), 100-200 mg (ALC)/day

Divided doses before meals

Special Conditions

Memory	150-300 mg/day (PS), 500-2,000 mg/day (ALC)
Physical stress	150-300 mg/day (PS)
Mood	150-300 mg/day (PS)
Alzheimer's Disease	150-300 mg/day (PS), 500-2,000 mg/day (ALC)
Peripheral neuropathy	150-300 mg/day (PS), 500-2,000 mg/day (ALC)

20

Branched Chain Amino Acids: Building Blocks for Strength and the Musculoskeletal System

Long before the appearance of life, the earth was awash in a primeval soup of simple chemicals like water and ammonia. At some mysterious point that soup began to form more complex molecules—perhaps triggered by ultraviolet light or sparks of lightning. Those molecules are called amino acids. Life itself was still a long way off, but even now, billions of years later, amino acids are the key to our survival. Why? Because, like bricks that form a house, they are the building blocks for protein—from meat and legumes to fish to eggs. We couldn't survive without them.

Amino acids are also enormously efficient and versatile nutraceuticals: they can act as fuel for the body, as precursors for most of the major neurotransmitters, as antiviral substances, and even as immune system stimulants. There are eight essential and sixteen nonessential amino acids in the body. We cannot make the eight essential amino acids ourselves, and our very survival depends on our frequent intake of them. Often, we can manufacture the other sixteen amino acids, though sometimes we can't make enough and may need to supplement them.

I think of all amino acids as the alphabet of the body: out of them we make many of the words our brain and body use to communicate with each other. Small chains of amino acids are known as peptides. Opiates are one example, and the brain chemical serotonin is another. Our bodies are literally studded with peptide receptors. They have been found to regulate mood and even behavior. In fact, Candace Pert, Ph.D., author of the book *Molecules of Emotion*, writes quite bluntly: "Peptides are the biochemical correlate of emotion." In other words, they are the way our body creates and regulates emotion. Longer chains of amino acids are just as important: they form the proteins that have built our bodies, particularly our muscles.

We often don't realize how much we need amino acids. Consider that every ten seconds our bone marrow makes 25 million red blood cells and every ten days our body replaces most of our white cells. This constant generating of new cells could not occur without amino acids.

Perhaps the most versatile are a group of three essential amino acids known as branched chain amino acids (BCAAs)—they are valine, leucine, and isoleucine. They are so named because of their similar chemical structure, which includes a carbon chain that branches. Although each one can function alone, they often work together. They make up a full 50 percent of the essential amino acids in our daily food supply.

I feel these substances have been overlooked in nutritional medicine. Until recently, the healing impact of amino acids has not been understood, and research into their effects has only gotten attention in the last ten years. BCAAs as a group are a bit complicated to study, since as a group of three they have an effect, yet each has individual effects as well. They are a unique class of nutrients. Our body relies on BCAAs in several absolutely crucial ways, perhaps most importantly for preserving muscles. Our skeletal muscles also use BCAAs as an energy source. In fact, BCAAs combined with weight-loss diets may actually help us firm up faster. But BCAAs also help to protect us from stress, repair the body after surgery, heal cirrhosis of the liver, and even in some cases help fitful sleeping or insomnia. BCAAs have also been studied in other arenas, although the research is preliminary: for example, BCAAs have been used in cases of the devastating neurological disease amyotrophic lateral sclerosis, or Lou Gehrig's disease, which leads to slow paralysis and death. They may even help in some cases of diabetes, as well as in treating the mood disorders associated with PMS.

Here's just a sampling of the studies proving the benefits of supplements of BCAAs all over the body:

- BCAAs protect the liver from damage. A study in animals found that BCAAs could protect the liver from the poisonous solvent called carbon tetrachloride.

- BCAAs can aid in weight-loss programs. When competitive wrestlers were given BCAAs and put on a weight-loss diet, they lost 34 percent more stomach fat than wrestlers who didn't take BCAAs.

- BCAAs can treat sleep apnea, one of the most common and dangerous sleep disorders, in which the sleeper periodically stops breathing. One study in 1994 showed that BCAAs make breathing easier; when children were studied, BCAAs reduced the average number of apnea episodes each night from fifty-eight to eleven.

- BCAAs improve recovery rates and increase energy after surgery. In nine elderly patients who had coronary bypass operations, BCAA supplements improved patients' fatigue.

- In other preliminary studies, doses of 10 grams of leucine daily helped sufferers of Parkinson's disease, while another study of all three BCAAs found them to be helpful in Lou Gehrig's disease. Of the nine participants, eight reported benefits from BCAAs over the one-year period of this small but intriguing study: the subjects maintained their muscle strength and mobility. However, of the nine Lou Gehrig's disease sufferers who did not receive BCAAs, five lost their ability to walk.

- If taken on a daily basis, BCAAs may improve athletic ability. Whether you're a runner, tennis player, or wrestler, BCAAs can build muscle tone, burn burdensome fat, and provide spurts of energy for high-intensity exercises like sprinting. Studies of marathon runners show they run faster and with greater endurance if they take BCAAs. The *British Journal of Sports Medicine* found that in long-lasting interval sports like tennis, BCAAs are an important energy source. Other studies indicate that even when BCAAs don't improve performance, they lessen the individual's feeling of fatigue, making exercise "feel" easier.

Marathon Madness

Taylor Stevens was a sickly child who grew into a wiry adult prone to colds and illness. But despite—or perhaps because of—his weakness, Taylor had always aspired to be an athletic star. His particular goal was to run the New York Marathon—and finish near the top. Determined to build strength and speed from an early age, Taylor would jog laps around the school gym after elementary school let out, often stopping to puff on his asthma inhaler, which concerned his protective mother. He convinced his father to buy him a bench press and free weights for Christmas one year, so he could pump iron every night before bed.

Ultimately, his persistence paid off. By high school, Taylor had become a key sprinter on the track team and even won a track scholarship to a prestigious southern university. Although he never quite lost his asthma or his susceptibility to other respiratory illnesses, he was able to run consistently and cleanly in practically every race, earning the respect of teammates and rivals alike. And while he was never able to build muscle bulk, his thin, sturdy frame still served him well on the track, where he was expected to be agile and swift.

When Taylor moved to Manhattan after college graduation, it looked like his dreams of a strong finish in the New York Marathon were right on track. True to his hard-working nature, he trained so thoroughly from the first day he arrived in the city that he was able to run the marathon his very first year in the Big Apple. Unfortunately, he didn't do so well. While training, Taylor had contracted the flu several times and developed chronic fatigue syndrome. Needless to say, the experience had been much more grueling than necessary. Taylor was determined to run the marathon the next year and finish with a better time, but he knew that he would need help. Chained to allergy pills, inhalers, and nasal sprays as a kid, however, Taylor was adamantly opposed to taking miracle drugs or steroids, and he hoped that better nutrition might improve his marathon mileage. He called me to see if there were natural alternatives for a struggling athlete in need of strength.

As it turns out, there was quite a lot. I tailored a special program for Taylor to address every part of the body that is impacted by rigorous training. My program included free radical fighters such as vitamins E and C, N-acetyl cysteine (which is helpful for respiratory function), lipoic acid (a powerful antioxidant that is both water and fat soluble), and a proper diet high in complex carbohydrates, including whole-grain pastas and rice. These carbohydrates help the muscles store energy in the form of a sugar called glycogen. Marathon runners have a high need for this sugar, and it seems to enhance their performance. This is especially important in sports in which endurance is important. I also included immune-boosting nutrients such as astragalus and echinacea, and glutamine—it is well-known that intensive exercise can actually suppress the immune system, and studies have shown that marathon runners are at greater risk for upper respiratory infections due to depleted levels of glutamine.

I also included nutrients to help preserve muscle, and the key was BCAAs. Research suggests that BCAAs can provide the competitive edge that he was lacking. I'd seen a study in the *British Journal of Sports Medicine* that tested eight nationally ranked tennis players. Exercise caused a 14 percent decrease in BCAAs, and it was found that supplements can actually replenish your stores. Other studies have shown that during intense exercise BCAAs are used up by muscles, and in one study five men who exercised to the point of exhaustion showed falling blood levels of BCAAs. Boosting Taylor's BCAAs could potentially protect him from tiring quickly and losing strength. These athletic amino acids also helped Taylor increase his endurance, diminishing the wheezing and breathlessness that he often experienced due to his asthma and frequent colds. One study showed that BCAAs worked better than a solution containing all amino acids in increasing the ability to breathe in healthy individuals. In another series of studies, BCAAs were shown to help premature babies breathe more easily. How do BCAAs enhance breathing? It seems they actually decrease the amount of carbon dioxide in your blood, which means that your lungs don't have to work as hard to blow out as much.

A few months before the next marathon, Taylor reported that training was much more productive than it had been the year before. He was able to run progressively faster and more continuously as the marathon grew nearer—and as his treatment plan continued—since he felt stronger and could go longer without losing his breath. By the time the marathon rolled around, he was confident enough, healthy enough, and energetic enough to perform well.

Exercise Your Heart

BCAAs protect all muscles—including the one that keeps us alive, the heart. An Israeli study of BCAAs in heart attacks found that BCAAs actually protected the heart against damage, enhanced recovery, and even improved heart function. That's why BCAAs were an essential treatment for Vic Trahane, a fifty-five-year-old radio announcer who first came to see me as a heart patient. His cardiologist had referred him to me for a nutritional consultation. In the past few years, he'd had several small attacks, and with a five-year-old boy to take care of, he was increasingly concerned about preventing any massive attacks headed his way. Unlike many patients with heart problems, and the stereotype of such individuals, Vic was neither sedentary nor overweight. As a matter of fact, Vic's heart problems were causing him to lose weight, strength, and muscle tone. Most people don't realize that even the thin and active can fall victim to heart disease; but genetic predispositions, high cholesterol, and high levels of homocysteine can lurk where we least expect them. Vic was actually an avid sportsman, filling his nights and weekends with pickup basketball games, squash, tennis, baseball, running, and boxing classes.

The mystery of Vic's heart attacks was revealed when I investigated his nutritional profile. Although he ate a fairly healthy low-fat diet replete with fruits and vegetables, he also ate bagels for breakfast every morning. His elevated triglyceride levels, a risk factor for heart disease, showed that he was probably sensitive to these carbohydrates. He also had high homocysteine levels, indicating a possible deficiency of B vitamins. Weak, tired, and rundown, Vic needed strength and nutritional fortification. In the months since the heart attacks began, he had lost fifteen pounds.

In addition to cutting down his carbs and boosting his B vitamin supplementation, I gave him magnesium and essential fatty acids like fish oils to help reduce the triglycerides, fats, and cholesterol that lead to heart disease. But to make sure that

Vic not only protected his heart from further damage but also regained his healthy muscle tone and athletic ability, I prescribed a trio of strength builders: BCAAs, whey, and creatine (see boxes). Numerous recent studies herald the abilities of creatine and whey in enhancing muscle performance and providing energy spurts necessary for weight training. A study from the Karolinska Institute in Sweden not only found that creatine improved the ability to build muscle but also suggested it as a novel treatment for cardiovascular disease.

This combination has proved effective. Vic slowly put on weight as his strength improved. As his muscles grew larger and more powerful, he regained his natural energy and athletic prowess. He is back to leaping tall buildings in a single bound, without his heart jumping in the way.

But BCAAs may do more than just protect muscles. They actually seem to make exercise more enjoyable by reducing the feeling of fatigue. One ingenious study tested cross-country runners on their ability to match words and colors both before and after a thirty-kilometer race. Half the runners were given a drink rich in carbohydrates, and half were given one rich in both carbohydrates and BCAAs. The runners who received BCAAs actually had improved test scores after exercise.

Exercisers report less mental fatigue after being given BCAAs. In a Scandinavian study, seven trained cyclists exercised for one hundred minutes, stopping every ten minutes to rate their mental fatigue. Some of the cyclists were given a placebo drink, and the others were given a drink enriched with BCAAs. The second group rated their fatigue as 15 percent lower.

It's fascinating, and a little mysterious. Although regular exercise is a known antidepressant (it boosts endorphins, the body's natural feel-good opiates), exercise also leads to a high concentration of serotonin in the brain. Serotonin can lead to a feeling of calm but can also cause drowsiness and sleepiness—which, for an athlete, may be a problem. BCAAs seem to prevent this.

Restful Sleep

BCAAs have helped some of my patients sleep more deeply and wake more rested. One patient, Liz Kramer, suffered from multiple chemical sensitivities and allergies. Though she ate carefully, avoiding foods to which she was sensitive, and lived in a clean air-filtered apartment, she found she was having trouble sleeping through the night.

"If I wake up at three or four," she said. "I can't go back to sleep for a few hours. Then I'm tired when I get to work. And this has been going on for months."

As editor of a national magazine, with only a small staff, Liz needed her sleep in order to keep her mind sharp and alert. She also complained that months of sleep deprivation had left her irritable and edgy and that she recently had been snapping at her colleagues.

It turned out that Liz was a victim of sleep apnea, a condition that causes sufferers to stop breathing momentarily during the night, often leading to snoring but sometimes leading to death by airway obstruction. Apnea is rare in young women and usually strikes older men who have loose flesh in the throat, which can lead to air blockage. Because apnea wakes individuals throughout the night, I knew that Liz would need some help making it through the night.

Because Liz was chemically sensitive, she refused to take sleeping medication. Even sleep-inducing herbs like valerian and kava left her feeling as if she had a "chemical hangover," she said. I suggested she try two capsules of branched chain amino acids, on an empty stomach before bedtime.

The next week she reported that, from the first night, she had slept without waking. "I don't know how they work, but they definitely do work. It's as if the sun has finally broken through the clouds. I'm feeling rested again."

Healing from Surgery

Anna Miller had been through a harrowing ordeal with breast cancer. At the age of thirty-four, she had been diagnosed with a malignant tumor in her left breast, and was eventually scheduled for a mastectomy. Although she knew surgery was inevitable, she came to me to see what she could do to make the surgery as painless and simple as possible.

Few patients realize that there are nutritional steps they can take before surgery to reduce complications and hasten recovery. With patients like Anna, I like to use a whole host of antioxidants such as vitamin E and carotenoids for a few weeks before the procedure. After surgery, I ask patients to continue with the antioxidants, which fight free radicals that can hinder skin from healing properly. This was part of the recovery program I prescribed for Anna. In addition, I asked Anna to use zinc and 250-500 milligrams of vitamin C daily to keep her body healthy while it worked to recover from the injury of the mastectomy. I also suggested that she apply aloe topically over her scar to soothe any pain and visible damage. Finally, I told her to take BCAAs to speed the healing process. BCAAs aren't just for athletes trying to improve performance; patients who receive BCAAs after surgery feel more energetic. This may simply be because BCAAs seem to reduce serotonin in the brain and thus make us feel less fatigued. When BCAAs have been given in intravenous form to malnourished surgical patients, they have recovered faster. In this case, BCAAs probably work by preventing the breakdown of muscle, since BCAAs are used by the body as fuel in starvation. The body of a malnourished, ill patient will be able to use BCAAs directly rather than breaking down muscle protein in order to "feed" itself.

No matter how one prepares for a procedure as life changing as breast surgery, it is certain to be traumatic. Anna had to resign herself to the idea of losing her breast, and she faced psychological issues of damaged self-image and stress about her fate. But with the help of BCAAs and other healing nutrients, she was able to focus more on learning to handle the life issues raised by breast cancer without having to worry about staying healthy.

Lose Weight, Not Muscle

BCAAs may be a safe way for wrestlers and body builders to lose weight without taking steroids or loading up on excessive protein powders. A study of twenty-five competitive wrestlers who went on a low-calorie diet for nineteen days found that the wrestlers who took BCAA supplements lost the most weight and had the greatest decrease in body fat. At the same time, their performance levels stayed constant, suggesting that BCAAs not only helped them on their diets but also kept muscles intact. Another study of sixteen individuals trekking for three straight weeks in the mountains found that all sixteen lost weight, but only those who took BCAAs actually had a gain in muscle mass.

Steroids are a dangerous—not to mention illegal—way to bulk up, and I am wholeheartedly against athletes using them for strength and muscle. BCAAs, on the other hand, are often a part of a program I use to enhance muscle gain and weight loss in my patients the safe and natural way. One of my patients, for example, was a 250-pound man who decided he wanted to be a wrestler. After years of following the sport and reading about the training regimen, Andy Jacobs was determined to try his hand at it. He certainly had the muscular build and short, stocky stature of a wrestler. There was an amateur competition in a month, but Andy would have to lose twenty pounds before he could meet the weight requirement. Luckily, knowing the dangers of weight-loss drugs and unwilling to commit himself to an unhealthy starvation diet, Andy came to me seeking a natural way to lose fat without sparing muscle. I've read frightening reports of wrestlers doing anything—including risking their lives—to get down to the right weight. This mindset needs to change. While athletic excellence is an admirable pursuit, it should not endanger health. Strict guidelines must be followed so aspiring wrestlers, gymnasts, and track stars don't die trying to achieve their best.

Having read the studies supporting BCAAs as a weight control tool for wrestlers, I decided to start him on daily doses of them under my guidance, to help him lose body fat and build muscle bulk. I also made sure that he drank plenty of fluids, since it's extremely important for athletes to stay hydrated in order to keep up energy and maintain strength. In the next month, Andy was able to lose almost fifteen pounds. In conjunction with a healthy diet and a heavy weight-training routine, Andy made it to the semifinals of his next wrestling tournament.

I recommend taking BCAAs during times of intense training and recovery for most athletes. Doses of 4 grams a day are often sufficient, but in cases of heavy training or for weight lifting as much as 6 grams a day can be used. For the occasional athlete, adding 2 grams a day is sufficient. As with most supplements, it's always a good idea to cycle your nutrient regimen and allow your body to balance itself and clear itself of any excess nutrients. A break of at least a few weeks, and up to a few months, is wise. This is particularly true if you are not chronically ill and just want to use supplements to enhance your performance or health. Remember, the body does have its own wisdom, and even the most powerful nutraceuticals are not necessarily recommended for daily use for months or years at a time.

Stay Strong

Because amino acids are the building blocks of every muscle, from our hearts to our biceps, they are a natural choice for aspiring athletes and hardened trainers hoping to build strength and lose unwanted fat. Especially with a regular exercise program and diet designed to build bulk, BCAAs can give the body energy and muscular protection necessary for many high-intensity sports. But because muscles keep all parts of our bodies going, BCAAs can help even those not aspiring for defined arms or an Olympic Gold. From keeping the heart pumping to facilitating a good night's sleep, BCAAs are your best bet for building strength and good health in energy-depleting situations from surgery to exercise training.

I LOVE LEUCINE

Leucine is a particularly interesting BCAA. It is the only amino acid that the body can use instead of glucose when fasting. It's actually an alternative energy source and can help maintain blood sugar levels. Leucine also seems to protect the liver. Low levels of leucine have been found in patients with liver disease.

Finally, some studies show that leucine stimulates the release of insulin. Insulin stimulates muscles to synthesize protein. Leucine actually promotes this protein synthesis and protects muscle. Leucine is also present in large amounts in pain-relieving peptides in the body known as enkephalins.

CURDS AND WHEY

In order to obtain extra amounts of BCAAs in your diet, you don't just have to take supplements. Whey protein, naturally found in human breast milk, is high in BCAAs, works to help build muscles, and is used by many bodybuilders. And it's actually good for your health: whey is composed of strange-sounding substances like alpha-lactoglobulin, beta-lactoglobulin, and, most important, immunoglobulins (such as IgG, IgA, and IgM). Immunoglobulins are a major source of your immune system's first line of defense. Whey is even rich in the building blocks for glutathione, which, as you may remember from chapter 7, is the liver's most powerful antioxidant. Glutathione levels have been shown to decrease with exercise, and a whey-rich diet has been shown to increase the level of glutathione in the livers of animals. Whey is rapidly absorbed by the body. Some physicians recommend a carbohydrate and whey protein drink to athletes after exercise. Perhaps the one concern about whey protein is for individuals with milk allergy.

HOW MUCH SHOULD I TAKE?

For General Health
See special conditions below, as needed
Divided doses before meals or bedtime.

Special Conditions

Sleep apnea/Insomnia	1,000-2,000 mg with water before bedtime
Post-surgery recovery	1,000-2,000 mg
Parkinson's	1,000-2,000 mg
Athletic performance	500-2,000 mg
Exercise-induced fatigue	500-2,000 mg
Heart disease/recovery	1,000-2,000 mg
Weight training	2-4 grams before exercise or in divided doses throughout the day

21

1) Red Clover
2) Dong Quai
3) Black Cohosh:

A Woman's Remedy—Menopause Hot Flashes

One out of three women experience PMS, or premenstrual syndrome, and for many women the symptoms can be crippling.

Take the case of Jane Blauer, a twenty-seven-year-old graduate student with agonizing menstrual cramps. Her PMS was so painful—and she lived in such dread of it—that it seemed to begin a week in advance. Bloating, headaches, excruciating cramps, breast tenderness, irritability, and violent mood swings heralded the arrival of her "monthly friend." Although naturally a compassionate, good-natured woman, Jane would become so cranky and withdrawn that her colleagues in the English department thought she was pretentious, condescending, and self-important. When suffering from PMS, she seemed unable to stop the caustic barbs flying out of her mouth. Because she figured that such monthly pain was to be her destiny, she never mentioned the condition to her physicians.

It was only when Jane came to see me about another health concern, her frequent colds, that I discovered her history of troubling PMS.

"Why don't you let me prescribe you some natural herbs and supplements to balance your menstrual cycle," I suggested.

Jane was silent for a moment, then looked at me with a mixture of hope, surprise, and bitterness.

"You mean there are things I could have been taking all along to stop my PMS?" she asked. "I'm not sure I believe you."

Like Jane, most women aren't told about nutrients they can take to relieve their monthly burden but only about pain-relieving drugs like Advil or Midol.

When I talked with Jane about her daily life, I realized that her diet may have been aggravating her PMS. She was always on the go or buried in a book, too preoccupied to worry about eating nutritious foods, instead grabbing whatever was most convenient: junk food. To enhance her paltry stipend as a graduate student, Jane worked nights at a local diner, where sodas, greasy burgers, and fries were readily available. Whether in class or reading in the library, Jane always found a vending machine that offered all too convenient and unhealthy replacements for good square meals. On weekends, she would sleep late and open her fridge, only to realize that she'd forgotten to go grocery shopping during the week. Somehow, though, there always seemed to be a stash of chocolate bars or ice cream in the freezer, and Jane would often munch on that in place of breakfast, lunch, or dinner.

This haphazard diet was probably one of the main causes of Jane's struggles with PMS. Although many women view themselves as helpless victims of the swirling hormones that drive the menstrual cycle, their lifestyle may play a large part in their suffering. Eating a nutritious diet packed with fruits, vegetables, essential fatty acids, calcium, and soy (which gently balances hormones) and eliminating sugar, salt, alcohol, and caffeine can go a long way toward reducing the cramps, headaches, and tenderness associated with PMS. Regular exercise can also help prevent PMS and, later in life, alleviate menopausal symptoms.

I implored Jane to start eating planned, balanced meals through the course of her day, augmenting her new diet with regular exercise, even if that simply meant brisk strolls across campus. I asked her to take magnesium for her headaches, primrose oil to balance her hormones, and flaxseed powder to cleanse her system.

Most important, to calm the careening hormones that were likely exacerbating her PMS, I gave her capsules of the dried root of black cohosh, a flowering plant that has long been a valued remedy for many ailments of the female reproductive system. From the pain of PMS to the struggle of childbirth and the discomfort of menopause, black cohosh is an herbal rescue remedy, normalizing the constantly fluctuating hormones that characterize a woman's monthly menstrual cycle.

Within six months, Jane had noticed a significant improvement in her symptoms. The first annoyance to disappear was her breast tenderness, followed quickly by her bloating. After a few more months, her cramps and finally even her mood swings were few and far between. Jane's friends and classmates began to think she was a completely different person and ultimately forgot what a crank she had once been. But Jane will always remember how hard it was to live life with PMS, and she continues to monitor her diet—and to take black cohosh.

Whether you're facing the perils of PMS or the monsters of menopause, black cohosh, red clover, and dong quai is the herb for women. When the intricate hormonal harmony of the menstrual cycle goes off-key, black cohosh is the herb that puts the reproductive system back in tune. It is there as a useful remedy to get you back in sync with the natural rhythms of your own body.

Managing the Menstrual Cycle

Perhaps the best-known herb for to menopause is black cohosh. Black cohosh, an herb native to the woods and riverbanks of North America, is a perennial plant capped with a plume of white flowers that often grows to eight feet. It was used early in our country's history by Native Americans and colonists as a natural medicine seemingly tailored for women and their biological needs. From menstrual cramps, dysmenorrhea (painful menstruation), and amenorrhea (missed periods) to childbirth, gynecological disorders, and menopausal hot flashes, black cohosh has long been prized as an important herb for women in every stage of their reproductive life.

Although black cohosh appears to be a strange name for a delicate white bloom, it's the knotted dark root of the plant that exerts its powers. In this root lie three phytoestrogenic compounds, or plant estrogens, which work together to mimic the effects of estrogens that are created in the body and govern women's menstrual cycles by binding to receptors in our reproductive organs. A German study confirmed that black cohosh has hormonelike properties.

While the exact hormonal causes of the symptoms of PMS and menopause, such as irritability, cramps, and hot flashes, are still unknown, it's safe to say that black cohosh makes periods—and the menopausal lack thereof—a much less painful proposition by balancing the fluxing hormones involved in the monthly reproductive cycle. This member of the buttercup family may relieve the pain and discomfort of "female problems" by reducing the amounts of luteinizing hormone (LH) circulating through the body. LH is a midcycle hormone, and hot flashes, in particular, seem to correlate with surges of LH. A review in the journal *Planta Medica* reports that black cohosh decreased the rise in LH associated with menopause in both animal and human studies.

Research shows that black cohosh extracts were used as early as 1940 to soothe premenstrual, dysmenorrheal, or menopausal symptoms. It can also diminish labor pains, pre—and postchildbirth discomfort, pelvic disturbances, and uterine problems. But black cohosh isn't strictly a remedy for the trials of the reproductive cycle. Studies such as the review in the *British Herbal Compendium* reveal that this dried root was traditionally—and is currently—used to treat rheumatism, rheumatoid arthritis, high blood pressure, low-grade depression, and tinnitus. It can also expel mucus from the lungs, relieve spasmodic conditions like recurrent coughs, and induce sedation.

Although a valued ancient remedy of the Native Americans, today black cohosh is most commonly used in Europe; it's been incorporated into clinical medicine in Germany since the 1950s. The German Commission E, which regulates and sets the world standard for use of herbs, has approved this dried root for use in fighting premenstrual discomfort, dysmenorrhea, and menopausal conditions. There are three standardized extracts of black cohosh sold on the market and used as natural alternatives to synthetic hormone-replacement therapy, which stimulate estrogen receptors in the body to combat diseases like osteoporosis. The most widely used and studied extract of black cohosh weakly binds with these receptors, unlike synthetic hormones, which bind more aggressively and can cause breast or endometrial cancer over the long term. Black cohosh has an excellent safety record in Germany and has been shown in several studies to produce better results than conjugated estrogens in relieving common menopausal symptoms such as hot flashes, vaginal atrophy, depression, and anxiety. It may also help with the mood swings, depression, and tension of PMS.

In combination with other nutrients, such as chaste berry and magnesium, that work at hormone receptors in the body to ease them through the menstrual and reproductive process, black cohosh is truly a woman's helper. I have found that many common hormonal problems can resolve themselves with the aid of black cohosh. It should be taken daily throughout the cycle, and usually within a few months will have helped a woman get back in sync with her own natural, healthy hormonal rhythms.

Understanding PMS

Whether you're a young woman just learning to live with PMS or a more mature woman settling into menopause, the dizzying dance of hormones waltzing through the body each month, driven by the music of the menstrual cycle, can wreak havoc with your mental and physical well-being.

Premenstrual syndrome is a recurrent condition that usually occurs in the week or two before menstruation. This part of the menstrual cycle is known as the luteal phase, just after the monthly egg has been released from the ovaries and the corpus luteum (egg sac) remains in its place. The corpus luteum is of special importance since it stimulates the production of estrogen and progesterone and stimulates the uterine lining to build up and thicken in preparation for the egg, in the event that pregnancy occurs and the egg implants into the lining. If this hormone production is not timed precisely—if, for example, progesterone production is delayed an extra day or too much estrogen is released—abnormal menstrual cycles, increased blood loss, or PMS symptoms may result. There is a seemingly endless list of symptoms associated with PMS, everything from irritability, depression, and altered sex drive to cramps, abdominal bloating, and backaches. It can also lead to acne, cravings, bowel movement dysfunction, worsening respiratory function in asthmatics, and joint pain.

For many years, PMS was not even recognized as a real medical condition. Even now, some people deride it as an imaginary illness, an excuse for complaints or mood swings. For many women, however, the symptoms of PMS are all too real. The physical and emotional problems resulting from PMS vary from woman to woman, and their intensity waxes and wanes through the reproductive years, often diminishing after childbirth, although some women never lose these symptoms. Unfortunately, because PMS is often misdiagnosed or dismissed, many women fail to get properly treated for their symptoms. At one point, a system was devised to categorize different types of PMS; PMS A was associated with anxiety, PMS H with bloating and hyperhydration, PMS D with depression, and PMS C with carbohydrate cravings. I don't find these classifications useful, however, since most cases of PMS I see incorporate many of these symptoms, the predominant problems being cravings, depression, and weight gain.

Although PMS has been identified as a monthly medical phenomenon since the 1930s, its cause is still unknown. Researchers surmise that its roots are an interplay between hormones, diet, psychological factors, genetics, and underlying medical conditions. Some doctors believe that PMS stems from ovarian dysfunction. Other researchers have proposed that PMS arises from a neurotransmitter imbalance, such as a deficit of serotonin, a thyroid imbalance, a testosterone deficiency, or an inadequate production of essential fatty acids. Some scientists suggest that yet another trigger for PMS might be the excess of harsh, synthetic estrogens found in the environment, from pesticides and plastics to meat and produce. The causes may be wide and varying, and we still haven't even begun to tease them out into a definite cause-and-effect relationship.

Often antidepressants such as Prozac or benzodiazepines like Valium are prescribed for PMS sufferers, but these drugs can be harmful and unnecessary. When I see symptoms of PMS, I first try to rule out other health concerns, such as hypothyroidism or depression unrelated to or exacerbating PMS. The most common causes for PMS-like symptoms I see include excess estrogen coursing through the body, decreased progesterone levels, thyroid dysfunction, nutrient deficiencies, and liver toxicity. Frequent alcohol intake, medications, imbalanced intestinal flora, and low fiber intake can increase discomfort. When these imbalances are corrected, often symptoms including cramps and depression improve.

The Perils of PMS

Most women with PMS experience a defined set of symptoms every month like clockwork, and they can predict the onset of one symptom almost to the day. Elaine Carrington, a thirty-four-year-old fashion designer, could set her watch by the onset of PMS. Exactly a week before her period would begin, a cluster of acne would pop up on her chin. A few days later, without fail, she would experience flulike feelings, hot flashes, insomnia, sudden depression, and severe cramps: in short, all the classic symptoms of PMS. These problems would last until the third day of her period, then disappear without a trace.

But each month, they disrupted her life. Unable to sleep, she would stumble into

HORMONE HELPERS

There are many of other nutrients that excel at the very same thing. Not all of these nutrients will work for every woman, so don't give up hope if you've tried one and failed to see the results: there may be another hormone helper better suited to your specific menstrual problem and body type.

Chaste Berry: Found in Europe, this plant earned its name because it was used to suppress libido. However, it's also a star at suppressing PMS. A review in the *Journal of Obstetrics and Gynecology* noted that it had improved symptoms in 90 percent of the subjects studied. Numerous European studies also validate its effects. Chaste berry seems to work on the hypothalamus and the pituitary gland in the brain to reduce an overabundance of prolactin or to fix a lack of progesterone. Because amenorrhea, the absence of a menstrual cycle, is caused by prolactin excess, I have also used chaste berry for patients to restore their periods. The plant often comes as a tincture, and patients can start on about ten drops a day and increase the dose up to about forty drops a day if necessary—until their symptoms resolve.

Dong Quai: Extremely popular in Asia, where it is second only to ginseng, dong quai is an invaluable part of my natural approach to easing the pain of both PMS and menopause. This plant is most effective two weeks before a period and can help during menstruation to relieve dysmenorrhea. Dong quai can also be used to promote uterine relaxation during pregnancy to facilitate labor. Dosage: 500 milligrams twice a day.

Licorice: Like chaste berry, licorice seems to enhance the production of progesterone and probably lowers amounts of estrogen by competing with the hormone at estrogen receptors. Because licorice may block aldosterone, an enzyme that blocks the breakdown of progesterone, high doses may lead to aldosterone excess, which can cause increased blood pressure and water retention. Thus, I don't recommend this particular nutrient for patients with hypertension or renal disease. Dosage: 100 milligrams twice a day.

Magnesium: A magnesium deficiency is a strong causative factor for PMS, reported a study in the *International Nutrition Clinical Reviews*. Perhaps this is why magnesium is one of my favorite remedies for the cramps associated with PMS. A 1991 study in the *Journal of Obstetrics and Gynecology* showed that magnesium also improved the foul mood often associated with PMS, and a study in the *Journal of Reproductive Medicine* found that about 95 percent of patients with PMS studied showed a reduction in symptoms like weight gain and breast tenderness. I recommend 200 milligrams of magnesium daily.

B Vitamins: The B vitamins, instrumental in fighting heart disease and preventing birth defects, are also remarkably effective in treating PMS. Studies in the *British Journal of Obstetrics and Gynecology* and the *Journal of the American College of Nutrition* confirm that B_6 has been used in numerous trials to relieve PMS symptoms like water retention. A 1987 study also showed that B_6 improved sociability and cognitive performance in women with PMS; 200 to 600 milligrams daily seems to elevate progesterone levels and lower estrogen. Dosage: Start with 50 milligrams daily.

Red Clover: One of my favorite natural remedy for women. A recent study from New York University showed that red clover had about thirty times the amount of natural estrogen as soy, a well-reputed hormone balancer. Red clover also seemed to diminish hot flashes in each of the twenty-five women studied. Dosage: As a tincture—20 drops daily in warm water.

Vitamin E: This vitamin has also shown promise in alleviating weight gain, breast tenderness, and other symptoms of PMS. The *Journal of the American College of Nutrition* found that 400 units daily reduced symptoms by 33 percent.

work exhausted. She would often arrive late, since her cramps would keep her curled up in bed until she could muster the strength to get up and get ready. The last doctor she'd seen had tried sleep medications for her symptoms, but her problems continued. Finally, she resigned herself to a life of monthly pain. At work, her friends commiserated with her, sharing their own PMS war stories, and she decided that if every other woman could handle it, so could she.

But she didn't have to. For the past few years, I'd treated Elaine for allergies, and she'd responded quite well to these natural treatments. When she offhandedly mentioned her PMS one month, ruefully joking about it, I suggested that we try a number of herbs to treat her debilitating symptoms. Figuring that her discomfort couldn't get any worse, Elaine told me that she was agreeable.

First, I prescribed red clover, to balance out the abnormal hormone surges that may cause PMS. Two other plants that are soothing treatments for menstrual distress are dong quai and licorice extract (see box on page 290), and I suggested that she try these as well. She began her anti-PMS regimen right after her next period, taking it faithfully every day but slightly doubtful that it would work. As her next period rolled around, she braced herself for the acne and cramps. In fact, her first fashion show was scheduled for the week before it was due, and she was dreading the pain, sleeplessness, and mood swings she'd have to endure while trying to produce the event.

But as the debut of her collection approached, Elaine became so immersed in organizing the last-minute details and finishing her collection she didn't even notice that, for the first time since her teens, she wasn't hampered by PMS. She was soaring with exhilaration, wearing a grin on her face, and cramp free, and if she had insomnia, it was only because she lay awake, planning each detail of the show so that it would go without a hitch. The show was a major success, and Elaine was basking in the glow of praise from friends and critics alike.

"When I first realized that I hadn't gotten cramps or acne or headaches, I thought I must be pregnant," she told me. "I can't believe how wonderful it feels to live completely free of PMS."

It was truly remarkable that her symptoms had disappeared in a single month. But study after study proves the efficacy of black cohosh and its companion nutrients in treating PMS. Elaine has recommended these supplements to her friends in the fashion world. As she said to me, "Why should any woman have to live in constant pain?"

Menopause

Menopause is defined as the date of a woman's last menstrual cycle and can be determined as such when a woman hasn't had her period for six months.

Hot flashes are probably the symptom most identified with menopause, although this time in a mature woman's life involves a constellation of physical and emotional changes. Most menopausal women experience hot flashes, and while some suffer them only occasionally, others have them twenty or more times a day. The obvious rise in body heat associated with hot flashes is often accompanied by anxiety, rapid heart rate, flushed skin, and profuse sweating. The feelings of heat occur primarily in the upper chest, neck, head, and shoulders, as well as the hands. The episodes themselves last about five minutes each, although variations occur. The progression of a hot flash begins with an increase in blood flow to the skin, causing flushing and a rise in temperature. The eventual reduction in body temperature often causes a chill afterward. Some women may also feel anxious, queasy, or uncomfortable after a hot flash.

Although hot flashes are the most common reason that women seek medical attention during menopause, other symptoms include insomnia and reduced sexual desire. The risk of medical problems like heart disease and osteoporosis also increases at this time in life.

We don't understand all the causes for menopausal symptoms; however, we do know that they are linked to a decrease in the production of estrogen. All of the female reproductive hormones, like LH and FSH (follicle stimulating hormone) probably play a role. For this reason, hormone-replacement therapy has been the standard treatment for hot flashes and the long-term problems associated with menopause. However, there has been increasing concern over this therapy, since the high levels of estrogen it employs lead to a high risk of uterine and breast cancer. There are, however, a number of alternative treatment possibilities that do not lead to these harmful results. Soy food, which can take on a natural anti-estrogenic or weak estrogenic effect, depending on whether there is too much or too little estrogen in the body, can balance our hormones. Changes in diet are particularly important to easing the body through menopause; flaxseed, fiber, and soy can restore the body to its optimal state. Proinflammatory foods like red meat can also aggravate symptoms. Finally, making sure that liver detoxification is proceeding properly will flush out any compounds that may be leading to menopausal symptoms.

Menopause and Blood Pressure

Although Nora Samuels, fifty-six, had gone through menopause six long years ago, she was still suffering hot flashes. She had initially tried hormone-replacement therapy, but the medications had made her feel even worse than she had before she began treatment. Over the years, her symptoms had even increased. If her hot flashes let up, Nora still felt fatigued and weary. Also after menopause, she found her blood pressure had gone up and a long-dormant problem with asthma had resurfaced. Finally, her husband complained that her sex drive had dropped considerably over the past few years.

When she asked me why menopause could have such seemingly random effects on the rest of her health, I explained that estrogen receptors are everywhere in the body, including blood vessels. Menopause causes high blood pressure when these receptors are no longer stimulated, due to the lack of hormones produced at this time. Estrogen is also a natural anti-inflammatory agent, so menopause can cause inflammation, aggravating asthma.

I put Nora on a comprehensive program of natural herbs containing phytoestrogenic compounds like black cohosh and dong quai. I also put her on foods like flaxseed and tofu, which can reduce the symptoms of menopause while helping to protect the body from uterine and breast cancer.

After about six months, I tested Nora's blood pressure and found that it was notably lower than before. Her breathing was also much easier, and tests of pulmonary function showed much improvement. She also liked the switch from hormone-replacement therapy to small oral doses of natural supplements; she felt more energetic, as if she weren't taking medication at all. Finally, this herbal combination lessened the intensity of her hot flashes. While they didn't entirely disappear, they diminished to just one or two a day, which she found much more manageable.

PMS, Menopause, and Depression

Most women don't think about menopause until it actually occurs; it's one of those conditions that is banished from conversation until it strikes, and even then endured in silence. Carolyn Matthews, however, was a forty-six-year-old art gallery owner who was intensely worried about the onset of menopause.

"I know it's going to hit me one of these days," she said, "and I know it's going to be horrible."

Carolyn had already faced a traumatic bout with breast cancer, had undergone a mastectomy, and was receiving localized radiation therapy to prevent further damage. Because she knew that hormone-replacement therapy, the common treatment for serious menopausal symptoms, can cause or aggravate breast cancer, she refused to take such treatment.

Soon, Carolyn began to sink into depression, probably stemming from years of living with the ordeal of breast cancer and her fear of menopause. The mood alterations she suffered due to PMS didn't help her emotional stability, either. Luckily, I'd seen a number of studies showing that black cohosh and St. John's wort, an increasingly popular natural antidepressant, work particularly well together. A report in the *Quarterly Review of Natural Medicine* heartily endorses this combination in treating both the physical and emotional aspects of menopause. A German study showed that, of 812 menopausal women, 81 percent deemed the duo of black cohosh and St. John's wort "very good" or "good." Ninety percent noted a diminishment of their symptoms, including irritability, tension, fear, hot flashes, and insomnia. I also suggested that Carolyn eat broccoli and drink green tea, to prevent cancer.

Almost immediately, Carolyn began to feel more tranquil and optimistic. Of course, the mere act of taking these natural, research-proven supplements might have initially eased her mind. But the first physical evidence of their effectiveness was the virtual disappearance of her PMS-related cravings and headaches. By the time her period ceased and menopause set in, Carolyn felt mentally and physically prepared for any symptoms coming her way. At first, she experienced a series of persistent hot flashes. She kept taking her hormone-balancing nutrients, however, and six weeks after the onset of hot flashes, she began to notice a decrease in the number of flashes she sweated out per day. Now, two years after she first experienced her symptoms, Carolyn rarely gets hot flashes. Thanks to a host of complementary herbs, she has made the transition from PMS to menopause easily and relatively painlessly. Energetic and dedicated to her art gallery, Carolyn is able to put her stressful medical history behind her and focus on the joys in life.

Menopause and Arthritis

Many times, menopause can be masked as other medical conditions. When Maria Tamerin first came to my office, she complained of the joint pain and arthritis not uncommon among women in their fifties. Upon taking her medical history, however, I found that she had recently gone through menopause. Like most menopausal women, Maria hadn't realized that joint ailments and menopause are often related. Although she was taking a natural supplement targeted toward arthritic joints, glucosamine, the nutrient wasn't really helping her, which again suggested menopause as an underlying cause of the condition.

Maria had told her gynecologist that she had been experiencing hot flashes, and although he gave her estrogen replacement pills for her symptoms, she was worried about tampering with her hormone levels and never took the medication. I soon found that her medical history held other factors complicating her health. Heart disease, for example, ran in her family, and she was concerned about developing the condition. Her cholesterol was a steady 240, and her diet wasn't worrisome, though her fondness for bagels and cream cheese was something she needed to keep in check. While Maria was generally healthy, her joint pain and hot flashes were beginning to get her down, and she found herself succumbing to a mild depression. Finally, constipation was slowing her down and making her irritable.

When Maria came to me, seeking a milder alternative to estrogen replacement, my first order of business was to provide symptomatic relief of her hot flashes, using black cohosh, red clover, and dong quai. A daily soy drink that contains the phytoestrogen genistein also compensated for her depleting hormones. Essential fatty acids in the form of fish oil, invaluable to practically everyone to fend off myriad illnesses from asthma to heart disease, would help her arthritis. Finally, for her constipation, I suggested that she take 1 tablespoon of flaxseed powder in 8 ounces of water daily to cleanse her gastrointestinal system.

After two months, Maria was thrilled to notice a reduction in the stiffness in her hands, elbows, and fingers. She no longer had to rely on friends or family members to carry objects or open doors for her. Her hot flashes gradually began to diminish, her cholesterol went down to 220, and her HDL cholesterol profile improved from moderate to low risk. Although her hot flashes do trouble her from time to time, the dangers of synthetic or conjugated hormone-replacement therapy are too great in her eyes, and she continues to choose the natural alternative.

A Woman's Choice

Women's hormones are an intricate, delicate, and incredibly complex symphony—a symphony that is needed in order to carry out the miraculous feat of conception, pregnancy, childbirth, and nursing a newborn baby. This ever-shifting symphony can easily be thrown out of whack. To come back into balance, nature offers us a cornucopia of healing herbs. Each has its own particular gift to offer: black cohosh, red clover, and dong quai are the herbs that offers gentle plant hormones to balance

HOW MUCH SHOULD I TAKE?

Black Cohosh
For General Health
See special conditions below, as needed, after meals in one or divided doses

Special Conditions

PMS	500-1,000 mg/day
Menopause	500-2,000 mg/day
Dysmenorrhea	500-1,000 mg/day

Red Clover

PMS	40 mg
Hot flashes	40 mgs

problems like PMS and menopausal symptoms. It is the best known of all the women's herbs and has a long tradition of use in folk healing. Studies support its ability to balance hormones.

Herbs like chaste berry, dong quai, and even vitamins like magnesium and calcium play an important role in easing some of the symptoms of hormone imbalance.

And finally, like isoflavones found—in soy—are being studied now for their remarkable ability to help protect against hormone-related cancers.

The world of nutraceuticals has much to offer women—harmonizing the intricate symphony that the reproductive system must play each day and helping women offer the greatest gift of all: new human life.

Word of Caution

Recent studies have questioned the use of black cohosh for the treatment of hot flashes. Herbal supplements can vary widely in their active ingredients. Always choose the best supplements and talk to your physician before starting any nutritional program. Women with a family history of cancer or who may be at risk for cancer should avoid estrogen-containing herbs.

22

Saw Palmetto: A Man's Best Friend Prostate Health

Some medical conditions are embarrassing to talk about. Sexual impotence. Flagging libido. And problems of the prostate.

Though many patients come to me with these conditions, they are reluctant to discuss them frankly. That's a shame, because prostate problems—known as benign prostatic hypertrophy (BPH)—are one of the most common conditions facing middle-aged and elderly men. Fifty percent of men under the age of 60 and 90 percent of men by the age of eighty fall victim to BPH—alarmingly high numbers for an ailment that is kept so hush-hush in our society. The frequent urination, reduced sexual ability, that result from BPH are a serious matter, but apparently not life-threatening enough for men to admit to their friends, or even their physicians. Amid all this secrecy, surgery to correct this condition is performed on four hundred thousand men every year—second only to cataract operations. There is even evidence that this condition can begin much earlier in life. Ten percent of men in their twenties and thirties are reported to have BPH. When I devoted an hour of my weekly radio show to benign prostatic hypertrophy, it turned out to be one of the busiest hours I've ever hosted. As soon as I mentioned the word "prostate," the phones lit up with men, protected by the anonymity of radio, seeking prescriptive advice about how to cope with this frustrating condition.

There is, however, good news. This condition is often treatable with natural supplements. Often there is no need for drugs, which can have side effects.

One of my patients, Robert Jones, a prolific well-known writer, was reluctant to admit that he was having prostate problems. At fifty-five, Robert was as fit as he had ever been. He was an avid long-distance bicyclist who pedaled scenic hills and valleys every weekend. He was eating well, in great shape, and going to bed early every night. But despite a healthy lifestyle, he woke up exhausted every morning—what might have been a good night's sleep was interrupted by his need to urinate frequently in the middle of the night.

Robert resolved to bear his nightly needs without complaint. By the end of the year, however, he had to admit that a problem as seemingly minor as frequent urination was ruining his life. Robert, who had been divorced for almost a decade, had begun to date an actress. Unfortunately, he not only found himself getting out of bed six times a night to use the bathroom but also noticed that sexually he was not performing as well as he wanted to. Robert was disappointed and frustrated, despite her insistence that he had no cause for worry.

Together, Robert's urologist and I confirmed that he did have an enlarged prostate. Once the diagnosis was made, I knew that there was one special plant extract that could restore Robert's peace and sense of masculinity. This nutrient is known as saw palmetto.

Prostate Balm from an Exotic Palm

After six weeks of taking the recommended dose of this single healing plant—450 milligrams twice a day—Robert began to remember the pleasure of a luxury he had been deprived of for two years: uninterrupted sleep. Although he still woke up with the urge to urinate once or twice a night, this was a dramatic and welcome improvement. Not only did his fatigue dissipate and his writing quality improve, but his libido strengthened as well. This boost may have been due to the extra rest and confidence he gained, but who knows? The supplements he was taking may well have had some sexual benefits in addition to the prostatic relief they gave. Happy in work, satisfied in bed, Robert owes his peace of mind to a little tree called the saw palmetto.

Saw palmetto, also known as *Serenoa repens*, is a dwarf palm tree native to the Atlantic coast of the United States and found in sunny southern climes, from South Carolina down to Florida. The active ingredient in saw palmetto comes not from its strong trunk or its broad green leaves but from a specific fat-soluble extract found in the tree's berries. Although there are several nutrients that are particularly good at soothing the prostate gland, such as stinging nettle, zinc, and pumpkinseed oil, saw palmetto remains the star among all of these.

Palmetto berries have long been used for healing purposes. Hundreds of years ago, it is believed, Native Americans consumed saw palmetto berries as part of their normal diet as a tonic for general male health. Rumor has it that they were also an effective aphrodisiac. Herbalists noted that the plant seemed to improve urinary tract problems and even helped women with mammary gland disorders and cystic breasts. In the 1960s, French researchers first began to examine the red berries of the saw palmetto and its chemical composition and confirmed its ability to mildly stimulate the libido and reduce prostatic hypertrophy. Currently, both the French and German governments approve the use of this extract to treat BPH. Both alone and in synchrony with other natural supplements, saw palmetto is a proven balm for the irritating, often embarrassing symptoms of BPH. Numerous studies show that palmetto extract is a dynamo at treating the enlarged prostate. One series of controlled clinical trials, for example, demonstrated that saw palmetto was able to reduce nocturia (excessive nighttime urination) by up to 74 percent. The high urinary frequency during the daytime associated with BPH was reduced by up to 43 percent, and urinary flow rate was increased by up to 50 percent. As befits a natural supplement, side effects are only rarely reported, with no known contraindications to long-term use of the plant. Considering how common BPH is in this country, saw palmetto is truly man's best friend.

What BPH Means to You

So what is this mysterious BPH, this rarely discussed condition that plagues men, making the natural act of urination a scary and humiliating proposition?

The prostate is a walnut-shaped male genital gland that sits at the base of the penis, right below the bladder. It surrounds the first inch of the urethra, the thin tube that carries urine to the bladder. The milky fluid which it emits is part of the semen that shoots out when men ejaculate. BPH occurs when the prostate grows enlarged or swollen. Common symptoms include frequent urination, urinary urgency, burning while urinating, and "dribbling," all of which stem from the blockage of the bladder and urethra due to the enlarged prostate. As the bladder gets squeezed smaller and smaller, it thickens, leaving less room to store urine and causing the urgent and persistent need to urinate.

Meanwhile, the urethra also narrows, impeding urine flow and leading to the dribbling of excess fluid out of the bladder at inopportune moments. If the bladder continues to get more and more blocked, more serious problems can occur, such as urine remaining trapped in the bladder. In time, the obstructed bladder can weaken severely, leading to infection, residual urine flow, and back pressure on the kidneys. If not stopped soon enough, there are two drastic treatments for BPH: TURP and prostatectomy. TURP stands for transurethral resection of the prostate; it is actually the second most common surgical procedure in America, with cataract surgery in first place. TURP involves boring a hole through the enlarged prostate. A prostatectomy involves removing the prostate. Sound painful? It's also expensive. Billions of dollars are spent on these surgeries and on medications every year.

Compared to a malignancy or prostate cancer, BPH is not the worst health fate. But when I learned about it in medical school, I resolved to do whatever I could to avoid it.

There are several theories about the cause of BPH. Some believe that persistent infection may cause an enlarged prostate, since bacteria from the urethra can easily infect the gland and thrive without any blood supply to help fight them off. These pesky bacteria may cause some of the swelling involved in BPH. Others believe that fluctuations in bodily hormone levels may trigger prostatic hypertrophy. Testosterone levels decrease as men age. Meanwhile, other hormones like FSH, LH, and estradiol take over and may promote testosterone's transformation to an extremely active form called dihydrotestosterone (DHT). DHT overstimulates the prostate and causes an explosive growth of prostate cells. In addition, it increases the absorption of testosterone in the prostate, enhancing its conversion to DHT while reducing the prostate's ability to excrete it, further encouraging the uncontrollable growth of cells.

Even if you have all of the symptoms of BPH, it's best to be diagnosed properly by a physician. A urologist will administer a diagnostic test and have you undergo a digital exam, pressing down on your prostate to determine how swollen it is. If you are diagnosed with BPH, most urologists will recommend two choices: drugs or surgery. Those were the only viable options for treatment, until now.

Saw palmetto is a safe, gentle, and noninvasive way to cure BPH. It seems that a fat-soluble extract of palmetto berries prevents the harmful conversion of testosterone to DHT, by blocking the chemical 5-alpha reductase, which is necessary to the process.

Men with BPH do not have an increased risk of prostate cancer; however, 10 percent of men who have had TURP for BPH have been found to have prostate cancer. Prostate cancer is the most common cancer among men and their leading cause of death except for lung cancer. One out of every 10 men will be diagnosed with cancer before the age of eighty-five, and even more will have it without realizing it. In 1996, 132,000 new cases of prostate cancer were diagnosed, and 33,000 men died from it. For reasons unknown, black men are at greater risk than white men for this scarily ubiquitous illness. Between 1973 and 1993 the number of diagnosed cases of prostate cancer increased by 103 percent.

Like BPH, late prostate cancer can cause severe pain, bladder outlet obstruction, diminished force of urine stream, and urinary frequency, especially during the night, due to reduced bladder capacity. Prostate cancer, like other cancers, can spread cancerous cells all over the body, decreasing chances of survival. And now is the time to worry about it: a report in a 1997 *Health Policy* newsletter noted a decadelong increase in prostate cancer. Genes may play a role in this disease; in 1995, a gene called HPCl that strongly predisposes men to prostate cancer was discovered. As in the case of breast cancer, susceptibility might possibly be passed from one generation to the next. The location of the prostate gland allows doctors to feel it through the rectum, enabling them to palpate the area where most tumors occur. Unfortunately, in the very early stages of cancer, there are often no symptoms to look for. If symptoms do occur, they usually suggest prostate enlargement or infection. A thorough set of medical procedures, however, can lead to the diagnosis of prostate cancer. In the past, tests were not accurate enough, or they detected the cancer too late. One blood test checked for prostatic acid phosphatase, which is elevated in patients whose prostate cancer has already spread.

Today, techniques for weeding out cancer are much more effective. The newest test is called a PSA, for prostate-specific antigen, a protein that is unique to the prostate. It is the most useful marker for the diagnosis and management of prostate cancer. This antigen can also be elevated in conditions such as BPH. A new test called the free PSA is believed to be more sensitive than the PSA for detecting prostate cancer. To confirm a test diagnosis, a needle biopsy and sonography are performed, during which a small sample of tissue from the prostate is removed and examined. Finally, further evaluations are conducted to prove that any cancer indicated actually exists. Unfortunately, natural extracts like saw palmetto have not been proven as effective in treating prostate cancer as BPH. My hope is that further research of the palmetto plant will offer some better defense against cancer in the future. In the meantime, there is hope for the natural prevention and treatment of cancer. Nutrients such as modified citrus pectin, which is a grapefruit extract, and genistein, a soy isoflavone known to have balancing hormonal properties, as described in chapter 5, are already showing great promise in fighting tumor cells. Perhaps one day, saw palmetto will join these ranks.

Flooding His Engine

Alfred Newton may not have understood much about DHT, testosterone, or the intricate hormonal workings of the body; but when it came to all things automotive, he was an expert. Alfred owned a car restoration company, and it was his job to turn classic automobiles from the 1940s and 1950s, vehicles that had seen better days, into shiny new collector's items. Day after day he spent in his shop, waxing T-birds and making old Chrysler engines purr like newborn kittens. One of his favorite projects was a 1958 Gull Wing Mercedes Roadster that he had recently restored to its former glory. Alfred was proud of his workmanship and had pictures of all the antique autos he had restored to life.

His problem? He was in need of a little restoration himself. Often tired, Alfred felt like he was running out of gas, and his sex drive was shutting down. One of the first symptoms of aging that he detailed to me was the increased frequency of urination he experienced both day and night. Unlike most people, however, Alfred was particularly annoyed by the hindrance his leaky bladder caused during daylight hours; because he was so passionate about his work, it was difficult for him to take numerous bathroom breaks while he was tuning one of his babies. He had long had problems with prostatitis, in which the prostate becomes inflamed due to infection, which required long bouts with antibiotics. Worried about overusing medications, Alfred turned to me for a natural approach to his problem.

There were several ways to get Alfred back to his auto obsession without further interruption from his prostate. First of all, after questioning him about his diet, I found that he was a real meat-and-potatoes kind of guy. I asked him to switch to a vegetarian diet, which would be gentler on his system. I also changed his drinking patterns, which most people don't think about but which can have quite an influence on health. Alfred, for example, heeded the traditional advice to drink eight cups of water a day, and he usually gulped them down in the morning with breakfast. Unfortunately, this goal is rather unrealistic for many men, especially those with faulty prostates, since they'd be running for the restroom twenty-five times a day! I told Alfred to drink mostly in the middle or end of the day to avoid disturbing his work for bathroom breaks.

Even without any help from supplements, these dietary changes were powerful enough to lessen the number of times he felt the urge to urinate each day. But the clincher was saw palmetto. Three weeks after I started him on a regimen of 450 milligrams twice a day, Alfred noticed that the number of bathroom visits necessary each day had been cut by at least half, without the help of any additional medical treatment. He even noticed differences in the quality of his urine stream. Alfred's was much more forceful, resulting in less of the constant residual dripping of urine that had made him extremely embarrassed in front of others. In fact, a yearlong study in Hungary unequivocally demonstrated that 320 milligrams daily of saw palmetto led to a reduction of residual urine and a strengthened urinary flow rate.

Alfred was satisfied with the major decrease in daily disturbances, and he found it rather remarkable that a simple plant extract could so change his quality of life. He is back to tinkering with his vintage autos, happily immersed in his work with few interruptions.

Saw Palmetto and the Bathroom Blues

Christopher Shine was an advertising executive who had made himself a fortune on Madison Avenue, wheeling, dealing, and reeling clients into hiring him for their biggest accounts. Not that he needed the fortune, really—he came from a family whose wealth had been dug out of the silver mines long ago. Despite being the heir to the family fortune and having a successful career, Christopher had problems. It's often said that as long as you have your health, nothing else matters; Christopher had everything but his health. Christopher suffered from what I call urinary tract syndrome, which resulted in too-frequent restroom breaks—an inconvenience in his busy days. Christopher traveled a great deal, which meant he often found himself in train stations and airports with crowded, dirty restrooms.

When Christopher went to get a physical, lab tests revealed that he had excess bacteria in his urine. For this, he was treated with antibiotics. Still, his symptoms never quite went away. His doctor then diagnosed him with benign prostatic hypertrophy and prescribed Hytrin, an antihypertensive drug that has been shown to alleviate nocturia as well as having the benefit of lowering blood pressure. Unfortunately, Christopher had an extremely adverse reaction to this drug. He suddenly started feeling tired and dizzy all the time; his blood pressure was already low, and Hytrin just lowered it further, leading to his lethargy. Finally, he came to see me for some natural relief to his watery distress.

Christopher's symptoms were a clear sign that his prostate needed work, and it would take mild supplements and gentle changes to repair it effectively. I decided that saw palmetto was the obvious choice for treatment, and not just because of his ever-present urge to urinate. Christopher was balding, which is often associated with prostate difficulties. However, I have seen no studies to suggest that saw palmetto may help balding. Tests showed that he had an elevated cholesterol count, which can be a marker of prostate abnormalities. His PSA levels were also above normal, which seriously concerned him, since PSAs are indicators of prostate weakness.

"Could . . . could I have cancer?" he asked me, bewildered that his frequent urination could be not just an annoyance but a sign of deadly disease. In his world of girls, glamour, and the good life, mortality had never been a concern. Until now.

"The chances are very slim," I reassured him. "More likely, you have an infection, which we will be able to treat with natural plant extracts and dietary modifications."

First, I eliminated sugar and alcohol, which seem to create unnecessary grief for individuals with prostate difficulties, from his diet. Christopher resisted sobriety strongly at first, since taking clients out for drinks and attending lavish cocktail parties were fixtures in his life. Still, when faced with a life of seeing the bathroom more than family and friends, he decided that the move was worth it. Next, I put him on a slew of supplements to heal his ailing prostate. Saw palmetto is the perfect solution for prostate problems, but there are other herbs and nutrients that, when combined with the palmetto plant, make it an even more effective treatment. *Pygeum africanum*, for example, is traditionally used in Africa to treat urinary tract symptoms, and stinging nettle appears to block the binding of DHT to receptors in the prostate. Pumpkinseed oil is yet another extract known to help the prostate—I recommend 1 gram twice a day. I prescribed a combination of all these nutrients to Christopher, and at first, despite this onslaught of supplements, he noticed no change in his bathroom behavior. After about a month, however, he slowly noticed that the number of times he needed to urinate during the day and night was decreasing. A year later, Christopher only needed to visit the bathroom at most once a night.

Saw Palmetto: A True Story

Fred Reynolds, thirty-two, was new to New York from the sunny state of South Carolina. Although he had moved up north for a glitzy job as the photo editor of a famous men's magazine, the exciting career move did nothing to incite in him a love for the Big Apple. He missed the warm weather, the friendly folks, and the lush green plantations of his home state. To make things worse, Fred began feeling a strange sensation in his stomach area soon after he began his new job. Every morning, he woke up with a persistent pressure on his bladder. By the end of the day, Fred would feel painfully full, no matter how little he had to drink or eat or how frequently he relieved himself. After much urging from his parents back home, Fred consulted a urologist. After a number of tests, his doctor diagnosed him with BPH. Luckily, his prostate was not cancerous, but blood tests showed that his PSA levels were at 7, which is high; the normal level is below 5. Furthermore, statistics on PSA levels and prostate cancer risk suggest that any patients younger than 75 with a PSA greater than 10 should be biopsied routinely. Patients with PSA values between 4 and 10 should be observed carefully, and if their values increase by 20 percent or more after a year of follow-up monitoring, they should also be biopsied.

Because such high PSA levels in a man of Fred's age indicated a higher-than-normal likelihood of prostate cancer, I was very concerned about Fred's health. A firm believer in the powers of herbs and extracts, he had come to me seeking treatment after the serious verdict issued by his urologist.

"I know my condition is pretty bad. My doctor explained everything about PSA levels to me and how dangerous mine are," said Fred. "Is there anything that natural supplements can do for me?"

"There is," I reassured him. "But first, we need to conduct some more tests."

Through ultrasound and biopsy we confirmed no presence of cancer, but I was still concerned. I put him on a high soy diet, since soy's phytochemicals can block receptors from excess hormone stimulation, and this can protect against hormone-related cancers. I also declared war against his PSA levels, zapping them with such prostate-friendly nutrients as zinc, essential fatty acids, amino acids—including alanine, glycine, and glutamic acid—pumpkinseed oil, and, of course, saw palmetto. Zinc, which is involved in numerous biochemical processes such as the formation of sperm, is concentrated in the prostate more than any other organ in the body. Zinc helps by enhancing the immune system, which fights infections. It also blocks enzymes that can cause cancer. Essential fatty acids can also inhibit prostatic cellular growth.

Although saw palmetto's ability to control the bothersome symptoms of BPH are duly noted and admired, the plant's mechanism of action is still in dispute. Many postulate that, like zinc, saw palmetto blocks 5-alpha reductase and the binding of DHT to prostate receptors, a hypothesis supported by in vitro studies. Others believe that it must have a nonhormonal method of attack, backed up by a study of twenty men in Italy who took saw palmetto for thirty days and experienced reduced BPH symptoms but no accompanying hormone difference. However saw palmetto works, it has been proved effective as a prostate wonder nutrient, especially in concert with other soothing supplements.

After three months on this regimen, I retested Fred's blood and happily found that his PSA levels had gone down to a normal state. Meanwhile, he noticed that the pressure on his bladder had lessened for the cancer danger zone, he will continue to stay on my high-risk list, and I will continue to monitor his progress. High PSA levels are scary harbingers of prostate danger, and the diseases and medical conditions they predict are so serious that Fred may not be out of the woods yet. His symptoms did improve remarkably, and for now he's feeling great. So great, in fact, that he's even beginning to feel at home in the big city.

Trust in Saw Palmetto

Most men reaching the later years of their lives will inevitably run into problems with the prostate gland. Keeping the prostate healthy and happy is a priority that should not be underestimated. By using saw palmetto and its companion nutrients, you can certainly keep the embarrassments of never-ending urination urges and slow flow to a minimum. In all seriousness, however, you may save yourself from pain and help protect against cancer through these supplements.

Keep in mind that saw palmetto treatment requires time and patience. Results may not appear until up to a year after the first pill is taken, although many men see a reduction in prostate size, pain, and blockage within four to six weeks. Saw palmetto can carry men through tough and trying times. It may seem like a simple plant extract, but it is truly a man's best friend.

After the age of fifty, men should consider using saw palmetto, particularly if they notice some of the symptoms discussed in this chapter. If you've been diagnosed with BPH, this is a perfect way to start. Men should seek medical advice prior to undergoing any therapy. And always consider supplements as part of an overall comprehensive approach to health.

HOW MUCH SHOULD I TAKE?

For General Health

If over 50 (male) or have a family history of BPH: 450 mg/day

Special Conditions

Benign Prostatic Hypertrophy	900-1,800 mg/day

23

Nutrients of the Future

Nutraceutical-based medical care is the future of medicine, and I'm proud to be a part of it. Typically, patients come to see me after seeing several other physicians without satisfactory results. I put them on a program of supplements, adjust their diet, and watch their lives change. At such times, I feel I am a witness to an extraordinary event. Not long ago I saw a thirty-five-year-old man with a history of migraine headaches; I treated him with something as simple as magnesium, the herb feverfew, and, for his allergies, nettle and quercetin, and within two weeks he reported that his headaches had disappeared. As a doctor, it's indescribably thrilling to witness such swift and beneficial changes. Nutritional medicine may still be the road less traveled, but, as Robert Frost said, in the end, traveling that road has made all the difference.

We are just at the beginning of the nutraceutical revolution. Within the world of nutritional medicine exist ever more powerful compounds yet to be discovered.

That is one reason why I became very interested in researching truly innovative alternative treatments. One of those was a cancer preventive extract of shark liver oil. You can't get much more esoteric than oil from the liver of Greenland sharks, but I was fascinated by the twenty years of studies that had been conducted on it and its ability to prevent malignancies.

Shark Oil: Can It Fight Cancer?

Originally discovered in 1922, shark liver oil extract contains compounds called alkylglycerols, which have also been found in breast milk and in bone marrow. The main source for these compounds is found in sharks around the deep, cold waters of Greenland. When cervical cancer was studied in 1986 there was a 29 percent regression in tumor growth in those patients taking 250 milligrams of alkylglycerols a day. In 1977, Astrid Brohult published a study in *Acta Obstetricia et Gynecologica Scandinavica* reporting how 250 milligrams per day of shark oil given one week prior to radiation therapy for cervical cancer reduced tissue injury, and another study in 1986 reported reduced mortality rates and improved immune response. Alkylglycerols have also been studied as a treatment for childhood leukemia. In the *Proceedings of the American Meeting of Cancer Research* in 1992 it was reported that leukemia prevents the immune system from properly forming white blood cells, but with this oil they seem to "mature" to a proper form more easily.

Shark liver oil is just one of many interesting, healing oils that have been studied of late. The preventive role for various fats—or lipids—in cancer has been suggested by studies on everything from omega-3 fatty acids to monounsaturated fats such as those in olive oil. The membranes of cancer cells actually change when they are exposed to different types of fat. It appears that certain physical properties of the cell membrane are altered. For instance, omega-3s tend to be anti-inflammatory and seem to slow down all inflammatory changes in the cell. Cancer cells may be stimulated by inflammatory chemicals, and oils that inhibit inflammation may help our immune system fight cancer.

The idea that a tumor cell could be altered so easily by an oil was fascinating to me. This is the fascination of all nutraceuticals, of course—not only are they versatile and powerful in and of themselves, but if we understand how they work, they may open the door to a host of other treatments and medicines. Here is a situation where you can literally change a cancer cell's very composition and perhaps potentially make it more susceptible to chemotherapy. If you rely on both nutraceuticals and modern medicine, you are offering your body a fuller spectrum of medical care.

I had long wanted to conduct my own research on alkylglycerols, but there was very little interest in the benefits of natural therapies for cancer in this country. I looked abroad and was extremely fortunate to receive a grant from the Royal Academy at the Karolinska Institute in Sweden. We took tumor samples from nine cancer patients who were undergoing surgery, and we cultured their cancer cells. Using a special technique called fluorescent cytoprint assay, we were able to cultivate tumor cells, grow them in individual petri dishes, and treat them with combinations of chemotherapy and shark oil.

This, by the way, is how cancer research begins: with studies in petri dishes, called in vitro studies. If the results are encouraging, the studies will be repeated, and then eventually the substance will be tested in laboratory animals to see if it is safe and still effective. Countless times, unfortunately, the results in animals are far different from those in a petri dish—either the substance is toxic to a living organism or it gets broken down and changed by the body before it can reach the cancer cells. In the case of shark oil extracts, we already know that they are well tolerated by humans and that oils taken orally do tend to get absorbed into the fatty membranes of cells. Alkylglycerols are actually a compound found in shark oil.

My particular study is now complete, and the initial results are impressive: in all of the patient cultures tested, alkylglycerols enhanced the effect of chemotherapy. Six patients' cancer cell counts dropped dramatically, with over 90 percent of the tumors in the cell culture eradicated; three others showed increases in sensitivity to the chemotherapy, above 50 percent.

What accounts for such a dramatic turnaround? Tumor cells, it turns out, concentrate alkylglycerols at a rate ten to one hundred times higher than normal tissue. The catch? Tumor cells may lack the enzyme to break down this compound. In a sense, the compound clogs and chokes them, making it more difficult for the cancer cells to replicate. Other studies suggest that alkylglycerols stimulate the immune system, which can then target tumor cells more effectively. We don't have all the answers yet, but the questions these compounds raise serve as clues in one of the most exciting treasure hunts around. Further studies on shark liver oil and cancer are now under way at the Karolinska Institute. Hopefully this will spur others to help fund research.

What does this mean for real-life cancer patients? In the big picture, it means we are beginning to understand what cancer cells depend upon and are learning how to pretreat them with natural compounds that they find very difficult to remove from their system. From substances that inhibit new blood vessel growth—including nutrients such as genistein and drugs such as endostatin, which has shown remarkable results in animal studies—to substances like perillyl alcohol, an extract of lavender that is being studied by the National Cancer Institute and other laboratories for its ability to reverse both pancreatic and breast cancer, we are on the verge of a breakthrough in treating cancer. Once we understand its weaknesses, we can use our regular arsenal of chemotherapy and radiation along with high-powered nutrition to deal the final one-two blow. Specifically, it means that I recommend to all my cancer patients a cocktail of fatty acids and oils that include flaxseed oil, fish oil, olive oil, and shark liver oil. All have been shown to have cancer-preventive effects.

Shark oil is only the beginning of the next wave of nutraceuticals. I'd like to let you in on some other equally promising nutrients of the future—nutraceuticals that may help prevent cancer, help you lose weight, protect against heart disease and diabetes, and enhance overall immunity. These nutrients are on the cutting edge of the nutraceutical revolution, and some of them are just beginning to be used by forward-looking physicians. I was able to show similar results for fish oils contains EPA and DHA as well.

Modified Citrus Pectin Cancer Prevention

A new and interesting cancer fighter is known as modified citrus pectin (MCP)—a soluble component of plant fiber derived from the peel and pulp of citrus fruits such as oranges and tangerines. Ordinary pectin is a complex carbohydrate molecule found in almost all plants. It is recognized for its ability to gel (as in the making of jams) but is not absorbed into the bloodstream because of its long molecular chain. For MCP, a special manufacturing process creates a shorter molecular chain.

MCP may work by preventing cancer cells from metastasizing, which occurs when malignant cells spread throughout the body, first detaching themselves from the original tumor and, like seeds blown on the wind, traveling through the bloodstream until they find another site on which to touch down, fasten themselves, and begin dividing and multiplying. Metastasis is the gravest danger a cancer patient can face: if a tumor were simply to stay where it originated, it might cause some local damage but would probably not kill us and could be surgically removed, usually with few if any complications.

We want to attack cancer at several levels—not only through oils such as alkylglycerols but through other nutrients that can disable the weaponry of malignant cells. Studies suggest that MCP may work like a special bait that attracts migrating cancer cells and renders them harmless. In one study of melanoma in mice, published in the *Journal of the National Cancer Institute*, MCP reduced metastasis by an astonishing 90 percent. And in a report of the proceedings of the annual meeting of the American Association of Cancer Researchers, MCP was reported to have stopped a wide variety of different malignant cells from successful metastisization. MCP actually interferes with metastasis of any kind, it seems, by preventing free-floating cancer cells from adhering to tissue.

It appears that MCP attracts cancer cells and binds with them before they get a chance to fasten themselves to healthy cells. Cancer cells contain a substance called galactin. Galactin looks for its counterpart, galactose, a sugar that fits neatly into the galactin receptors. Many cells contain galactose, but MCP is particularly high in this substance. Because it contains so much galactose, it can attract the outlaw cancer cells, bind to them, and then render them harmless. Cancer cells bound to galactose are then no longer on the hunt for something to stick to, having found a kind of "decoy" food. They have been tricked by their own clever chemistry. The cancer cell doesn't appear to "care" whether it is binding to MCP or a human cell, because it's simply "hungry" and on the hunt for galactose. A 1992 study in the *Journal of the National Cancer Institute* reported that when melanoma cells were grown in the laboratory and injected into mice, a group of mice that had received

MCP had a 90 percent reduction in metastasis, and the group that did not receive MCP had an up to threefold increase in the appearance of lung tumor colonies per mouse.

MCP is a carbohydrate, and carbohydrates are usually broken down into simple sugars before absorption. Can MCP pass through the digestive process unharmed, into the blood where it's needed? Not always. Apparently not all MCPs are alike. The size of the molecule matters: it must be small enough to be absorbed yet large enough to have enough binding sites to attract the cancer cell. Research by Kenneth Pienta, MD, at Wayne State University, has set specifications for the most effective size; companies whose products follow this standard can be found on the World Wide Web. Search to make sure that the company follows Dr. Pienta's recommendations.

Calcium D-glucarate
Stop Cancer Before It Starts

Calcium d-glucarate stopping cancer before it starts. Another approach to preventing cancer is to stop it before it starts. One promising nutrient may achieve this by helping the liver detoxify hormones, which can often promote tumor growth. You may recall our discussions of the herb milk thistle, which helped protect the liver, and of the nutrient N-acetyl cysteine (NAC), which protected and preserved the liver's most powerful antioxidant, glutathione.

Now, another revolutionary nutraceutical may offer additional help: calcium d-glucarate, which is found in certain fruits and vegetables and acts as a potent inhibitor of an enzyme known as beta-glucuronidase. This enzyme is created by bacteria in the colon and can be harmful to us because it undoes the work of the liver. The liver often takes potentially toxic compounds, binds them safely to neutral compounds, and passes them on to the digestive system for excretion. A healthy liver, for instance, is able to take excess hormones and bind them to substances called glucuronides. When these bound molecules encounter the enzyme beta-glucuronidase, they are cleaved apart, and the estrogen is once again free to circulate. The liver will have to double its workload and once again bind up the free estrogen; but if it's too overworked, that excess estrogen will be free to promote and stimulate tumor growth. Calcium d-glucarate may prevent this by inhibiting the potentially dangerous beta-glucuronidase. This compound is so promising that the National Cancer Institute has begun a study of calcium glucarate in patients at high risk for breast cancer. It is a promising natural substance with no known toxicity and supports the cleansing and detoxification of the body.

Pycnogenol, Grapeskin, and Green Tea

To enhance general immunity and, once again, possibly protect against cancer, there are three important cutting-edge nutraceuticals, and one of them can even be sipped in the afternoon.

The first, pycnogenol, is a patented blend of bioflavonoids derived from pine bark. Bioflavonoids work synergistically with vitamin C, strengthening the walls of capillaries, helping to quench allergies and inflammation, working to maintain healthy skin, and protecting against cancer.

Pycnogenol is an especially potent blend of bioflavonoids. The use of this compound as a healing agent probably stretches back to the beginnings of Native American medicine. Native Americans discovered that a tea brewed from the bark and needles of certain evergreen trees cured scurvy. Later, Dr. Albert Szent-Gyorgyi, who was awarded the Nobel Prize in 1937 for isolating vitamin C, noted that the crude extracts from lemon juice were more effective against scurvy than pure vitamin C, and he later determined that this was because of the presence of bioflavonoids.

A rich variety of flavonoids are found in evergreen trees. The most potent of these flavonoids—such as catechins and proanthocyanidins—are strong free radical fighters. One 1992 study in the journal *Cancer Research* found that catechins have potent anticancer effects. Cancer of the pharynx, breast, colon, and brain have all been inhibited by flavonoids.

The versatility and far-reaching benefits of pycnogenol make it one of the main bioflavonoid combinations I rely on most heavily in my practice. Everything from allergies to heart disease can be helped by pycnogenol, which protects the body at a cellular level.

Another important flavonoid, made from the skin of grapes, is resveratrol. It's a relatively newly discovered compound that is believed to be the active healthful ingredient in grapeskin and red wine. It's a flavonoid that seems to protect the heart and also has been found to inhibit cancer formation. In 1997, *Science* reported that resveratrol prevented all three stages of cancer growth (initiation, promotion, and progression). This substance inhibits the clumping of white blood cells known as platelets. As you'll recall from our discussion of ginkgo—which has the same effect on platelets—this is important in correcting allergies and in protecting us from heart disease.

Very few white wines contain resveratrol. Red wine, however, has high levels, particularly wines from the Pinot Noir grapes (irrespective of the country or region of origin). Rather than try to consume these flavonoids in the form of wine—and risk the adverse health effects of alcohol—I recommend resveratrol supplements to patients who are at risk for heart disease or cancer. Starting doses are from 25 milligrams to 50 milligrams a day and are now found in a number of formulations.

Finally, a simple, tasty, and age-old beverage, green tea, has potent, health-enhancing flavonoids. All teas (except herbal teas) are made from the leaf of *Camellia sinensis*, and tea leaves contain a variety of complex compounds, many of which are beneficial to health. Green tea seems to protect against several cancers and heart disease. This is good news since, after water, tea is the most popular beverage in the world.

Tea was originally grown in the highlands of Asia but now is grown in Russia, South America, Africa, and Turkey as well. Black tea is dried, crushed, fermented, and then dried again. Green teas are not crushed and oxidized. Instead they are steamed, then rolled and dried.

A cup of green tea contains about 400 milligrams of polyphenols, which are highly beneficial to our health. One of these polyphenols, known as EGCG (epigallocatechin gallate), is a more potent antioxidant than vitamin C or vitamin E. Green tea drinkers have a reduced risk of colorectal and pancreatic cancer. Studies have found it even reduces cholesterol and liver toxicity.

I drink a few cups of green tea daily, and I recommend it to my patients. It's a pleasant light beverage that can be sipped throughout the day with marvelous health benefits.

Licorice for Ulcers

People the world over love the smell and taste of licorice: the root itself was found buried with King Tut in his tomb and was used as a medicine in ancient Egypt. In China circa 3000 BC, licorice was included in religious ceremonies. For many of us, black licorice whips and twirls were a memorable treat of childhood.

There's ample reason for the popularity of the root (*Glycyrrhiza glabra*). First of all, it's potent and almost pungent, yet sweet. Second, it contains powerful flavonoids and substances that make it a fine healing agent, including the cortisonelike substance glycyrrhizin, which unfortunately can cause side effects like bloating and hypertension. Precisely because it can increase blood pressure, glycyrrhizin can actually be helpful in cases of chronic fatigue syndrome, which is often associated with continual low blood pressure and a mild deficiency in natural cortisone. A review in the *Quarterly Review of Natural Medicine* found that licorice dissolved in milk helped CFS patients increase their stamina and energy.

Licorice has other healing properties as well. An extract of licorice called deglycyrrhizinated licorice or DGL is a good antiulcer compound. It has been shown in studies to be as effective as the prescription medication Tagamet. In Europe, it's the most popular treatment for ulcers. Unlike most ulcer medications, which reduce stomach acid, DGL actually stimulates both the body's normal defense mechanisms and the mucus-secreting cells in the stomach. Mucus protects the lining of the stomach, allowing it to heal.

One patient came in to me with chronic ulcers that were not due to *H. pylori*, the bacteria known to be the most common cause of ulcers. (Many people with *H. pylori* don't end up with ulcers, which suggests that there are other mechanisms at work.) For this particular patient, I recommended the drug Pepcid, which reduces acid, and I also asked her to begin a daily program of DGL and aloe vera (which heals the stomach lining). She returned two weeks later and reported that she felt great. I said, "Wonderful, let's stop the Pepcid and just keep you on the DGL and aloe." She sighed and said, "I have a confession. I never did take the Pepcid or the aloe. I just took the DGL the whole time, and it did the trick." I now use DGL as a first-line treatment in many cases of ulcers or gastritis.

Lipoic Acid: A Diabetic's Friend

Many health problems can be traced to excess sugar in the diet, because sugar itself can promote free radical damage, particularly in diabetics, just as oxygen can. Both are fuel for the body and primary sources of energy, but both need to be balanced by a strong antioxidant defense system. Alpha lipoic acid, also known as thioctic acid, is the only antioxidant that is both water and fat soluble, which means that it's easily available to all areas of the body. It helps quench free radical damage caused by sugars and it is used by the mitochondria, the little energy powerhouses in every cell. The mitochondria help transform glucose into energy, and lipoic acid is crucial in this transformation.

Lipoic acid helps the liver. It can actually restore the liver's most powerful antioxidant, glutathione. This nutrient is very important for diabetics, and as Richard Passwater, Ph.D., a nutrition expert, says, "It would not be an exaggeration to call it a blessing." Lipoic acid helps to normalize blood sugar and protect blood vessels against the damage that excess sugar can cause. Free radical damage caused by high blood sugar leads to diabetic complications such as cataracts, heart disease, and nerve damage. It has been effective in treating peripheral neuropathy in diabetics—a condition where nerve damage causes the feet and sometimes the hands to become numb. Since diabetes strikes one in every twenty Americans and is the third leading cause of death, lipoic acid is good and important news in the world of nutraceutical medicine.

Diabetes is not the only condition lipoic acid helps. German research has shown that it can protect against cancer and heart disease. This nutrient can help restore and recycle vitamin E, another powerful antioxidant. Lipoic acid actually functions in the cell interior—because it is a small molecule, it readily passes through the cell membrane and can quench free radicals not just in the bloodstream but in the very heart of the cell, thus protecting our DNA from damage and possible mutation.

I recommend this nutraceutical to all my diabetic patients, as well as those suffering from heart disease and those with the kind of chronic health problems that produce inflammation and free radical damage (such as chronic asthma and arthritis).

CLA: A Fat that Fights Cancer, Heart Disease, and Weight Gain

A strange thing happened in 1979. An extract from hamburger was found to inhibit tumors in mice. In 1987, this extract was identified as conjugated linoleic acid (CLA). It belongs to the omega-6 fatty acid family. After nearly twenty years of research on this designer fat, we've found out that it inhibits breast cancer in laboratory animals as well as plaque formation in the arteries. We've also found that CLA may reduce body fat and increase lean body mass.

How does it work? We aren't quite sure. It seems that CLA may modulate fat metabolism in the liver. It also may stop fat from being deposited in the body, increase the actual breakdown of fat in cells, and increase the utilization of fat for energy. One clinical trial over a period of ninety days produced an average of 4.3 percent reduction in body fat.

CLA is not the only nutraceutical in our weight-loss arsenal. A compound called hydroxycitric acid (HCA) also seems to help curb weight gain. It's found in the highest concentrations in a South Asian tree called *Garcinia cambogia* and is actually a digestive aid. In 1970, Hoffman La Roche, a drug company, began to investigate HCA and found that it reduces our body's conversion of carbohydrate to fat. It also lowers the production of cholesterol and may even suppress the appetite. How does HCA work? During and after meals, calories that are not used for energy are stored in the liver and muscles as glycogen, which is a source of energy for the body. When glycogen stores become filled, the liver sends out signals to the brain indicating we are full, effectively sating the appetite during a meal. If we continue to eat anyway, however, the glycogen is turned into fat. The conversion of carbohydrates into fat requires an enzyme called ATP-citrate lyase. HCA works by temporarily inhibiting this enzyme, which essentially means it blocks the fat production.

Yet another weight-loss nutraceutical is known as pyruvate. Pyruvate is an essential part of energy production in the body. It actually improves the action of insulin and is one of the end products of glucose metabolism. Pyruvate actually sets the body's "idle" at a higher level. People with a weight problem generally have a low "idle" level—a slower metabolism than normal. They also seem to store the energy in food more efficiently than thin people.

Ronald T. Stanko, MD, at the University of Pittsburgh Medical Center, studied fourteen obese women on a one-thousand-calorie liquid diet for three weeks. Half of the women were also given 36 grams of pyruvate daily. Those taking pyruvate lost 37 percent more weight (13 versus 9.5 pounds) and 48 percent more fat (8.8 versus 5.9 pounds) than the control group. Pyruvate also facilitates weight loss by regulating thyroid hormone. In animal studies, pyruvate raised thyroid hormone levels by as much as 14 percent; thyroid regulates metabolism, and a faster metabolism helps burn fat. Pyruvate might even increase endurance: a study of ten active college students (all male) found they had a 20 percent increase in endurance after seven days on the supplement. Best of all, pyruvate fights body fat without compromising valuable muscle mass.

All these nutrients are promising, and they each work in different ways. I often administer them in various combinations for my patients with weight problems.

Arginine: Natural Vasodilator

In 1992, nitric oxide was named molecule of the year by *Science* magazine. This was because of its widespread function in the body: it controls blood pressure, functions as a neurotransmitter, helps the body to fight tumors, and regulates blood clotting. It was hypothesized that this gas was actually a major neurotransmitter and that it regulates blood pressure by dilating blood vessels. Furthermore, when there is too little nitric oxide in the mucosal lining of the gut, individuals are susceptible to yeast infections in the digestive system. The gas actually seems to kill many pathogens. When nitric oxide is produced in excess, however, it can be damaging to the body, cause harmful inflammation, and, in the most serious conditions, send the body into a state of shock that leads to the collapse of all the blood vessels and death. Nitric oxide, therefore, is both a healing and potentially harmful compound in our body.

There are now tests being developed that will establish how much nitric oxide a person has in his or her body and which individuals might benefit from taking supplements to increase nitric oxide. One of these tests measures the amount of nitrates eliminated in the urine. If a person has high urinary nitrates, they may have high amounts of nitric oxide in their body.

Arginine, a common and useful amino acid, can increase nitric oxide in the body. Supplementing the diet with arginine, in doses of 1 or 2 grams a day, has been found to stimulate the body's synthesis of nitric oxide. When taking arginine, however, it's important to add a cocktail of antioxidants—since, as stated, too much nitric oxide leads to inflammation.

Arginine is present in most proteins, including meats, nuts, milk, cheese, and eggs. Arginine deficiency can result in hair loss, constipation, a delay in the healing of wounds, and liver disease.

Arginine is essential to the metabolism of ammonia that is generated from protein breakdown. At a dose of more than 3 grams daily, it has been shown to stimulate the pituitary gland to produce and secrete human growth hormone in young males. Human growth hormone helps in muscle building, leading to increased muscle strength and tone. Arginine also stimulates thymus activity, and the thymus is the gland that produces the immune system's all important T-cells. It also helps the body heal from wounds. Some research has shown that high doses of arginine may increase male fertility by increasing sperm production and motility.

Perhaps most interesting is arginine's possible impact on sexual function. For men who are not yet ready to try a drug like Viagra, this amino acid can make erections easier to achieve. A 1984 study of fifteen men taking nearly 3,000 milligrams a day for two weeks found that six of the older men had more frequent erections while on the supplement. In 1997, another study found that men who took arginine were more likely to attain erections.

Arginine may also be helpful for a painful condition that some women suffer from called interstitial cystitis. This is a chronic inflammation of the bladder that does not seem linked to overt infection. Women who took 1.5 grams of the amino acid daily for six months experienced significant relief from pain and discomfort.

When St. John's Wort Doesn't Work

What if you're depressed and you can't tolerate the side effects of medications, but the antidepressant herb St. John's wort hasn't done the trick for you either? An unusual nutrient known as SAMe (S-adenosylmethionine) has been shown to be unusually effective in treating depression. SAMe is manufactured from the amino acid methionine. When it is changed into SAMe, it has an extra methyl molecule available—and methyl molecules are very important in many critical reactions in the body. They are especially important in the brain.

SAMe is crucial for the brain to manufacture neurotransmitters, and when depressed patients are given SAMe, they have increased levels of important brain chemicals like dopamine and serotonin—both of which are implicated in depression.

SAMe also helps improve what is known as the "binding" of neurotransmitters, or their ability to fasten to receptors on brain cells. So it actually improves the effectiveness of brain neurotransmitters.

In one Scandinavian study in 1990, twenty patients with major depression were treated with SAMe. Nine patients responded to SAMe, including two who had been unresponsive to any other medications. I find that particularly promising. Another 1994 study compared SAMe to the antidepressant desipramine (Norpramin) in twenty-six patients. At the end of four weeks, 62 percent of the SAMe patients and 50 percent of the desipramine patients improved. There was also an odd twist to this study: in both groups, the patients who improved had measurable increases of SAMe in their blood. This is tantalizing evidence that SAMe is somehow linked to depression. Researchers have speculated that SAMe might work in various ways—that it might influence neurotransmitters like norepinephrine or dopamine or that it might work like some monoamine oxidase inhibitors (MAOs).

There are no reported side effects in studies of SAMe so far, and studies have used from 400 to 800 milligrams daily. However, it can be hard to find a stable source of SAMe, and even then, the nutrient can be expensive. Since deficiencies of B_{12} and folate are linked to decreases in the concentration of SAMe in the nervous system, SAMe might be boosted by giving these nutrients, along with the amino acid methionine. In addition, the nutrient trimethylglycine can also enhance levels of SAMe.

These are just a few of the amazing vitamins, minerals, essential oils and amino acids out there. This is truly the beginning of a bold new era. We have truly married science with nutrition, and we are beginning to peer into the cell to watch how even phytochemicals work.

Nutraceuticals offer viable alternatives to drugs and certain traditional medications, by acting as natural medicines. Sometimes we will want to combine nutrition with medication; many other times nutrition alone will suffice. Either way, we are on a path that will lead us to an era of effective preventive medicine. As recently as a decade ago physicians such as myself could do no more than recommend a few vitamins and minerals. Our new understanding of everything from the chemicals in broccoli sprouts to the healing fatty acids in fish is so increasingly precise that we can now target disease with ever greater accuracy.

With this book, The Vitamin Prescription for Life you have taken the first step towards good health. You have the beginnings of a nutraceutical program for life, one that will keep your heart healthy, help prevent cancer, strengthen your bones help you think better, boost your mood, balance your hormones, and keep your liver functioning well. This is a program you and your doctor can tailor to your own specific needs. It's an opportunity that simply was not available when I started in my practice. Take the promise of the Vitamin Prescription and make the most of it. And remember, any prescription is just the beginning. The rest is in your hands.

Addendum

The best way to experience The Vitamin Prescription For Life is through your diet. As Hippocrates said, "Let food be your medicine and your medicine food."

Dawn Perry, a personal chef, cooking instructor and certified holistic health counselor has put together a list of wonderful recipes that are filled with powerful nutraceuticals. Dawn was trained at the California Culinary Academy in San Francisco and the Institute for Integrative Nutrition in New York City. Each of the delicious recipes below contain specific nutraeuticals such as resveratrol, Indole-3-carbinols, Omega-3 fatty acids , lycopene, and lutein. I have personally tested and enjoyed every delicious meal.

SPRING

Roasted Beet Salad with Orange

1 pound red or gold beets (about 4 medium)
2 tablespoons plus 2 teaspoons extra virgin olive oil
Salt and pepper
1 orange, peeled and segmented, plus ¼ cup freshly squeezed orange juice
1 small shallot, minced
2 teaspoons red wine vinegar

Preheat oven to 400. Trim tops from beets and discard. Place beets in the center of a large piece of aluminum foil. Drizzle with 2 teaspoons olive oil and season with salt and pepper. Wrap foil over beets and seal. Place foil packet on a baking sheet and roast until beets are tender when pierced with a knife, 50-60 minutes depending on the size of the beets. Let beets cool until easy to handle. Using a paper towel, rub skin from beets and discard. Cut into wedges and place in a medium bowl. Add oranges, orange juice, shallot, vinegar and remaining 2 tablespoons olive oil. Season with salt and pepper and toss well to combine. Salad can be made up to a day ahead. Serves 4

Roasted Turnips and Radishes

1 bunch radishes, tops removed, quartered
3 medium turnips, peeled and cut into ¾-inch pieces
4 teaspoons extra virgin olive oil
Salt and pepper
1 tablespoon lemon juice (about half a juicy lemon)

Preheat oven to 400. On a large rimmed baking sheet toss radishes and turnips with olive oil and season generously with salt and pepper. Roast in the middle of the oven until golden and tender, shaking the pan a couple of times throughout, 25-30 minutes. Squeeze lemon juice all over vegetables. Season with more salt and pepper if desired. Serve warm. Serves 3-4

Pea and Greens Soup

2 teaspoons extra virgin olive oil
1 large shallot, minced
1 bag (10 ounces) frozen peas
salt and pepper
1 ¾ cup vegetable broth
5 ounces dark greens such as spinach or arugula
handful fresh mint leaves

In a medium soup-pot, heat oil over medium-high. Add shallot and cook until slightly softened, about 3 minutes. Add peas, vegetable broth and 1 ½ cups water and season with salt and pepper. Bring to a boil, reduce to simmer and cook 3 minutes. Remove from heat and add the greens. Cover the pot and set aside until greens are wilted, about 5 minutes. Working in batches, transfer mixture to a blender, add mint and puree until smooth. Season with salt and pepper and serve hot or transfer to refrigerator to chill and serve cold. Serves 4-6

Braised Leeks

6 medium leeks
1 ¼ cup chicken or vegetable broth
4 sprigs fresh thyme
salt and pepper
2 tablespoons unsalted butter, cut into ½-inch cubes

Preheat oven to 400. Trim roots and dark green tops from leeks. Split each leek lengthwise and run under cool water, gently separating the layers to rinse away any sand or grit. Arrange leeks snuggly in an oven-safe baking dish. Add broth and season with salt and pepper. Top with thyme sprigs and dot with butter. Cover dish tightly with aluminum foil and bake in center of oven until leeks are tender when pierced with the tip of a sharp knife, about 25 minutes. Remove foil and bake until leeks begin to turn golden, 25-30 minutes longer. Serve warm. Serves 4

Roasted Tofu and Broccoli

1 pound extra firm tofu, cut into 5 3/4-inch slabs
2 tablespoons soy sauce
1 1/2 teaspoons toasted sesame oil
1 1/2 teaspoons grapeseed oil
1 tablespoon honey
1 large head broccoli, cut into large florets

Place 3 sheets of paper towel on a cutting board. Arrange tofu slabs in one layer and place 3 more sheets of paper towel on top. Place a baking sheet or dish on top of the paper towel and a few cans or a heavy tea kettle on top. This will draw some of the moisture out of the tofu. Let rest 15 minutes.

Preheat oven to 400. Cut drained tofu into cubes. In a large bowl combine soy sauce, oils and honey. Stir to dissolve honey and season with salt and pepper. Add tofu cubes and broccoli florets to bowl and toss gently to coat. Transfer tofu, broccoli and any extra marinade to a rimmed baking sheet and shake to arrange in a single layer. Roast, shaking the pan halfway through, until tofu is golden and broccoli is tender, about 20 minutes. Serves 4.

Flax-berry Smoothie

1/2 cup silken tofu
1 cup frozen berries
1 cup cranberry juice
1 tablespoon flax seed
2 tablespoons honey
Combine all ingredients in a blender and puree until smooth. Serves 2

Halibut,Brown Rice and Vegetable Packets

4 6-ounce filets halibut or other firm-fleshed white fish
2 cups cooked brown rice or barley
1 small leek, halved lengthwise, rinsed and sliced thin crosswise
1 carrot, peeled and cut into matchsticks
1 shallot, thinly sliced
salt and pepper
3 tablespoons extra virgin olive oil
1 lemon, thinly sliced
4 sprigs fresh thyme

Preheat oven to 425. Rinse fish filets and pat them dry. Line four large sheets of aluminum foil with 4 large sheets of parchment paper. Divide the rice or barley equally among the pieces of parchment. Top rice with equal amounts leek, carrot and shallot and place fish filets on top; season with salt and pepper and drizzle with olive oil. Top each piece of fish with a few lemon slices and a sprig of thyme. Fold up the sides of the foil and parchment and crimp all the edges to make a tight seal. Place the packets on a baking sheet and bake until puffed and fish is cooked through, 12-15 minutes depending on the thickness of the fish. Carefully open the packets and serve immediately. Serves 4

SUMMER

3 Bean Salad

6 ounces green beans, trimmed and cut into 1-inch pieces
1 15-ounce can kidney beans, rinsed and drained
1 15-ounce can garbanzo beans, rinsed and drained

2 teaspoons whole grain mustard
2 tablespoons cider vinegar
2 tablespoons extra-virgin olive oil
small handful chopped fresh herbs such as parsley, dill or basil
1 small shallot, minced
1 garlic clove, minced
pinch red pepper flake (optional)
salt and pepper

Bring a pot of salted water to a boil. Drop in green beans and cook until beans are crisp-tender and bright green, about 2 minutes. Drain beans and run under cold water to stop them from cooking. In a large bowl combine green beans with remaining ingredients and season to taste with salt and pepper. Let sit 30 minutes before serving, tossing occasionally. Salad can be made up to 2 days ahead. Serves 4-6

Green Tea Lemonade with Fresh Mint

1 1/2 cup brewed green tea, cooled
1/4 cup freshly squeezed lemon juice
2 tablespoons agave nectar
4 sprigs fresh mint

In a large pitcher, combine tea, lemon juice and agave nectar. Stir well to dissolve agave. Serve tea over ice, garnished with mint. Serves 2.

Slow-Roasted Plum Tomatoes

1 pound plum tomatoes (about 10), halved
2 tablespoons extra-virgin olive oil
salt and pepper
1/2 teaspoon dried oregano

Preheat oven to 300. Place tomatoes on a rimmed baking sheet and toss with oil. Arrange tomatoes cut side up and season with salt and pepper. Sprinkle with oregano and roast until collapsed and slightly shriveled, 2 hours. Serve hot, room temperature or cold. Serves 4.

Cucumbers in Herbed Yogurt

1 medium cucumber, peeled, halved and seeded
1 cup plain lowfat yogurt (preferably Greek)
2 tablespoons finely chopped dill, mint or cilantro
1 garlic clove, minced or pressed
salt and pepper

In a medium bowl, combine all ingredients and stir well to combine. Season to taste with salt and pepper. Can be made up to a day ahead. Serves 4.

Quinoa and Black Bean Salad
1 cup quinoa
salt and pepper
1 ear corn, shucked
1 15-ounce can black beans, rinsed and drained
1 tomato, seeded and chopped
1 jalapeno, minced
small handful finely chopped cilantro
1 tablespoon lime juice (from about 1/2 a juicy lime)
1 tablespoon olive oil
2 teaspoons red wine vinegar

In a medium pot, bring 1 1/2 cups water to a boil. Season with salt and pepper and add quinoa. Return to a boil and reduce heat to simmer. Cover and cook until water is absorbed, about 12 minutes. Remove from heat and let rest, covered, 5 minutes. Fluff with a fork and transfer to a medium bowl.

While quinoa cooks, roast corn over a gas flame or under the broil until lightly charred on all sides. Cut kernels from corn cob and add to bowl with quinoa. Add beans and remaining ingredients to bowl and toss to combine. Season with salt and pepper and serve. Can be made up to a day ahead. Serves 4.

Spinach Salad with Berries, Walnuts and Walnut Vinaigrette

1 tablespoon red wine or raspberry vinegar
2 tablespoons walnut oil
salt and pepper
10 ounces baby spinach, washed and spun dry
6 ounces blackberries, rinsed
6 ounces strawberries, rinsed, hulled and quartered

1/2 cup toasted walnuts, coarsely chopped
4 ounces fresh goat cheese, crumbled (optional)

In a large bowl, whisk together vinegar and oil and season with salt and pepper. Add spinach, berries and walnuts and toss gently to combine. Season with more salt and pepper and top with goat cheese if desired. Serves 4

Shaved Zucchini Salad

4 medium zucchini, shaved or cut into thin coins (preferably on a mandolin)
zest and juice of 1 lemon
salt and pepper
1/4-1/2 teaspoon red pepper flakes
3 tablespoons extra virgin olive oil
small handful fresh herbs such as basil, tarragon or oregano

In a large bowl, combine zucchini, lemon zest and juice, and season with salt and pepper. Let sit 10 minutes. Just before serving, arrange on a platter or place in a large bowl and top with red pepper flakes, drizzle with olive oil and sprinkle with herbs. Serve at room temperature. Serves 4

Honey-Roasted Figs

16 fresh figs
3 tablespoons best quality honey
coarse sea salt

Preheat oven to 400. Place figs in a shallow baking dish and drizzle with honey. Roast until figs have just burst, 15-20 minutes. Sprinkle with sea salt and serve warm or at room temperature. Serves 4

Early FALL

Mashed Yams with Orange and Cinnamon

1 pound garnet or jewel yams, peeled and cut into chunks
salt
¼ cup freshly squeezed orange juice
1 tablespoon unsalted butter or olive oil
½ teaspoon ground cinnamon

Place yams in a medium pot and cover with cold water by 1 inch. Add a large pinch of salt and place pot over medium-high heat; bring to a boil. Reduce to a simmer and cook until yams are easily mashed against the side of the pot. Drain yams and return to pot. Add orange juice, butter or oil and cinnamon and mash with a whisk until mostly smooth. Season with more salt and cinnamon if desired. Serve warm.Serves 4

Roasted Cauliflower with Capers, Currants and Pine nuts

1 head cauliflower, separated into florets
3 tablespoons extra virgin olive oil
salt and pepper
1 tablespoon capers, rinsed
3 tablespoons currants or golden raisins
2 tablespoons toasted pine nuts
2 teaspoons red wine vinegar
small handful chopped flat leaf parsley

Preheat oven to 400. On a rimmed baking sheet, toss cauliflower with 2 tablespoons olive oil and season with salt and pepper. Roast until tender and golden brown, about 20 minutes. shaking the pan halfway through. While cauliflower roasts, combine remaining ingredients in a large bowl. Add the hot cauliflower to the bowl and toss well to combine. Season with salt and pepper and serve warm or at room temperature. Serves 4

Shaved Brussels Sprouts Salad with Lemon and Parmesan

1 pound Brussels sprouts, ends trimmed
½ cup grated Parmesan
zest and juice of 1 lemon
3 tablespoons extra virgin olive oil
salt and pepper
small handful chopped fresh flat leaf parsley and/or basil

In a food processor fitted with the grater attachment, shred Brussels sprouts a few at a time. Alternately, halve sprouts and slice as thinly as possible. Transfer shaved sprouts to a large bowl and add remaining ingredients. Toss well to combine and let sit at least 15 minutes before serving. Serves 4-6

Late Fall

Turkey Cutlets with Cranberry Chutney

1 pound turkey or chicken cutlets
salt and pepper
1 teaspoon grapeseed oil
1 large shallot, minced
2 teaspoons minced fresh ginger
8 ounces fresh or frozen cranberries
½ cup freshly squeezed orange juice
3 tablespoons honey

Season cutlets on both sides with salt and pepper. In a large, shallow pan, heat oil over medium high. Working in batches, cook cutlets until browned on both sides and cooked through, 2-3 minutes per side depending on thickness. Transfer cooked cutlets to a baking sheet and tent with aluminum foil to keep warm. Add shallot to pan and sauté until beginning to soften, 3-5 minutes. Add ginger and cook until fragrant, another minute. Add cranberries, orange juice and honey and bring to a boil. Reduce heat slightly and let simmer rapidly until reduced and syrupy, about 5 minutes. Season with salt and pepper and serve alongside turkey. Serves 4

Poached Pears in Red Wine

4 pears, pealed, halved and cored
1/2 bottle red wine
1/2 cup agave nectar
1 cinnamon stick
3 whole cloves
2 teaspoons blackpeppercorns

In a large pot, combine all ingredients and bring to a boil. Reduce to a gentle simmer and cook, stirring occasionally and flipping pears every five minutes, until pears are easily pierced with the tip of a sharp knife, 15-20 minutes. Remove pears to a bowl with a slotted spoon and raise heat to high. Boil red wine mixture until reduced and slightly syrupy, about 15 minutes. Spoon red-wine syrup over pears and serve warm, room temperature or cold. Serves 4.

Gingery Butternut Squash and Apple Soup

1 small butternut squash, peeled
2 tablespoons unsalted butter or olive oil
1 large yellow onion, finely chopped
salt and pepper
1 apple, peeled, cored and chopped
1 tablespoon minced fresh ginger
4 cups vegetable or chicken broth
1 teaspoon white vinegar

Halve squash and using a spoon, remove seeds and place them in a small pot. Cover with 2 cups cold water and bring to a boil. Reduce heat and simmer 15 minutes. Strain squash broth and set aside; discard seeds. Cut squash into 1 inch chunks.

In a large soup pot, melt butter or heat oil over medium high. Add onion and season with salt and pepper. Cook, stirring often, until softened, about 5 minutes. Add apple and ginger and cook until fragrant, 1-2 minutes. Add squash, squash broth and vegetable or chicken broth and season with salt and pepper. Bring to a boil, reduce heat, and simmer, partially covered until squash and apples are tender, about 20 minutes. Working in batches, transfer soup to a blender and puree until smooth. Return to pot and add vinegar. Season with salt and pepper and serve. Serves 6.

Roasted Carrots and Parsnips with Green Olives

1 pound carrots, peeled and cut into 2-inch chunks
1 pound parsnips, peeled and cut into 2-inch chunks
1/4 cup olive oil
small handful chopped flat leaf parsley
1/4 cup green olives, pitted and coarsely chopped
1 tablespoon fresh lemon juice (from 1/2 a juicy lemon)
salt and pepper

Preheat oven to 400. Place carrots and parsnips on a rimmed baking sheet. Toss with 2 tablespoons olive oil and season generously with salt and pepper. Roast, shaking pan occasionally, until golden brown and tender, 30 minutes. While vegetables are roasting, combine remaining 2 tablespoons olive oil, parsley, olives and lemon juice and season with salt and pepper. Serve roasted vegetables with olive-relish. Serves 4.

WINTER

Wild Rice Salad

1 cup wild rice
salt and pepper
2 stalks celery, thinly sliced crosswise
small handful pistachios, roughly chopped
small handful dried cherries
1 tablespoon extra virgin olive oil
small handful chopped flat-leaf parsley
1 tablespoon freshly squeezed lemon juice

In a medium pot, bring 2 cups water and ½ teaspoon salt to a boil. Add rice and stir to incorporate. Reduce heat to a simmer and cover. Cook until rice is tender and water is absorbed, about 1 hour. Remove pot from heat and let sit, covered, 10 minutes. Transfer rice to a medium bowl and stir in remaining ingredients. Season to taste with salt and pepper. Can be made up to a day in advance. Serves 4-6

Chocolate-Nut Oatmeal

2/3 cup rolled oats (not quick-cooking)
¼ teaspoon cinnamon (optional)
pinch salt
small handful chopped toasted almonds or pecans
½-1 ounce best quality dark chocolate (70-85% cocoa), chopped

In a medium pot, bring 2 cups water to a boil. Add oats, a pinch of salt and cinnamon if using. Reduce heat to medium and simmer until mixture is thickened and oats are tender, about5 minutes. Stir in nuts and divide between 2 bowls. Top with chocolate and another pinch salt if desired. Serve immediately.Serves 2

Raw Kale Salad with Pomegranate

1 bunch lacinato kale, washed well, ribs removed and leaves sliced crosswise into 1/4-inch ribbons
2 tablespoons freshly squeezed lemon juice (about 1 juicy lemon)
3 tablespoons extra-virgin olive oil
small handful grated Parmesan
small handful chopped toasted walnuts (optional)
small handful pomegranate seeds or dried cranberries
salt and pepper

In a large bowl, combine kale with remaining ingredients and toss well. Let stand at room temperature 15-20 minutes or until kale is just starting to wilt. Serves 4

Maple-Mustard Glazed Salmon

2 tablespoons whole grain mustard
2 tablespoons pure maple syrup
salt and pepper
4 6-ounce filets wild salmon

Preheat oven to 450. In a small bowl combine mustard and maple syrup and season with salt and pepper. Line a rimmed baking sheet with parchment paper and arrange fish on top. Season fish with salt and pepper and spoon mustard-maple mixture evenly over each of the filets. Roast until fish is just cooked through and glaze is bubbling, 10-12 minutes depending on the thickness of the fish. Serves 4

Grapefruit, Avocado and Arugula Salad

1 large pink grapefruit
1 bunch arugula, trimmed and washed
small handful pomegranate seeds (optional)
1 ripe avocado, sliced about ¼-inch thick
juice of half a lemon
2 tablespoons extra virgin olive oil
salt and pepper

Using a sharp knife cut ends from grapefruit. Standing the fruit on one of the flat sides and following the curve of the fruit, carefully cut away the peel and pith and discard. Slice grapefruit crosswise into ¼-inch thick slices. Arrange slices in an even layer on a large platter. Toss arugula with lemon juice olive oil and season with salt and pepper. Arrange arugula on top of grapefruit slices and top with pomegranate seeds if using and avocado slices. Season all over with salt and pepper. Serve immediately. Serves 4

Spiced Roasted Pumpkin

1 small pumpkin or acorn squash, split, seeded and cut into 1 1/2-inch wedges
1/2 teaspoon cinnamon
1/4 teaspoon cayenne pepper
1/4 teaspoon ground coriander
3 tablespoons extra virgin olive oil
salt and pepper

Preheat oven to 400. On a rimmed baking sheet, toss pumpkin with spices and olive oil and season generously with salt and pepper. Roast until tender and golden brown, flipping pieces over halfway through, about 35-40 minutes total. Serves 4-6

Supplement Companies that provide Quality Nutraceuticals

COMPANY	ADDRESS	PHONE NUMBER
ADH HEALTH PRODUCTS	215 North Route 303 Congers, NY 10920	Phone: (845) 268-0027
ALLERGY RESEARCH GROUP	2300 North Loop Road Alameda, CA 94502	Phone: (800) 545-9960
CARDIOVASCULAR RESEARCH	1061 Shary Circle Concord, CA 94518	Phone: (925) 827-2636
DOUGLAS LABORATORIES	600 Boyce Road Pittsburgh, PA 15205	Phone: (800) 245-4440
EMERSON ECOLOGICS	7 Commerce Drive Bedford, NH 03110	Phone: (800) 654-4432
HEALTHY ORIGINS	P.O. Box 12615 Pittsburgh, PA 15241	Phone: (888) 228-6650
HERBS, ETC	1340 Rufina Circle Santa Fe, NM 87507	Phone: (800) 634-3727
JARROW FORMULAS	1824 So. Robertson Blvd Los Angeles, CA 90035	Phone: (800) 726-0886
METAGENICS	100 Avenida La Pata San Clemente, CA 92673	Phone: (800) 638-2848
MMS PRO	Springville, Utah 84663	Phone: (800) 240-9912
NATURE'S WAY	Springville, Utah 84663	Phone: (800) 9NATURE
PURE ENCAPSULATIONS	490 Boston Post Road Sudbury, MA 01776	Phone: (800) 753-2277
RELIANCE	500 Memorial Drive Somerset, NJ 08873	Phone: (800) 848-0089
SCHIFF	2002 South 5070 West Salt Lake City, UT 84104	Phone: (800) 526-6251

References

Chapter 3. Magnesium

Ascherio, A., Rimm, E. B., Giovannucci, E. L., et al. "A prospective study of nutritional factors and hypertension among U.S. men." *Circulation* (1992) 86(5):1475-84.

Bhargava, B., Chandra, S., Agarwal, V. V., et al. "Adjunctive magnesium infusion therapy in acute myocardial infarction." *Int J Cardiol* (1995) 52(2):95-9.

Bloch, H., Silverman, R., Mancherje, N., et al. "Intravenous magnesium sulfate as an adjunct in the treatment of acute asthma." *Chest* (1995) 107(6):1576-81.

Cairns, C. B., Kraft, M. "Magnesium attenuates the neutrophil respiratory burst in adult asthmatic patients." *Acad Emerg Med* (1996) 3(12):1093-7.

Ciarallo, L., Sauer, A. H., Shannon, M. W. "Intravenous magnesium therapy for moderate to severe pediatric asthma: results of a randomized, placebo-controlled trial." *J Pediatr* (1996) 129(6):809-14.

Dahle, L. O., Berg, G., Hammar, M., et al. "The effect of oral magnesium substitution on pregnancy-induced leg cramps." *Am J Obstet Gynecol* (1995) 173(1):175-80.

Eibl, N. L., Kobb, H. P., Nowak, H. R., et al. "Hypomagnesemia in Type II diabetes: effect of a 3-month replacement therapy." *Diabetes Care* (1995) 18(2):188-92.

Facchinetti, F., Sances, G., Borella, P., et al. "Magnesium prophylaxis of menstrual migraine: effects on intracellular magnesium." *Headache* (1991) 31(5:298-301.

Falkner, D., Glauser, J., Allen, M. "Serum magnesium levels in asthmatic patients during acute exacerbations of asthma." *Am J Emerg Med* (1992) 10(1):1-3.

Frakes, M. A., Richardson, L. E., 2nd. "Magnesium sulfate therapy in certain emergency conditions." *Am J Emerg Med* (1997) 15(2):182-7.

Fulgoni V 3rd, Nicholls J, Reed A, Buckley R, Kafer K, Huth P, Dirienzo D. Miller GD. Dairy consumption and related nutrient intake in african-american adults and children in the United States: continuing survey of food intakes by individuals 1994-1996, 1998, and the national health and nutrition examination survey 1999-2000. J Am Diet Assoc. 2007 Feb;107(2):256-64.

Gallai, V., Sarchielli, P., Coata, G., et al. "Serum and salivary magnesium levels in migraine. Results in a group of juvenile patients." *Headache* (1992) 32(3):132-5.

Garber, A. J. "Magnesium utilization survey in selected patients with diabetes." *Clin Ther* (1996) 18(2):285-94.

Geleijnse, J. M., Witteman, J. C., Bak, A. A., et al. "Reduction in blood pressure with a low sodium, high potassium, high magnesium salt in older subjects with mild to moderate hypertension." *Br Med J* (1994) 309(6952):436-40.

Hill, J. M., Britton, J. "Effect of intravenous magnesium sulphate on airway calibre and airway reactivity to histamine in asthmatic subjects." *Br J Clin Pharmacol* (1996) 42(5):629-31.

Joachims, Z., Netzer, A., Ising, H., et al. "Oral magnesium supplementation as prophylaxis for noise-induced hearing loss: results of a double blind field study." *Schriftenr-Ver-Wasser-Boden Lufthyg* (1993) 88:503-16.

Mauskop, A., Altura, B. T., Cracco, R. Q., et al. "Intravenous magnesium sulphate relieves migraine attacks in patients with low serum ionized magnesium levels: a pilot study." *Clin Sci* (Colch) (1995) 89(6):633-6.

________. "Intravenous magnesium sulfate rapidly alleviates headaches of various types." *Headache* (1996) 36(3):154-60.

Mazzotta, G., Sarchielli, P., Alberti, A., et al. "Electromyographical ischemic test and intracellular and extracellular magnesium concentration in migraine and tension-type headache patients." *Headache* (1996) 36(6):357-61.

McCarty, M. F., Rubin, E. J. "Rationales for micronutrient supplementation in diabetes." *Med Hypotheses* (1984) 13(2):139-51.

McNamara, R. M., Spivey, W. H., Skobeloff, E., et al. "Intravenous magnesium sulfate in the management of acute respiratory failure complicating asthma." *Ann Emerg Med* (1989) 18(2):197-9.

Nadler, J. L., Malayan, S., Luong, H. "Intracellular free magnesium deficiency plays a key role in increased platelet reactivity in Type II diabetes mellitus." *Diabetes Care* (1992) 15(7):835-41.

Nannini, L. J., Jr., Hofer, D. "Effect of inhaled magnesium sulfate on sodium metabisulfite-induced bronchoconstriction in asthma." *Chest* (1997) 111(4):858-61.

Noppen, M., Vanmaele, L., Impens, N., et al. "Bronchodilating effect of intravenous magnesium sulfate in acute severe bronchial asthma." *Chest* (1990) 97(2):373-6.

Okayama, H., Aikawa, T., Okayama, M., et al. "Bronchodilating effect of intravenous magnesium sulfate in bronchial asthma." *JAMA* (1987) 257(8):1076-8.

Paolisso, G., Barbagallo, M. "Hypertension, diabetes mellitus, and insulin resistance: the role of intracellular magnesium." *Am J Hypertens* (1997) 10(3):346-55.

Peikert, A., Wilimzig, C., Kohne-Volland, R. "Prophylaxis of migraine with oral magnesium: results from a prospective multicenter, placebo-controlled and double-blind randomized study." *Cephalalgia* (1996) 16(4):257-63.

Ramadan, N. M., Halvorson, H., Vande-Linde, A., Levine, S. R., Helpern, J. A., Welch, K. M. "Low brain magnesium in migraine." *Headache* (1989) 29(7):416-9 (see comments in *Headache* [1990] 30(3):168).

Resnik, L. M., Barbagallo, M., Gupta, R. K., et al. "Ionic basis of hypertension in diabetes mellitus. Role of hyperglycemia." *Am J Hypertens* (1993) 6(5 pt 1):413-7.

Rude, R. K., Olerich, M. "Magnesium deficiency: possible role in osteoporosis associated with gluten-sensitive enteropathy." *Osteoporos Int* (1996) 6(6):453-61.

Sanjuliani, A. F., de-Abreu-Fagundes, V. G., Francischetti, E. A. "Effects of magnesium on blood pressure and intracellular ion levels of Brazilian hypertensive patients." *Int J Cardiol* (1996) 56(2):177-83.

Satake, K., Lee, J. D., Shimizu, H., et al. "Relation between severity of magnesium deficiency and frequency of anginal attacks in men with variant angina." *J Am Coll Cardiol* (1996) 28:897-902.

Skobeloff, E. M., Spivey, W. H., McNamara, R. M., et al. "Intravenous magnesium sulfate for the treatment of acute asthma in the emergency department." *JAMA* (1989) 262(9):1210-3.

Soriani, S., Arnaldi, C., De Carlo, L., Arcudi, D., Mazzotta, D., Battistella, P. A., Sartori, S., Abbasciano, V. "Serum and red blood cell magnesium levels in juvenile migraine patients." *Headache* (1995) 35(1):14-16.

Sueta, C. A., Clarke, S. W., Dunlap, S. H., et al. "Effect of acute magnesium administration on the frequency of ventricular arrhythmia in patients with heart failure." *Circulation* (1994) 89(2):660-6.

Sugiyama T, Xie D. Graham-Maar RC, Inoue K., Kobayashi Y, Stettler N. Dietary and lifestyle factors associated with blood pressure among U.S. adolescents. J Adolesc Health. 2007 Feb;40(2):166-72. Epub 2006 Nov 29.

Witteman, J. C., Grobbee, D. E., Derkx, F. H., et al. "Reduction of blood pressure with oral magnesium supplementation in women with mild to moderate hypertension." *Am J Clin Nutr* (1994) 60(1):129-35.

Chapter 4. Fish Oil

Arisaka, M., Arisaka, O., Yamashiro, Y. "Fatty acid and prostaglandin metabolism in children with diabetes mellitus. II. The effect of evening primrose oil supplementation on serum fatty acid and plasma prostaglandin levels." *Prostaglandins Leukot Essent Fatty Acids* (1991) 43(3):197-201.

Aslan, A., Triadafilopoulos, G. "Fish oil fatty acid supplementation in active ulcerative colitis: a double-blind, placebo-controlled, crossover study." *Am J Gastroenterol* (1992) 87(4):432-7.

Bagga, D., Ashley, J. M., Geffrey, S. P., et al. "Effects of a very low fat, high fiber diet on serum hormones and menstrual function: implications for breast cancer prevention." *Cancer* (1995) 76(12):2491-6.

Beil, F. U., Terres, W., Orgass, M., Greten, H. "Dietary fish oil lowers lipoprotein (a) in primary hypertriglyceridemia." *Atherosclerosis* (1991) 90:95-7.

Belch, J. J., Ansell, D., Madhok, R., et al. "Effects of altering dietary essential fatty acids on requirements for non-steroidal anti-inflammatory drugs in patients with rheumatoid arthritis: a double blind placebo controlled study." *Ann Rheum Dis* (1988) 47(2):96-104.

Boyd, N. F., Martin, L. J., Noffel, M., et al. "A meta-analysis of studies of dietary fat and breast cancer risk." *Br J Cancer* (1993) 68(3):627-36.

Bronsgeest-Schoute, H. C., van Gent, C. M., Luten, J. B., et al. "The effect of various intakes of omega-3 fatty acids on the blood lipid composition in healthy human subjects." *Am J Clin Nutr* (1981) 34:1752-7.

Brzeski, M., Madhok, R., Capell, H. A. "Evening primrose oil in patients with rheumatoid arthritis and side-effects of non-steroidal anti-inflammatory drugs." *Br J Rheumatol* (1991) 30(5):370-2.

Burns, C. P., Spector, A. A. "Effects of lipids on cancer therapy." *Nutr Rev* (1990) 48(6):233-40.

Clandinin, M. T., Jumpsen, J., Suh, M. "Relationship between fatty acid accretion, membrane composition, and biologic functions." *J Pediatr* (1994) 125(5 pt 2):S25-32.

Clifford, C., Kramer, B. "Diet as risk and therapy for cancer." *Med Clin North Am* (1993) 77(4):725-44.

Connolly, J. M., Rose, D. P. "Effects of fatty acids on invasion through reconstituted basement membrane ('matrigel') by a human breast cancer cell line." *Cancer Lett* (1993) 75(2):137-42.

Connor, W. E. "Do the n-3 fatty acids from fish prevent deaths from cardiovascular disease?" (editorial; comment) *Am J Clin Nutr* (1997) 66(1):188-9.

Connor, W. E., Prince, M. J., Ullmann, D., et al. "The hypotriglyceridemic effect of fish oil in adult-onset diabetes without adverse glucose control." *Ann N Y Acad Sci* (1993) 683:337-40.

Cunnane, S. C., Manku, M. S., Horrobin, D. F. "Abnormal essential fatty acid composition of tissue lipids in genetically diabetic mice is partially corrected by dietary linoleic and gamma-linolenic acids." *Br J Nutr* (1985) 53(3):449-58.

Dagnelie, P. C., Rietveld, T., Swart, G. R., et al. "Effect of dietary fish oil on blood levels of free fatty acids, ketone bodies and triacylglycerol in humans." *Lipids* (1994) 29:41-5.

Dusserre, E., Pulcini, T., Bourdillon, M. C., et al. "Omega-3 fatty acids in smooth muscle cell phospholipids increase membrane cholesterol efflux." *Lipids* (1995) 30(1):35-41.

Fiaccavento R, Carotenuto F, Minieri M, Masuelli L, Vecchini A, Bei R. Modesti A, Binaglia L. Fusco A, Bertoli A, Forte G, Carosella L, Di Nardo P. Alpha-linolenic acid-enriched diet prevents myocardial damage and expands longevity in cardiomyopathic hamsters. Am J Pathol. 2006 Dec;169(6):1913-24.

Giovannucci, E., Rimm, E. B., Colditz, G. A., et al. "A prospective study of dietary fat and risk of prostate cancer." *J Natl Cancer Inst* (1993) 85(19):1571-9.

Harris, W. S. "Fish oils and plasma lipid and lipoprotein metabolism in humans: a critical review." *J Lipid Res* (1989) 30:785-807.

Harris WS, Gonzales M. Laney N, Sastre A, Borkon AM. Effects of omega-3 fatty acids on heart rate in cardiac transplant recipients. Am J Cardiol. 2006 Nov 15;98(10):1393-5. Epub 2006 Oct 2.

Harris, W. S., Rambjor, G. S., Windsor, S. L., et al. "N-3 fatty acids and urinary excretion of nitric oxide metabolites in humans." *Am J Clin Nutr* (1997) 65(2):459-64.

Holm, L. E., Nordevang, E., Hjalmar, M. L., et al. "Treatment failure and dietary habits in women with breast cancer." *J Natl Cancer Inst* (1993) 85(1):32-6.

Katsouyanni, K., Trichopoulou, A., Stuver, S., et al. "The association of fat and other macronutrients with breast cancer: a case-control study from Greece." *Br J Cancer* (1994) 70(3):537-41.

Makrides, M., Neumann, M. A., Simmer, K., et al. "Erythrocyte fatty acids of term infants fed either breast milk, standard formula, or formula supplemented with long-chain polyunsaturates." *Lipids* (1995) 30(10):941-8.

Rabini, R. A., Fumelli, P., Galassi, R., et al. "Action of dietary polyunsaturated fatty acids on the fluidity of erythrocyte and platelet membrane in NIDDM." *Ann N Y Acad Sci* (1993) 683:371-2.

Risch, H. A., Jain, M., Marrett, L. D., Howe, G. R. "Dietary fat intake and risk of epithelial ovarian cancer." *J Natl Cancer Inst* (1994) 86(18):1409-15.

Sanders, T. A. B., Sullivan, D. R., Reeve, J., et al. "Triglyceride-lowering effect of marine polyunsaturates in patients with hypertriglyceridemia." *Arteriosclerosis* (1985) 5:459-65.

Sebokova, E., Garg, M. L., Wierzbicki, A., et al. "Alteration of the lipid composition of rat testicular plasma membranes by dietary (n-3) fatty acids changes the responsiveness of leydig cells and testosterone synthesis." *J Nutr* (1990) 120(6):610-8.

Shekelle, R. B., Missell, L. V., Paul O., et al. "Fish consumption and mortality from coronary heart disease." (letter) *N Engl J Med* (1985) 313:820.

Shu, X. O., Zheng, W., Potischman, N., et al. "A population-based case-control study of dietary factors and endometrial cancer in Shanghai, People's Republic of China." *Am J Epidemiol* (1993) 137(2):155-65.

Siscovick, D. S., Raghunathan, T. E., King, I., et al. "Dietary intake and cell membrane levels of long-chain n-3 polyunsaturated fatty acids and the risk of primary cardiac arrest." *JAMA* (1995) 274(17):1363-7.

Stenson, W. F., Cort, D., Rodgers, J., et al. "Dietary supplementation with fish oil in ulcerative colitis." *Ann Intern Med* (1992) 116(8):609-14.

Toft, I., Bonaa, K. H., Ingebretsen, O. C., et al. "Effects of n-3 polyunsaturated fatty acids on glucose homeostasis and blood pressure in essential hypertension. A randomized, controlled trial." *Ann Int Med* (1995) 123(12):911-8.

Trichopoulou, A., Katsouyanni, K., Stuver, S., et al. "Consumption of olive oil and specific food groups in relation to breast cancer risk in Greece." *J Natl Cancer Inst* (1995) 87(2):110-6.

Valdini, A. F., Glenn, M. A., Greenblatt, L., et al. "Efficacy of fish oil supplementation for treatment of moderate elevation of serum cholesterol." *J Fam Pract* (1990) 30:55-9.

van den Brandt, P. A., van't Veer, P., Goldbohm, R. A., et al. "A prospective cohort study on dietary fat and the risk of postmenopausal breast cancer." *Cancer Res* (1993) 53(1):75-82.

Vilaseca, J., Salas, A., Guarner, F., et al. "Dietary fish oil reduces progression of chronic inflammatory lesions in a rat model of granulomatous colitis." *Gut* (1990) 31(5):539-44.

von Schacky, C. "Prophylaxis of atherosclerosis with marine omega-3 fatty acids." *Ann Intern Med* (1987) 107:890-9.

Welch AA, Bingham SA, Ive J, Friesen MD, Wareham NJ, Riboli E, Khaw KT. Dietary fish intake and plasma phospholipid n-3 polyunsaturated fatty acid concentrations in men and women in the European Prospective Investigation into Cancer-Norfolk United Kingdom cohort. Am J Clin Nutr. 2006 Dec;84(6):1330-9.

Willett, W. C., Stampfer, M. J., Colditz, G. A., et al. "Relation of meat, fat, and fiber intake to the risk of colon cancer in a prospective study among women." *N Eng J Med* (1990) 323(24):1664-72.

Zhang, S., Folsom, A. R., Sellers, T. A., et al. "Better breast cancer survival for postmenopausal women who are less overweight and eat less fat." The Iowa Women's Health Study. *Cancer* (1995) 76(2):275-83.

Chapter 5. Genistein/Soy

Adlercreutz, C. H., Goldin, B. R., Gorbach, S. L., et al. "Soybean phytoestrogen intake and cancer risk." *J Nutr* (1995) 125(suppl 3):757S-70S.

Adlercreutz, C. H., Hamalainen, E., Gorbach, S. L., et al. "Dietary phyto-oestrogens and the menopause in Japan." *Lancet* (1992) 339:1233.

Adlercreutz, C. H., Honjo, H., Higashi, A., et al. "Urinary excretion of lignans and isoflavonoid phytoestrogens in Japanese men and women consuming a traditional Japanese diet." *Am J Clin Nutr* (1991) 54(6):1093-100.

Adlercreutz, C. H., Markkanen, H., Watanabe, S. "Plasma concentrations of phyto-oestrogens in Japanese men." *Lancet* (1993) 342:1209-10.

Anderson, J. W., Johnstone, B. M., Cook-Newell, M. E. "Meta-analysis of the effects of soy protein on serum lipids." *New Engl J Med* (1995) 333:276-82.

Barnes, S. "Effect of genistein on in vitro and in vivo models of cancer." *J Nutr* (1995) 125(suppl 3):777-83.

Cancellieri F, De Leo V, Genazzani AD, Nappi C, Parenti GL, Polatti F, Ragni N, Savoca S, Teglio L, Finelli F, Nichelatti M. Efficacy on menopausal neurovegetative symptoms and some plasma lipids blood levels of an herbal product containing isoflavones and other plant extracts. Maturitas. 2007 Jan 30; [Epub ahead of print]

Cassidy, A., Bingham, S., Setchell, K. R. "Biological effects of a diet rich in isoflavones on the menstrual cycle of premenopausal women." *Amer J Clin Nutr* (1994) 60(3):333-40.

Dwyer, J. T., Goldin, B. R., Saul, N. "Tofu and soy drinks contain phytoestrogens." *J Am Diet Assoc* (1994) 94(7):739-43.

Felson, D. T., Zhang, Y., Hannan, M. T., et al. "The effect of postmenopausal estrogen therapy on bone density in elderly women." *N Engl J Med* (1993) 329(16):1141-6.

Holt, S. "A soya-based dietary supplement to lower blood cholesterol and promote cardiovascular health." *Alternative and Complementary Therapies* (1995) Nov-Dec:373-6.

Kalu, D. N., Masoro, E. J., Yu, B. P., et al. "Modulation of age-related hyperparathyroidism and senile bone loss in Fischer rats by soy protein and food restriction." *Endocrinology* (1988) 122(5):1847-54.

Kirkman, L. M., et al. "Urinary lignan and isoflavonoid excretion in men and women consuming vegetable and soy diets." *Nutr Cancer* (1995) 24:1-12.

Kováa, A. B. "Efficacy of ipriflavone in the prevention and treatment of postmenopausal osteoporosis." *Agents Actions* (1994) 41:86-7.

Lee, H. P., et al. "Dietary effects on breast-cancer risk in Singapore." *Lancet* (1991) 337:1197-200.

Martin, P. M., Horwitz, K. B., Ryan, D. S., et al. "Phytoestrogen interaction with estrogen receptors in human breast cancer cells." *Endocrinology* (1978) 103(5):1860-7.

Manjanatha MG, Shelton S, Bishop ME, Lyn-Cook LE, Aidoo A. Dietary effects of soy isoflavones daidzein and genistein on 7,12-dimethylbenz [a]anthracene-induced mammary mutagenesis and carcinogenesis in ovariectomized Big Blue transgenic rats. Carcinogenesis. 2006 Dec;27(12):2555-64.

Messina, M. "Modern applications for an ancient bean: soybeans and the prevention and treatment of chronic disease." *J Nutr* (1995) 125(suppl 3):567S-69S.

Messina, M., Barnes, S. "The role of soy products in reducing the risk of cancer." *J Natl Cancer Inst* (1991) 83(8):541-6.

Messina, M. J., Persky V., Setchell, K. D., et al. "Soy intake and cancer risk: a review of the in vitro and in vivo data." *Nutr Cancer* (1994) 21:113-31.

Occhiuto F, Pasquale RD, Guglielmo G, Palumbo DR, Zangla G, Samperi S, Renzo A. Circosta C. Effects of phytoestrogenic isoflavones from red clover (Trifolium pratense L.) on experimental osteoporosis. Phytother Res. 2007 Feb;21(2):130-4.

Pelletier, X., Belbraouet, S., Mirabel, D., et al. "A diet moderately enriched in phytosterols lowers plasma cholesterol concentrations in normocholesterolemic humans." *Ann Nutr Metab* (1995) 39:291-5.

Sammartino A, Tommaselli GA, Gargano V, di Carlo C, Attianese W, Nappi C. Short-term effects of a combination of isoflavones, lignans and Cimicifuga racemosa on climacteric-related symptoms in postmenopausal women: a double-blind, randomized, placebo-controlled trial. Gynecol Endocrinol. 2006 Nov;22(11):646-50.

Shaw, N. S., Chin, C. J., Pan, W. H. "A vegetarian diet rich in soybean products compromises iron status in young students." *J Nutr* (1995) 125(2):212-9.

Smith, D. C., Prentice, R., Thompson, D. J., et al. "Association of exogenous estrogen and endometrial carcinoma." *N Engl J Med* (1975) 293:1164-7.

Sung, M. K., Kendall, C. W., Koo, M. M., et al. "Effect of soybean saponins and gypsophilla saponin on growth and viability of colon carcinoma cells in culture." *Nutr Cancer* (1995) 23:259-70.

Tavani, A., La Vecchia, C. "Fruit and vegetable consumption and cancer risk in a Mediterranean population." *Am J Clin Nutr* (1995) 61(suppl 6):1374S-77S.

Tikkanen, M. J., Wahala, K., Ojala, S., et al. "Effect of soybean phytoestrogen intake on low density lipoprotein oxidation resistance." *Proc Natl Acad Sci USA* (1998) 95(6):3106-10.

Wang, T. T., Sathyamoorthy, N., Phang, J. M. "Molecular effects of genistein on estrogen receptor mediated pathways." *Carcinogenesis* (1996) 17(2):271-5.

Xu, X., Harris, K. S., Wang, H. J., et al. "Bioavailability of soybean isoflavones depends upon gut microflora in women." *J Nutr* (1995) 125(9):2307-15.

Ziel, H. K., Finkle, W. D. "Increased risk of endometrial carcinoma among users of conjugated estrogens." *N Engl J Med* (1975) 293:1167-70.

Chapter 6. Coenzyme Q10

Ames, B., Shigenaga, M. K., Hagen, T. M. "Oxidants, antioxidants, and the degenerative diseases of aging." *Proc Natl Acad Sci USA* (1993) 90:7918.

Atar, D., Mortensen, S. A., Flachs, H., et al. "Coenzyme Q10 protects ischemic myocardium in an open chest swine model." *Clin Investig* (1993) 71:S103-11.

Baggio, E., Gandini, R., Plancher, A. C., et al. "Italian multicenter study on the efficacy of coenzyme Q_{10} as adjunctive therapy in heart failure (interim analysis)." *Clin Invest* (1993) 71:S145-49.

Beal, M. F., Matthews, R. T., Tieleman, A., et al. "Coenzyme Q_{10} attenuates the 1-methyl-4-phenyl-1,2,3, tetrahydropyridine (MPTP) induced loss of striatal dopamine and dopaminergic axons in aged mice." *Brain Res* (1998) 783(1):109-14.

Belardinelli R, Mucaj A, Lacalaprice F, Solenghi M, Seddaiu G, Principi F, Tiano L, Littarru GP. Coenzyme Q10 and exercise training in chronic heart failure. Eur Heart J. 2006 Nov;27(22):2675-81. Epub 2006 Aug 1.

Belardinelli R, Mucaj A, Lacalaprice F, Solenghi M, Principi F, Tiano L, Littarru GP. Coenzyme Q10 improves contractility of dysfunctional myocardium in chronic heart failure. Biofactors. 2005;25(1-4):117-26. Review. No abstract available.

Bendahan, D., Desnuelle, C., Vanuxem, D., et al. "31P NMR spectroscopy and ergometer exercise test as evidence for muscle oxidative performance improvement with coenzyme Q in mitochondrial myopathies." *Neurology* (1992) 42(6):1203-8.

Chello, M., Mastroroberto, P., Romano, R., et al. "Protection by coenzyme Q_{10} from myocardial reperfusion injury during coronary artery bypass grafting." *Ann Thorac Surg* (1994) 58(5):1427-32.

Digiesi, V., Cantini, F., Brodbeck, B. "Effect of coenzyme Q_{10} on essential hypertension." *Curr Ther Res* (1990) 47:841-5.

Folkers, K., Langsjoen, P., Willis, R., et al. "Lovastatin decreases coenzyme Q levels in humans." *Proc Natl Acad Sci* (1990) 87:8931-4.

Folkers, K., Vadhanavikit, S., Mortensen, S. A. "Biochemical rationale and myocardial tissue data on the effective therapy of cardiomyopathy with coenzyme Q_{10} "*Proc Natl Acad Sci* (1985) 82:901-4.

Folkers, K., Wolaniuk, J., Simonsen, R., et al. "Biochemical rationale and the cardiac response of patients with muscle disease to therapy with coenzyme Q_{10}." *Proc Natl Acad Sci* (1985) 82:4513-6.

Fujimoto, S., Kurihara, N., Hirata, K., Takeda, T. "Effects of coenzyme Q_{10} administration on pulmonary function and exercise performance in patients with chronic lung diseases." *Clin Investig* (1993) 17(suppl 8):S162-66.

Hanaki, Y. "Coenzyme Q10 and coronary artery disease." *Clin Investig* (1993) 71:S112-S115.

Jameson, S. "Statistical data support prediction of death within six months at low levels of coenzyme Q_{10} and other entities." *Clin Investig* (1993) 71:S137-9.

Judy, W. V. "Myocardial preservation by therapy with coenzyme Q_{10} during heart surgery." *Clin Investig* (1993) 71:S155-61.

Kamikawa, T., Kobayashi, A., Yamashita, T., et al. "Effects of coenzyme Q_{10} on exercise tolerance in chronic stable angina pectoris." *Am J Cardiol* (1985) 56:247-51.

Karlsson, J., Diamant, B., Folkers, K. "Exercise-limiting factors in respiratory distress." *Respiration* (1992) 59 (suppl 2): 18-23.

Karlsson, J., Diamant, B., Folkers, K., et al. "Muscle fibre types, ubiquinone content and exercise capacity in hypertension and effort angina." *Ann Med* (1991) 23(3):339-44.

Langsjoen, P. H., Langsjoen, P. H., Folkers, K. "Long-term efficacy and safety of coenzyme Q_{10} therapy for idiopathic dilated cardiomyopathy." *Am J Cardiol* (1990) 65:521-3.

Langsjoen PH, Langsjoen JO, Langsjoen AM, Lucas LA. Treatment of statin adverse effects with supplemental Coenzyme Q10 and statin drug discontinuation. Biofactors. 2005;25(1-4):147-52.

Levin, B. "Coenzyme Q: clinical monograph." *Quar Rev Natural Medicine* (Fall 1994): 235-49.

Littarru, G. P., Nakamura, R., Ho, L., et al. "Deficiency of coenzyme Q_{10} in gingival tissue from patients with periodontal disease," *Proc Natl Acad Sci* (1971) 68:2332-5.

Morisco, C., Trimarco, B., Condorelli, M. "Effect of coenzyme Q_{10} in patients with congestive heart failure: a long-term multicenter randomized study." *Clin Invest* (1993) 71:S134-36.

Sander S, Coleman CI, Patel AA, Kluger J, White CM. The impact of coenzyme Q10 on systolic function in patients with chronic heart failure. J Card Fail. 2006 Aug;12(6):464-72.

Witt, E. H., Reznick, A. Z., Viguie, C. A., et al. "Exercise, oxidative damage and effects of antioxidant manipulation." *J Nutr* (1992) 122 (suppl 3): 766-73.

Ylikoski, T., Piirainen, J., Hanninen, O., et al. "The effect of coenzyme Q_{10} on the exercise performance of cross-country skiers." *Mol Aspects Med* (1997) (suppl 18): S283-90.

Chapter 7. Milk Thistle

Agarwal, R., Lahiri, M., Mohan, R. R., et al. "Stage specific antitumor promoting potential of silymarin in mouse skin." (meeting abstract) *Proc Annu Meet Am Assoc Cancer Res* (1996) 37:1893.

Alarcon de la Lastra, A. C., Martin, M. J., Motilva, V., et al. "Gastroprotection induced by silymarin, the hepatoprotective principle of Silybum marianum in ischemia-reperfusion mucosal injury: role of neutrophils." *Planta Med* (1995) 61(2):116-9.

Boijk, G., Stroedter, L., Herbst, H., et al. "Silymarin retards collagen accumulation in early and advanced biliary fibrosis secondary to complete bile duct obliteration in rats." *Hepatology* (1997) 26(3):643-9.

Campos, R., Garrido, A., et al. "Silybin dihemisuccinate protects against glutathione depletion and lipid peroxidation induced by acetaminophen on rat liver." *Planta Med* (1989) 55:417-9.

Crocenzi FA, Roma MG. Silymarin as a new hepatoprotective agent in experimental cholestasis: new possibilities for an ancient medication. Curr Med Chem. 2006;13(9):1055-74. Review.

Das SK, Vasudevan DM. Protective effects of silymarin, a milk thistle (Silybium marianum) derivative on ethanol-induced oxidative stress in liver. Indian J Biochem Biophys. 2006 Oct;43(5):306-11.

Dehmlow, C., Erhard, J., de Groot, H. "Inhibition of Kupffer cell functions as an explanation for the hepatoprotective properties of silibinin." *Hepatology* (1996) 23(4):749-54.

Ferenci, P., Dragosics, B., Dittrich, H., et al. "Randomized controlled trial of silymarin treatment in patients with cirrhosis of the liver." *J Hepatol* (1989) 9(1):105-13.

Flaig TW, Gustafson DL, Su LJ, Zirrolli JA, Crighton F, Harrison GS, Pierson AS, Agarwal R, Glode LM. A phase I and pharmacokinetic study of silybin-phytosome in prostate cancer patients. Invest New Drugs. 2007 Apr;25(2):139-46. Epub 2006 Nov 1.

Flora, K., Hahn, M., Rosen, H., et al. "Milk thistle (Silybum marianum) for the therapy of liver disease." *Am J Gastroenterol* (1998) 93(2):139-43.

Hoh C, Boocock D, Marczylo T, Singh R, Berry DP, Dennison AR, Hemingway D, Miller A, West K, Euden S, Garcea G, Farmer PB, Steward WP, Gescher AJ. Pilot study of oral silibinin, a putative chemopreventive agent, in colorectal cancer patients: silibinin levels in plasma, colorectum, and liver and their pharmacodynamic consequences. Clin Cancer Res. 2006 May 1;12(9):2944-50.

Katiyar, S. K., Korman, N. J., Mukhtar, H., et al. "Protective effects of silymarin against photocarcinogenesis in a mouse skin model." *J Natl Cancer Inst* (1997) 89(8):556-66.

Krecman, V., Skottova, N., Walterova, D., et al. "Silymarin inhibits the development of diet-induced hypercholesterolemia in rats." *Planta Med* (1998) 64(2):138-42.

Lang, I., Nekam, K., Deak, G., et al. "Immunomodulatory and hepatoprotective effects of in vivo treatment with free radical scavengers." *Ital J Gastroenterol* (1990) 22:283-7.

Muriel, P., Mourelle, M. "Prevention by silymarin of membrane alteration in acute CC14 liver damage." *J Appl Toxicol* (1990) 10(4):275-9.

Pietrangelo, A., Borella, F., Casalgrandi, G., et al. "Antioxidant activity of silybin in vivo during long-term iron overload in rats." *Gastroenterology* (1995) 109(6):1941-9.

Salmi, H. A., Sarna, S. "Effect of silymarin on chemical, functional, and morphological alterations of the liver, a double-blind controlled study." *Scand J Gastroenterol* (1982) 17(4):517-21.

Valenzuela, A., Aspillaga, M., et al. "Selectivity of silymarin on the increase of the glutathione content in different tissues of the rat." *Planta Med* (1989) 55:420-2.

Velussi, M., Cernigoi, A. M., De Monte, A., et al. "Long-term (12 months) treatment with an antioxidant drug (silymarin) is effective on hyperinsulinemia, exogenous insulin need and malondialdehyde levels in cirrhotic diabetec patients." *J Hepatol* (1997) 26(4):871-9.

Zhou B, Wu LJ, Tashiro S, Onodera S, Uchiumi F, Ikejima T. Silibinin protects rat cardiac myocyte from isoproterenol-induced DNA damage independent on regulation of cell cycle. Biol Pharm Bull. 2006 Sep;29(9):1900-5.

Zi, X., Grasso, A. W., Kung, H. J., et al. "A flavonoid antioxidant, silymarin, inhibits activation of erbB1 signaling and induces cyclin-dependent kinase inhibitors, G1 arrest, and anticarcinogenic effects in human prostate carcinoma DU145 cells." *Cancer Res* (1998) 58(9):1920-9.

Zi, X., Mukhtar, H., Agarwal, R. "Novel cancer chemopreventive effects of a flavonoid antioxidant silymarin: inhibition of mRNA expression of an endogenous tumor promoter TNF alpha." *Biochem Biophys Res Commun* (1997) 239(1):334-9.

Chapter 8. Probiotics

Andre, C., Andre, F., Colin, L., et al. "Measurement of intestinal permeability to mannitol and lactulose as a means of diagnosing food allergy and evaluating therapeutic effectiveness of disodium cromoglycate." *Ann Allergy* (1987) 59(5 pt 2):127-30.

Berg, R., Bernasconi, P., Fowler, D., et al. "Inhibiton of *Candida albicans* translocation from the gastrointestinal tract of mice by oral administration of *Saccharomyces boulardii*." *J Infect Dis* (1993) 168:1314-8.

Bernet, M. F., Brassart, D., Neeser, J. R., Servin, A. L. "*Lactobacillus acidophilus* LA 1 binds to human intestinal lines and inhibits cell attachment and cell invasion by enterovirulent bacteria." *Gut* (1994) 35:483-9.

Bjarnason, I., Peters, T. J., Wise, R. J. "The leaky gut of alcoholism: possible route of entry for toxic compounds." *Lancet* (1984) 1(8370):179-82.

Bleichner, G., Blehaut, H., Mentec, H., et al. "*Saccharomyces boulardii* prevents diarrhea in critically ill tube-fed patients. A multicenter, randomized, double-blind placebo-controlled trial." *Intensive Care Med* (1997) 23(5):517-23.

Casey PG, Gardiner GE, Casey G, Bradshaw B, Lawlor PG, Lynch Pb. Leonard FC, Stanton C, Ross RP, Fitzgerald GF, Hill C. A FIVE-STRAIN PROBIOTIC COMBINATION REDUCES PATHOGEN SHEDDING AND ALLEVIATES DISEASE SIGNS IN PIGS CHALLENGED WITH SALMONELLA TYPHIMURIUM. Appl Environ Microbiol. 2007 Jan 19; [Epub ahead of print]

Colombel, J. R., Cortot, A., Neut, C., et al. "Yoghurt with Bifidobacterium longum reduces erythromycin-induced gastrointestinal effects." (letter) *Lancet* (1987) 2(8549):43.

Dias, R. S., Bambirra, E. A., Silva, M. E., et al. "Protective effect of *Saccharomyces Boulardii* on the establishment of various strains of 'candida' in the digestive tract of gnotobiotic mice." *Ann Microbiol* (1982) 133:491-501.

Elmer, G. W., Surawicz, C. M., McFarland, L. V. "Biotherapeutic agents. A neglected modality for the treatment and prevention of selected intestinal and vaginal infections." *JAMA* (1996) 275(11):870-6.

Fuller, R. "Probiotics in human medicine." *Gut* (1991) 32(4):439-42.

Fuller, R., Gibson, G. R. "Modification of the intestinal microflora using probiotics and prebiotics." *Scand J Gastroenterol Suppl* (1997) 222:28-31.

Gibson, G. R., Beatty, E. R., Wang, X., et al. "Selective stimulation of bifidobacteria in the human colon by oligofructose and insulin." *Gastroenterology* (1995) 108(4):975-82.

Heczko PB, Strus M. Kochan P. Critical evaluation of probiotic activity of lactic acid bacteria and their effects. J Physiol Pharmacol. 2006 Nov;57 Suppl 9:5-12.

Hiller, S. L., Krohn, M. A., Rabe, L. K., et al. "The normal vaginal flora, H_2O_2 producing lactobacilli and bacterial vaginosis in pregnant women." *Clin Infect Dis* (1993) 16 (suppl 4):S273-81.

Hilton, E., Isenberg, H. D., Alpertstein, P., et al. "Ingestion of *Lactobacilli acidophilus* as prophylaxis for candidal vaginitis." *Ann Intern Med* (1992) 116:353-7.

Hollander, D., Vadheim, C. M., Brettholz, E., et al. "Increased intestinal permeability in patients with Crohn's disease and their relatives: a possible etiologic factor." *Ann Intern Med* (1986) 105(6):883-5.

Isolauri, E., Juntamen, M., Rautanen, T., et al. "A human Lactobacillus strain (*Lactobacillus casei* SP strain GG) promotes recovery from acute diarrhea in children." *Pediatrics* (1991) 88:90-7.

Kjeldsen-Kragh, J., Haugen, M., Borchgrevink, C. F., et al. "Controlled trial of fasting and one-year vegetarian diet in rheumatoid arthritis." *Lancet* (1991) 338:899-902.

Larsen, B. "Vaginal flora in health and disease." *Clin Obstet Gynecol* (1993) 36:107-21.

Mao, Y., Nobaek, S., Kasravi, B., et al. "The effects of Lactobacillus strains and oat fiber on methoxtrexate-induced interocolitis in rats." *Gastroenterology* (1996) 111(2):334-44.

Mach T. Clinical usefulness of probiotics in inflammatory bowel diseases. J Physiol Pharmacol. 2006 Nov;57 Suppl 9:23-33.

Mills, J. A. "Do bacteria cause chronic polyarthritis?" *N Engl J Med* (1989) 320(4):245-6.

Peltonen, R., Kjeldsen-Kragh, J., Haugen, M., et al. "Changes of faecal flora in rheumatoid arthritis during fasting and one-year vegetarian diet." *Br J Rheumatol* (1994) 33:638-43.

Reid, G., Bruce, A. W., Cook, R. L., et al. "Effect on urogenital flora of antibiotic therapy for urinary tract infection." *Sand J Infect Dis* (1990) 22:43-7.

Reid, G., Bruce, A. W., Taylor, M. "Influence of three-day antimicrobial therapy and *Lactobacillus* vaginal suppositories on recurrence of urinary tract infections." *Clin Ther* (1992) 14:11-6.

Reid, G., Cook, R. L., Bruce, A. W. "Examination of strains of lactobacilli for properties that may influence bacterial interference in the urinary tract." *J Urol* (1987) 138(2):330-5.

Salminen S, Isolauri E. Intestinal colonization, microbiota, and probiotics. J Pediatr. 2006 Nov;149(5 Suppl):S115-20.

Tepper, R. E., Simon, D., Brandt, L. J., et al. "Intestinal permeability in patients infected with human immunodeficiency virus." *Am J Gastroenterol* (1994) 89:878-82.

Thomason, J. L., Gelbart, S. M., Scaglione, N. J. "Bacterial vaginosis: current review with indications for asymptomatic therapy." *Am J Obstet Gynecol* (1991) 165:1210-17.

Tong JL, Ran ZH, Shen J, Zhang CX, Xiao SD. Meta-analysis: the effect of supplementation with probiotics on eradication rates and adverse events during Helicobacter pylori eradication therapy. Aliment Pharmacol Ther. 2007 Jan 15;25(2):155-68.

Witsell, D. L., Garret, C. G., Yarbrough, W. G., et al. "Effect of lactobacillus acidophilus on antibiotic-associated gastrointestinal morbidity: a prospective randomized trial." *J Otolaryngol* (1995) 24(4):230-3.

Chapter 9. Glutamine

Aukrust, P., Svardal, A. M., Muller, F., et al. "Increased levels of oxidized glutathione in CD4+ lymphocytes associated with disturbed intracellular redox balance in human immunodeficiency virus type 1 infection." *Blood* (1995) 86(1):258-67.

Bell SG. Immunomodulation. Part IV: Glutamine. Neonatal Netw. 2006 Nov-Dec;25(6):439-43. Review.

Byrne, T. A., Persinger, R. L., Young, L. S., et al. "A new treatment for patients with short-bowel syndrome. Growth hormone, glutamine, and a modified diet." *Ann Surg* (1995) 222(3):243-54.

Curi, T. C., De Melo, M. P., De Azevedo, R. B., et al. "Glutamine utilization by rat neutrophils: presence of phosphate-dependent glutamininase." *Am J Physiol* (1997) 273(4 pt 1):C1124-29.

Devreker, F., Winston, R. M., Hardy, K. "Glutamine improves human preimplantation development in vitro." *Fertil Steril* (1998) 69(2):293-9.

Droge, W., Holm, E. "Role of cysteine and glutathione in HIV infection and other diseases associated with muscle wasting and immunological dysfunction." *FASEB J* (1997) 11(13):1077-89.

Fahr, M. J., Kornbluth, J., Blossom, S., et al. "Glutamine enhances immunoregulation of tumor growth." Harry M. Vars Research Award. *J Parenter Enteral Nutr* (1994) 18(6):471-6.

Flynn, W. J., Jr., Gosche, J. R., Garrison, R. N. "Intestinal blood flow is restored with glutamine or glucose suffusion after hemorrhage." *J Surg Res* (1992) 52(5):499-504.

Furukawa, S., Saito, H., Fukatsu, K., et al. "Glutamine-enhanced bacterial killing by neutrophils from postoperative patients." *Nutrition* (1997) 13(10):863-9.

Gianotti, L., Alexander, J. W., Gennari, R., et al. "Oral glutamine decreases bacterial translocation and improves survival in experimental gut-origin sepsis." *J Parenter Enteral Nutr* (1995) 19 (1):69-74.

Grant, J. P., Snyder, P. J. "Use of L-glutamine in total parenteral nutrition." *J Surg Res* (1988) 44(5):506-13.

Hack, V., Weiss, C., Friedmann, B., et al. "Decreased plasma glutamine level and CD4+ T cell number in response to eight weeks of anaerobic training." *Am J Physiol* (1997) 272(5 pt 1):E788-95.

Harward, T. R., Coe, D., Souba, W. W., et al. "Glutamine preserves gut glutathione levels during intestinal ischemia/reperfusion." *J Surg Res* (1994) 56(4):351-5.

Holecek M, Muthny T, Kovarik M, Sispera L. Simultaneous infusion of glutamine and branched-chain amino acids (BCAA) to septic rats does not have more favorable effect on protein synthesis in muscle, l iver, and small intestine than separate infusions. JPEN J Parenter Enteral Nutr. 2006 Nov-Dec;30(6):467-73.

Houdijk, A. P., Teerlink, T., Bloemers, F. W., et al. "Gut endotoxin restriction prevents catabolic changes in glutamine metabolism after surgery in the bile duct-ligated rat." *Ann Surg* (1997) 225(4):391-400.

Keast, D., Arstein, D., Harper, W., et al. "Depression of plasma glutamine concentration after exercise stress and its possible influence on the immune system." *Med J Aust* (1995) 162(1):15-8.

Klimberg, V. S., Kornbluth, J., Cao, Y., et al. "Glutamine suppresses PGE2 synthesis and breast cancer growth." *J Surg Res* (1996) 63(1):293-7.

Klimberg, V. S., McClellan, J. L. "Glutamine, cancer, and its therapy." *Am J Surg* (1996) 172(5):418-24.

Klimberg, V. S., Pappas, A. A., Nwokedi, E., et al. "Effect of supplemental glutamine on methotrexate concentrations in tumors." *Arch Surg* (1992) 127(11):1317-20.

Klimberg, V. S., Salloum, R. M., Kasper, M., et al. "Oral glutamine accelerates healing of the small intestine and improves outcome after whole abdominal radiation." *Arch Surg* (1990) 125(8):1040-5.

Klimberg, V. S., Souba, W. W., Dolson, D. J., et al. "Prophylactic glutamine protects the intestinal mucosa from radiation injury." *Cancer* (1990) 66(1):62-8.

Lacey, J. M., Wilmore, D. W. "Is glutamine a conditionally essential amino acid?" *Nutr Rev* (1990) 48:299-309.

McAnena, O. J., Moore, F. A., Moore, E. E., Jones, T. N., Parrsons, P. "Selective uptake of glutamine in the gastrointestinal tract: confirmation in a human study." *Br J Surg* (1991) 78:480-2.

Newsholme, E. A., Calder, P. C. "The proposed role of glutamine in some cells of the immune system and speculative consequences for the whole animal." *Nutrition* (1997) 13(7-8):728-30.

Ogle, C. K., Ogle, J. D., Mao, J. X., et al. "Effect of glutamine on phagocytosis and bacterial killing by normal and pediatric burn patient neutrophils." *J Parenter Enteral Nutr* (1994) 18:128-33.

Rhoads, J. M., Argenzio, R. A., Chen, W., Rippe, R. A., et al. "L-glutamine stimulates intestinal cell proliferation and activates mitogen-activated protein kinases." *Am J Physiol* (1997) 272(5 pt 1): G943-53.

Rouse, K., Nwokedi, E., Woodliff, J. E., et al. "Glutamine enhances selectivity of chemotherapy through changes in glutathione metabolism." *Ann Surg* (1995) 221(4):420-6.

Rudman, D., Kutner, M. H., Rogers, C. M., et al. "Impaired growth hormone secretion in the adult population: relation to age and adiposity." *J Clin Invest* (1981) 67:1361-9.

Schimpl, G., Pesendorfer, P., Steinwender, G., et al. "Allopurinol and glutamine attenuate bacterial translocation in chronic portal hypertensive and common bile duct ligated growing rats." *Gut* (1996) 39(I):48-53.

Soondrum K, Hinds R. Management of intestinal failure. Indian J Pediatr. 2006 Oct;73(10):913-8. Review.

Smith, R. J. "Glutamine metabolism and its physiologic importance." *J Parenter Enteral Nutr* (1990) 14:40S-44S.

Souba, W. W. "Glutamine and cancer." *Ann Surg* (1993) 218:715-28.

Souba, W. W., Herskowitz, K., Klimberg, V. S., et al. "The effects of sepsis and endotoxemia on gut glutamine metabolism." *Ann Surg* (1990) 211(5):543-9; discussion 549-51.

Souba, W. W., Klimberg, V. S., Hautamaki, R. D., et al. "Oral glutamine reduces bacterial translocation following abdominal radiation." *J Surg Res* (1990) 4(1):1-5.

Souba, W. W., Klimberg, V. S., Plumley, D. A., et al. "The role of glutamine in maintaining a healthy gut and supporting the metabolic response to injury and infection." *J Surg Res* (1990) 48:383-91.

van der Hulst, R. R., van Kreel, B. K., von Meyenfeldt, M. F., et al. "Glutamine and the preservation of gut integrity." *Lancet* (1993) 341:1363-5.

van der Hulst, R. R., von Meyenfeldt, M. F., Deutz, N. E., et al. "Glutamine extraction by the gut is reduced in patients with depleted gastrointestinal cancer." *Ann Surg* (1997) 225(1):112-21.

van der Hulst, R. R., von Meyenfeldt, M. F., Soeters, P. B. "Glutamine: an essential amino acid for the gut." *Nutrition* (1996) 12(suppl 11-12):S78-81.

Welbourne, T. C. "Increased plasma bicarbonate and growth hormone after an oral glutamine load." *Am J Clin Nutr* (1995) 61:1058-61.

Welbourne, T. C., King, A., Horton, K. "Enteral glutamine supports hepatic glutathione efflux during inflammation." *J Nutr Biochem* (1993) 4:236-42.

Yoshida, S., Matsui, M., Shirouzu, Y., et al. "Effects of glutamine supplements and radiochemotherapy on systemic immune and gut barrier function in patients with advanced esophageal cancer." *Ann Surg* (1998) 227(4):485-91.

Zapata-Sirvent, R. L., Hansbrough, J. F., Ohara, M. M., et al. "Bacterial translocation in burned mice after administration of various diets including fiber- and glutamine-enriched enteral formulas." *Crit Care Med* (1994) 22(4):690-6.

Chapter 10. Flaxseed

Adlercreutz, H., Hockerstedt, K., Bannwart, C., et al. "Effect of dietary components, including lignans and phytoestrogens, on enterohepatic circulation and liver metabolism of estrogens and on sex hormone binding globulin (SHBG)." *J Steroid Biochem* (1987) 27(4-6):1135-44.

Adlercreutz, H., Mousavi, Y., Hockerstedt, K. "Diet and breast cancer." *Acta Oncol* (1992) 31(2):175-81.

Belch, J. J., Ansell, D., Madhok, R., et al. "Effects of altering dietary essential fatty acids on requirements for non-steroidal anti-inflammatory drugs in patients with rheumatoid arthritis: A double blind placebo controlled study." *Ann Rheum Dis* (1988):96-104.

Bierenbaum, M. L., Reichstein, R., Watkins, T. R. "Reducing atherogenic risk in hyperlipemic humans with flax seed supplementation: a preliminary report." *J Am Coll Nutr* (1993) 12(5):501-4.

Borriello, S. P., Setchell, K. D., Axelson, M., et al. "Production and metabolism of lignans by the human faecal flora." *J Appl Bacteriol* (1985) 58(1):37-43.

Cunnane, S. C., Ganguli, S., Menard, C., et al. "High alpha-linolenic acid flaxseed (Linum usitatissimum): some nutritional properties in humans." *Br J Nutr* (1993) 69(2):443-53.

Cunnane, S. C., Hamadeh, M. J., Liede, A. C., et al. "Nutritional attributes of traditional flaxseed in healthy young adults." *Am J Clin Nutr* (1995) 61(1):62-8.

de Lorgeril, M., Renaud, S., Mamelle, N., et al. "Mediterranean alpha-linolenic acid-rich diet in secondary prevention of coronary heart disease." *Lancet* (1994) 343:1454-9.

Ferrier, L. K., Caston, L. J., Leeson, S., et al. "Alpha-linolenic acid—and docosahexaenoic acid-enriched eggs from hens fed flaxseed: influence on blood lipids and platelet phospholipid fatty acids in humans." *Am J Clin Nutr* (1995) 62(1):81-6.

Holub, B. J. "Flaxseed: a potential treatment for lupus nephritis." *Kidney Int* (1994) 48(2):475-80.

Kelly, D. S. "Alpha-linolenic acid and immune response." *Nutrition* (1992) 8:215-7.

Kronberg SL, Barcelo-Coblijn G, Shin J, Lee K, Murphy EJ. Bovine muscle n-3 fatty acid content is increased with flaxseed feeding. Lipids. 2006 Nov;41(11):1059-68.

Lampe, J. W., Martini, M. C., Kurzer, M. S., et al. "Urinary lignan and isoflavonoid excretion in premenopausal women consuming flaxseed powder." *Am J Clin Nutr* (1994) 60:122-8.

Martin, M. E., Haourigui, M., Pelissero, C., et al. "Interactions between phytoestrogens and human sex steroid binding protein." *Life Sci* (1996) 58(5):429-36.

Nielsen, G. L., Faarvang, K. L., Thomsen, B. S., et al. "The effects of dietary supplementation with n-3 polyunsaturated fatty acids in patients with rheumatoid arthritis: a randomized, double-blind trial." *Eur J Clin Invest* (1992) 22(10):687-91.

Paschos GK, Magkos F, Panagiotakos DB, Votteas V, Zampelas A. Dietary supplementation with flaxseed oil lowers blood pressure in dyslipidaemic patients. Eur J Clin Nutr. 2007 Jan 31; [Epub ahead of print]

Prasad, K. "Dietary flax seed in prevention of hypercholesterolemic atherosclerosis." *Atherosclerosis* (1997) 132 (1):69-76.

Serraino, M. "Studies on the effect of flaxseed on colon and mammary carcinogenesis." *Diss Abstr Int [B]* (1993) 53(8):4041.

Serraino, M., Thompson, L. U. "The effect of flaxseed supplementation on early risk markers for mammary carcinogenesis." *Cancer Lett* (1991) 60(2):135-42.

________. "The effect of flaxseed on the initiation and promotional stages of mammary tumorigenesis." (meeting abstract) *FASEB J* (1991) 5(5):A928.

________. "Flaxseed supplementation and early markers of colon carcinogenesis." *Cancer Lett* (1992) 63:159-65.

Thompson, L. U., Rickard, S. E., Orcheson, L. J., et al. "Flaxseed and its lignan and oil components reduce mammary tumor growth at a late stage of carcinogenesis." *Carcinogenesis* (1996) 17(6):1373-6.

Thompson, L. U., Serraino, M. R. "Protective effect of flaxseed as suggested by risk markers for mammary carcinogenesis." (meeting abstract) *FASEB J* (1991) 5(5):A928.

Chapter 11. Homocysteine, B_6, B_{12}, and Folate

Anker, G., Lonning, P. E., Ueland, P. M., et al. "Plasma levels of the atherogenic amino acid homocysteine in post-menopausal women with breast cancer treated with tamoxifen." *Int J Cancer*. (1995) 60:365-8.

Beaumont, V., Malinow, M. R., Sexton, G., et al. "Hyperhomocyst(e)inemia, anti-estrogen antibodies and other risk factors for thrombosis in women on oral contraceptives." *Atherosclerosis* (1992) 94(2-3):147-52.

Boers, G. "Hyperhomocysteinaemia: A newly recognized risk factor for vascular disease." *Neth J Med* (1994) 4:34-41.

Bottiglieri, T. "Folate, vitamin B_{12}, and neuropsychiatric disorders." *Nutr Rev* (1996) 54(12):382-90.

Boushey, C. J., Beresford, S. A., Omenn, G. S., et al. "A quantitative assessment of plasma homocysteine as a risk factor for vascular disease: probable benefits of increasing folic acid intakes." *JAMA* (1995) 274:1049-57.

Brattstrom, L., Lindgren, A., Israelsson, B., et al. "Homocysteine and cysteine: determinants of plasma levels in middle-aged and elderly subjects." *J Intern Med* (1994) 236:633-41.

________. "Hyperhomocysteinaemia in stroke: prevalence, causes, and relationships to type of stroke and stroke risk factors." *Eur J Clin Invest* (1992) 22:214-21.

Chasen-Taber, L., Selhub, J., Rosenberg, I., et al. "A prospective study of folate and vitamin B6 and risk of myocardial infarction in U.S. physicians." *J Am Coll Nutr* (1996) 15:136-43.

Cheng, S. W., Ting, A. C., Wong, J. "Fasting total plasma homocysteine and atherosclerotic peripheral vascular disease." *Ann Vasc Surg* (1997) 11:217-23.

Clarke, R., Daly, L., Robinson, K., et al. "Hyperhomocysteinemia: an independent risk factor for vascular disease." *N Engl J Med* (1991) 324:1149-55.

Coull, B. M., Malinow, M. R., Beamer, N., et al. "Elevated plasma homocyst(e)ine concentration as a possible independent risk factor for stroke." *Stroke* (1990) 21:572-6.

Cravo, M. L., Gloria, L. M., Selhub, J., et al. "Hyperhomocysteinemia in chronic alcoholism: correlation with folate, vitamin B_{12}, and vitamin B_6 status." *Am J Clin Nutr* (1996) 63:220-4.

Den Heijer, M., Koster, T., Blom, H. J., et al. "Hyperhomocysteinemia as a risk factor for deep-vein thrombosis." *N Engl J Med* (1996) 334:759-62.

Dzielinska Z, Januszewicz A, Demkow M, Makowiecka-Ciesla M, Prejbisz A, Naruszewicz M, Nowicka G, Kadziela J, Zielinski T, Florczak E, Janas j,

Januszewicz M, Ruzyllo W. Cardiovascular risk factors in hypertensive patients with coronary artery disease and coexisting renal artery stenosis. J Hypertens. 2007 Mar;25(3):663-670.

Fallest-Strobl, P. C., Koch, D. D., Stein, J. H., et al. "Homocysteine: a new risk factor for atherosclerosis." *Am Fam Physician* (1997) 56(6):1607-12.

Franken, D., Boers, G., Blom, H., et al. "Treatment of mild hyperhomocysteinaemia in vascular disease patients." *Arterioscler Thromb Vasc Biol* (1994) 14:465-70.

Glueck, C. J., Shaw, P., Lang, J. E., et al. "Evidence that homocysteine is an independent risk factor for atherosclerosis in hyperlipidemic patients." *Am J Cardiol* (1995) 75:132-6.

Hultberg, B., Agardh, E., Anderson, A., et al. "Increased levels of plasma homocysteine are associated with nephropathy, but not severe retinopathy in Type 1 diabetes mellitus." *Scand J Clin Lab Invest* (1991) 51:277-82.

Landgren, F., Israelsson, B., Lindgren, A., et al. "Plasma homocysteine in acute myocardial infarction: homocysteine-lowering effect of folic acid." *J Int Med* (1995) 237:381-88.

Levitt, A. J., Karlinsky, H. "Folate, vitamin B_{12} and cognitive impairment in patients with Alzheimer's disease." *Acta Psychiatr Scand* (1992) 86:301-5.

Loehrer, F., Angst, C., Haefeli, W., et al. "Low whole-blood S-adenosylmethionine and correlation between 5-methyltetrahydrofolate and homocysteine in coronary artery disease." *Arterioscler Thromb Vasc Biol* (1996) 16:227-33.

Lussier-Cacan, S., Xhignesse, M., Piolot, A., et al. "Plasma total homocysteine in healthy subjects: sex-specific relation with biological traits." *Am J Clin Nutr* (1996) 64:587-93.

Malinow, M. R., Kang, S. S., Taylor, L. M., et al. "Prevalence of hyperhomocyst(e)inemia in patients with peripheral arterial occlusive disease." *Circulation* (1989) 79:1180-8.

McCully, K. S. "Vascular pathology of homocysteinemia: implications for the pathogenesis of arteriosclerosis." *Am J Pathol* (1996) 56:111-28.

Metz, J., Bell, A. H., Flicker, L., et al. "The significance of subnormal serum B12 concentration in older people: a case control study." *J Am Geriatr Soc* (1996):44:1355-61.

Molgaard, J., Malinow, M. R., Lassvik, C., et al. "Hyperhomocyst(e)inaemia: an independent risk factor for intermittent claudication." *J Intern Med* (1992) 231:273-9.

Munshi, M. N., Stone, A., Fink, L., et al. "Hyperhomocysteinemia following a methionine load in patients with non-insulin-dependent diabetes mellitus and macrovascular disease." *Metabolism* (1996) 45:133-5.

Neugebauer, S., Baba, T., Kurokawa, K., et al. "Defective homocysteine metabolism as a risk factor for diabetic retinopathy." *Lancet* (1997) 349:473-4.

Nygard, O., Nordrehaug, J. E., Refsum, H., et al. "Plasma homocysteine levels and mortality in patients with coronary artery disease." *N Engl J Med* (1997) 337(4): 230-6.

Nygard, O., Vollset, S. E., Refsum, H., et al. "Total plasma homocysteine and cardiovascular risk profile—the Hordaland Homocysteine Study." *JAMA* (1995) 274:1526-33.

Reynolds, E. H. "Multiple sclerosis and vitamin B_{12} metabolism." *J Neuroimmunol* (1992) 40(2-3):225-30.

Reynolds, E. H., Bottiglieri, T., Laundy, M., et al. "Vitamin B_{12} metabolism in multiple sclerosis." *Arch Neurol* (1992) 49:649-52.

Robinson, K., Mayer, E., Jacobsen, D. W. "Homocysteine and coronary artery disease." *Cleve Clin J Med* (1994) 61:438-50.

Ruiz JR, Sola R, Gonzalez-Gross M, Ortega FB, Vicente-Rodriguez G, Garcia-Fuentes M, Gutierrez A, Sjostrom M, Pietrzik K, Castillo MJ. Cardiovascular Fitness Is Negatively Associated With Homocysteine Levels in Female Adolescents. Arch Pediatr Adolesc Med. 2007 Feb;16(2):166-171.

Scholl, T. O., Hediger, M. L., Schall, J. I., et al. "Dietary and serum folate: their influence on the outcome of pregnancy." *Am J Clin Nutr* (1996) 63:520-5.

Stampfer, M. J., Malinow, M. R., Willett, W. C., et al. "A prospective study of plasma homocyst(e)ine and risk of myocardial infarction in U.S. physicians." *JAMA* (1992) 268:877-81.

Swain, R. "An update of vitamin B_{12} metabolism and deficiency states." *J Fam Pract* (1995) 41(6):595-600.

Tucker, K. L., Selhub, J., Wilson, P. W., et al. "Dietary intake pattern relates to plasma folate and homocysteine concentrations in the Framingham Heart Study." *J Nutr* (1996) 126:3025-31.

Ubbink, J., Vermaak, W., van der Merwe, et al. "Vitamin requirements for the treatment of hyperhomocysteinemia in humans." *J Nutr* (1994) 124:1927-33.

Vaccaro, O., Ingrosso, D., Rivellese, A., et al. "Moderate hyperhomocysteinaemia and retinopathy in insulin-dependent diabetes." (letter) *Lancet* (1997) 349:1102-3.

Vizzardi E, Nodari S, Fiorina C, Metra M, Dei Cas L. Plasma Homocysteine Levels and Late Outcome in Patients with Unstable Angina Cardiology. 2007 Feb 1;107(4):354-359 [Epub ahead of print]

Wald, N. J., Hackshaw, A. D., Stone, R., et al. "Blood folic acid and vitamin B_{12} in relation to neural tube defects." *Br J Obstet Gynaecol* (1996) 103(4):319-24.

Wenzler, E., Rademakers, A., Boers, G., et al. "Hyperhomocysteinemia in retinal artery and retinal vein occlusion." *Am J Ophthalmol* (1993) 11:162-7.

Wiklund, O., Fager, G., Andersson, A., et al. "N-Acetylcysteine treatment lowers plasma homocysteine but not serum lipoprotein (A) levels." *Atherosclerosis* (1996) 119: 99-106.

Chapter 12. Vitamin E

Bendich, A., Machlin, L. J. "Safety of oral intake of vitamin E." *Am J Clin Nutr* (1988) 48:612-9.

Black, P. N., Sharpe, S. "Dietary fat and asthma: is there a connection?" *Eur Respir J* (1997) 10:6-12.

Dieber-Rotheneder, M., Puhl, H., Waeg, G., Striegl, G., Esterbauer, H. "Effect of oral supplementation with d-alpha-tocopherol on the vitamin E content of human low density lipoproteins and resistance to oxidation." *J Lipid Res* (1991) 32(8): 1325-32.

Dietrich M, Traber MG, Jacques PF, Cross CE, Hu Y, Block G. Does gamma-tocopherol play a role in the primary prevention of heart disease and cancer? A review. J Am Coll Nutr. 2006 Aug;25(4):292-9. Review.

Elias, E., Muller, D. P., Scott, J. "Association of spinocerebellar disorders with cystic fibrosis or chronic childhood cholestasis and very low serum vitamin E." *Lancet* (1981) 2(8259):1319-21.

Esterbauer, H., Puhl, H., Dieber-Rotheneder, M., et al. "Effect of antioxidants on oxidative modification of LDL." *Ann Med* (1991) 23(5):573-81.

Gey, K. F., Brubacher, G. B., Ståhelin, H. B. "Plasma levels of antioxidant vitamins in relation to ischemic heart disease and cancer." *Am J Clin Nutr* (1987) 45:1368-77.

Goh, S. H., Hew, N. F., Norhanom, A. W., et al. "Inhibition of tumor promotion by various palm-oil tocotrienols." *Int J Cancer* (1994) 57(4):529-31.

Guthrie, N., Chambers, A. F., Gapor, A., et al. "In vitro inhibition of proliferation of receptor-positive MCF-7 human breast cancer cells by palm oil tocotrienols." *FASEB J* (1995) 9(4):A988.

Guthrie, N., Gapor, A., Chambers, A. F., et al. "Inhibition of proliferation of estrogen receptor-negative MDA-MB-435 and—positive MCF-7 human breast cancer cells by palm oil tocotrienols and tamoxifen, alone and in combination." *JN* (1997) 127(3):544S-48S.

Handelman, G. J., Packer, L., Cross, C. E. "Destruction of tocopherols, carotenoids, and retinol in human plasma by cigarette smoke." *Am J Clin Nutr* (1996) 63(4):559-65.

Hittner, H. M., Godio, L. B., Rudolph, A. J., et al. "Retrolental fibroplasia: efficacy of vitamin E in a double-blind clinical study of preterm infants." *N Engl J Med* (1981) 305(23):1365-71.

Kagan, V. E., Serbinova, E. A., Forte, T., et al. "Recycling of vitamin E in human low density lipoproteins." *J Lipid Res* (1992) 33:385-97.

Kamal-Eldin, A., Appelquist, L. A. "The chemistry and antioxidant properties of tocopherols and tocotrienols." *Lipids* (1996) 31(7):671-701.

Komiyama, K., Iizuka, K., Yamaoka, M., et al. "Studies on the biological activity of tocotrienols." *Chem Pharm Bull (Tokyo)* (1989) 37(5):1369-71.

Kushi, L. H., Folsom, A. R., Prineas, R. J., et al. "Dietary antioxidant vitamins and death from coronary heart disease in postmenopausal women." *N Engl J Med* (1996) 334(18):1156-62.

Leo, M. A., Rosman, A. S., Lieber, C. A. "Differential depletion of carotenoids and tocopherol in liver disease." *Hepatology* (1993) 17(6):977-86.

Menkes, M. S., Comstock, G. W., Vuilleumier, J. P., et al. "Serum beta-carotene, vitamins A and E, selenium, and the risk of lung cancer." *N Engl J Med* (1986) 315(20):1250-4.

Meydani, S. N., Meydani, M., Blumberg, J. B., et al. "Vitamin E supplementation and in vivo immune response in healthy elderly subjects: a randomized controlled trial." *JAMA* (1997) 277(17):1380-6.

Miwa, K., Miyagi, Y., Igawa, A., et al. "Vitamin E deficiency in variant angina." *Circulation* (1996) 94(1):14-8.

Nesaretnam, K., Guthrie, N., Chambers, A. F., et al. "Effect of tocotrienols on the growth of a human breast cancer cell line in culture." *Lipids* (1995) 30 (12):1139-43.

Ngah, W. Z., Jarien, Z., San, M. M., et al. "Effect of tocotrienols on hepatocarcinogenesis induced by 2-acetylaminofluorene in rats." *Am J Clin Nutr* (1991) 53(suppl 4):1076S-81S.

Novelli, G. P., Adembri, C., Gandini, E., et al. "Vitamin E protects human skeletal muscle from damage during surgical ischemia-reperfusion." *Am J Surg* (1997) 173:206-9.

Ohrvall, M., Tengblad, S., Vessby, B. "Lower tocopherol serum levels in subjects with abdominal adiposity." *J Intern Med* (1993) 234(1):53-60.

Packer, L. "Protective role of vitamin E in biological systems." *Am J Clin Nutr* (1991) 53: (Suppl):1050S-55S.

Parker, R. A., Pearce, B. C., Clark, R. W., et al. "Tocotrienols regulate cholesterol production in mammalian cells by post-transcriptional suppression of 3-hydroxy-3-methylglutaryl-coenzyme A reductase." *J Biol Chem* (1993) 268(15):11230-8.

Qureshi, A. A., Bradlow, B. A., Brace, L., et al. "Response of hypercholesterolemic subjects to administration of tocotrienols." *Lipids* (1995) 30(12):1171-7.

Rapola, J. M., Virtamo, J., Ripatti, S., et al. "Randomised trial of alpha-tocopherol and beta-carotene supplements on incidence of major coronary events in men with previous myocardial infarction." *Lancet* (1997) 349(9067):1715-20.

Rimm, E. B., Stampfer, M. J., Ascherio, A., et al. "Vitamin E consumption and the risk of coronary heart disease in men." *New Engl J Med* (1993) 328:1450-6.

Sano, M., Ernesto, C., Thomas, R. G., et al. "A controlled trial of selegiline, alpha-tocopherol, or both as treatment for Alzheimer's disease: the Alzheimer's Disease Cooperative Study." *N Engl J Med* (1997) 336(17):1216-22.

Sen CK, Khanna S, Roy S. Tocotrienols: Vitamin E beyond tocopherols. Life Sci. 2006 Mar 27;78(18):2088-98. Epub 2006 Feb 3. Review.

Sokol, R. J., Guggenheim, M. A., Iannaccone, S. T., et al. "Improved neurologic function after long-term correction of vitamin E deficiency in children with chronic cholestasis." *N Engl J Med* (1985) 313(25):1580-6.

Srivastava JK, Gupta S. Tocotrienol-rich fraction of palm oil induces cell cycle arrest and apoptosis selectively in human prostate cancer cells. Biochem Biophys Res Commun. 2006 Jul 28;346(2):447-53. Epub 2006 Jun 2.

Steinberg, D. "Antioxidants and atherosclerosis: a current assessment." *Circulation* (1991) 84:1420-5.

Stringer, M. D., Görög, P. G., Freeman, A., et al. "Lipid peroxides and atherosclerosis." *BMJ* (1989) 298(6669):281-4.

Thiele, J. J., Traber, M. G., Polefka, T. G., et al. "Ozone-exposure depletes vitamin E and induces lipid peroxidation in murine stratum corneum." *J Invest Dermatol* (1997) 108(5):753-7.

Tomeo, A. C., Geller, M., Watkins, T. R., et al. "Antioxidant effects of tocotrienols in patients with hyperlipidemia and carotid stenosis." *Lipids* (1995) 30(12):1179-83.

Traber, M. G., Sokol, R. J., Ringel, S. P., et al. "Lack of tocopherol in peripheral nerves of vitamin E-deficient patients with peripheral neuropathy." *N Engl J Med* (1987) 317(5):262-5.

Watkins, T., Lenz, P., Gapor, A., et al. "Gamma-tocotrienol as a hypocholesterolemic and antioxidant agent in rats fed atherogenic diets." *Lipids* (1993) 28(12):1113-8.

Weber, C., Podda, M., Rallis, M., et al. "Efficacy of topically applied tocopherols and tocotrienols in protection of murine skin from oxidative damage induced by UV-radiation." *Free Radic Biol Med* (1997) 22(5):761-9.

Chapter 13. Ginkgo

Boelsma E, Lamers RJ, Hendriks HF, van Nesselrooij JH, Roza L. Evidence of the regulatory effect of Ginkgo biloba extract on skin blood flow and study of its effects on urinary metabolites in healthy humans. Planta Med. 2004 Nov;70(11):1052-7.

Chen, X., Salwinski, S., Lee, T. J. "Extracts of *Ginkgo biloba* and ginsenosides exert cerebral vasorelaxation via a nitric oxide pathway." *Clin Exp Pharmacol Physiol* (1997) 24:958-9.

Doly, M. "Effect of Ginkgo biloba extract on the electrophysiology of the isolated diabetic rat retina." *Presse Med* (1986) 15(31):1480-3.

Drabaek, H., Petersen, J. R., Winberg, N., et al. "The effect of Ginkgo biloba extract in patients with intermittent claudication." *Ugeskrift Laeger* (1996) 158(27):3928-31.

Emerit, I., Oganesian, N., Sarkisian, T., et al. "Clastogenic factors in the plasma of Chernobyl accident recovery workers: anticlastogenic effect of Ginkgo biloba extract." *Radial Res* (1995) 144 (2):198-205.

Haramaki, N., Aggarwal, S., Kawabata, T., et al. "Effects of natural antioxidant Ginkgo biloba extract (Egb 761) on myocardial ischemia-reperfusion injury." *Free Rad Biol Med* (1994) 16:789-94.

Hofferberth, B. "[The effect of Ginkgo biloba extract on neurophysiological and psychometric measurement results in patients with psychotic organic brain syndrome: a double-blind study against placebo.]" *Arzveimittel-forschung* (1989) 39(8):918-22.

Holgers, K. M., Axelsson, A., Pringle, I. "Ginkgo biloba extract for the treatment of tinnitis." *Audiology* (1994) 33:85-92.

Itil, T., Martorano, D. "Natural substances in psychiatry (Ginkgo biloba in dementia)." *Psychopharmarcol Bull* (1995) 31(1):147-58.

Itil, T. M., Eralp, E., Tsambis, E., et al. "Central nervous system effects of *Ginkgo biloba*, a plant extract." *Am J Ther* (1996) 3:63-73.

Lan WJ, Zheng XX. Activity of Ginkgo biloba extract and quercetin on thrombomodulin expression and tissue-type plasminogen activator secretion by human umbilical vein endothelial cells. Biomed Environ Sci. 2006 Aug;19(4):249-53.

Le Bars, P. L., Katz, M. M., Berman, N., et al. "A placebo-controlled, double-blind, randomized trial of an extract of Ginkgo biloba for dementia." North American EGb Study Group. *JAMA* (1997) 278:1327-32.

Lebuisson, D. A., Leroy, L., Rigal, G. "Treatment of senile macular degeneration with Ginkgo biloba extract: a preliminary double-blind study versus placebo." *Presse Med* (1986) 15(31):1556-8.

Li, C. L., Wong, Y. Y. "The bioavailability of ginkgolides in Ginkgo biloba extracts." *Planta Med* (1997) 63(6):563-5.

Maitra, I., Marcocci, L., Droy-Lefaix, M. T., et al. "Peroxyl radical scavenging activity of Ginkgo biloba extract EGb 761." *Biochem Pharmacol* (1995) 49(11):1649-55.

Otamiri, T., Tagesson, C. "Ginkgo biloba extract prevents mucosal damage associated with small-intestinal ischaemia." *Scand J Gastroenterol* (1989) 24(6):666-70.

Oyama, Y., Chikahisa, L., Ueha, T., et al. "Ginkgo biloba extract protects brain neurons against oxidative stress induced by hydrogen peroxide." *Brain Research* (1996) 712(2):349-52.

Pietri, S., Seguin, J. R., d'Arbigny, P., et al. "*Ginkgo biloba* extract (Egb 761) pretreatment limits free radical-induced oxidative stress in patients undergoing coronary bypass surgery." *Cardiovasc Drugs Ther* (1997) 11:121-31.

Racagni, G., Brunello, N., Paoletti, R. "Variations of neuromediators in cerebral ageing: effects of Ginkgo biloba extract." *Presse Med* (1986) 15:1488-90.

Rong, Y., Geng, Z., Lau, B. H. "*Ginkgo biloba* attenuates oxidative stress in macrophages and endothelial cells." *Free Radic Biol Med* (1996) 20:121-7.

Schubert, H., Halama, P. "Depressive episode primarily unresponsive to therapy in elderly patients: efficacy of *Ginkgo biloba* extract (Egb 761) in combination with antidepressants." *Geriatr Forsch* (1993)3:45-53.

Sikora, R., Sohn, M., Deutz, F. J., et al. "Ginkgo biloba extract in the therapy of erectile dysfunction." (abstract) *J Urol* (1989) 141:188.

Smith, P. F., Maclennan, K., Darlington, C. L. "The neuroprotective properties of the *Ginkgo biloba* leaf: a review of the possible relationship to platelet-activating factor (PAF)." *J Ethnopharmacol* (1996) 50:131-9.

Taillandier, J., Ammar, A., Rabourdin, J. P., et al. "[Treatment of cerebral aging disorders with Ginkgo biloba extract. A longitudinal, multicentre, double-blind drug versus placebo study.]" *Presse Med* (1986) 15(31):1583-7.

Taylor, J. E. "Binding of neuromediators to their receptors in rat brain. Effect of chronic administration of Ginkgo biloba extract." *Presse Med* (1986) 15:1488-90.

Tosaki, A., Pali, T., Droy-Lefaix, M. T. "Effects of Ginkgo biloba extract and preconditioning on the diabetic rat myocardium." *Diabetologia* (1996) 39 (11):1255-62.

Trumbeckaite S, Bernatoniene J, Majiene D, Jakstas V, Savickas A, Toleikis A. Effect of Ginkgo biloba extract on the rat heart mitochondrial function. J Ethnopharmacol. 2006 Dec 28; [Epub ahead of print]

Chapter 14. N-Acetyl Cysteine and Glutathione

Akerlund, B., Jarstrand, C., Lindeke, B., et al. "Effect of N-acetylcysteine (NAC) treatment on HIV-1 infection: a double-blind placebo-controlled trial." *Eur J Clin Pharmacol* (1996) 50(6):457-61.

Ardissino, D., Merlini, P. A., Savonitto, S., et al. "Effect of transdermal nitroglycerin or N-acetylcysteine, or both, in the long-term treatment of unstable angina pectoris." *J Am Coll Cardiol* (1997) 29(5):941-7.

Bernard, G. R. "N-acetylcysteine in experimental and clinical acute lung injury." *Am J Med* (1991) 91(3C):54S-59S.

Boesgaard, S., Iversen, H. K., Wroblewski, H., et al. "Altered peripheral vasodilator profile of nitroglycerin during long-term infusion of N-acetylcysteine." *J Am Coll Cardiol* (1994) 23(1):163-9.

Bridgeman, M. M., Marsden, M., Selby, C., et al. "Effect of N-acetylcysteine on the concentrations of thiols in plasma, bronchoalveolar lavage fluid, and lung tissue." *Thorax* (1994) 49(7):670-5.

Buhl, R., Meyer, A., Vogelmeier, C. "Oxidant-protease interaction in the lung: prospects for antioxidant therapy." *Chest* (1996) 110(suppl 6):267S-72S.

Buhl, R., Vogelmeier, C., Critenden, M., et al. "Augmentation of glutathione in the fluid lining the epithelium of the lower respiratory tract by directly administering glutathione aerosol." *Proc Natl Acad Sci USA* (1990) 87(11):4063-7.

Burgunder, J. M., Varriale, A., Lauterburg, B. H. "Effect of N-acetylcysteine on plasma cysteine and glutathione following paracetamol administration." *Eur J Clin Pharmacol* (1989) 36:127-31.

Chiba, T., Takahashi, S., Sato, N., et al. "Fas-mediated apoptosis is modulated by intracellular glutathione in human T cells." *Eur J Immunol* (1996) 26(5):1164-9.

De Flora, S., Bennicelli, C., Camoirano, A., et al. "In vivo effects of N-acetylcysteine on glutathione metabolism and on the biotransformation of carcinogenic and/or mutagenic compounds." *Carcinogenesis* (1985) 6:1735-45.

Droge, W. "Cysteine and glutathione deficiency in AIDS patients: a rationale for the treatment with N-acetyl-cysteine." *Pharmacology* (1993) 46(2):61-5.

Flanagan, R. J., Meredith, T. J. "Use of N-acetyl-cysteine in clinical toxicology." *Am J Med* (1991) 91(3C):131S-9S.

Hercbergs, A., Brok-Simoni, F., Holtzman, F., et al. "Erythrocyte glutathione and tumor response to chemotherapy." *Lancet* (1992) 339(8801):1074-6.

Jaber R. Respiratory and allergic diseases: from upper respiratory tract infections to asthma. Prim Care. 2002 Jun;29(2):231-61. Review.

Janssen, Y. M., Heintz, N. H., Mossman, B. T. "Induction of c-fos and c-jun proto-oncogene expression by asbestos is ameliorated by N-acetyl-L-cysteine in mesothelial cells." *Cancer Res* (1995) 55(10):2085-9.

Julius, M., Lang, C. A., Gleiberman, L., et al. "Glutathione and morbidity in a community-based sample of elderly." *J Clin Epidemiol* (1994) 47(9):1021-6.

Kinscherf, R., Fischbach, T., Mihm, S., et al. "Effect of glutathione depletion and oral N-acetylcysteine treatment on CD4+ and CD8+ cells." *FASEB J* (1994) 8:448-451.

Livardjani, F., Lediga, M., Koppa, P., et al. "Lung and blood superoxide dismutase activity in mercury vapor exposed rats: effect of N-acetylcysteine treatment." *Toxicology* (1991) 66:289-95.

Lomaestro, B. M., Malone, M. "Glutathione in health and disease: pharmacotherapeutic issues." *Annals Pharmacother* (1995) 29:1263-73.

Lopez-Torres, M., Perez-Campo, R., Rojas, C., et al. "Simultaneous induction of SOD, glutathione reductase, GSH, and ascorbate in liver and kidney correlates with survival during aging." *Free Radic Biol Med* (1993) 15(2):133-42.

MacNee, W., Bridgeman, M. M., Marsden, M., et al. "The effects of N-acetylcysteine and glutathione on smoke-induced changes in lung phagocytes and epithelial cells." *Am J Med* (1991) 91(3C):60S-6S.

Morris, P. E., Bernard, G. R. "Significance of glutathione in lung disease and implications for therapy." *Am J Med Sci* (1994) 307(2):119-27.

Park SJ, Lee YC. Antioxidants as novel agents for asthma. Mini Rev Med Chem. 2006 Feb;6(2):235-40. Review.

Pastor, A., Collado, P. S., Almar, M., et al. "Antioxidant enzyme status in biliary obstructed rats: effects of N-acetylcysteine." *J Hepatol* (1997) 27:363-70.

Reid, M. B., Stokic, D. S., Koch, S. M., et al. "N-acetylcysteine inhibits muscle fatigue in humans." *J Clin Invest* (1994) 94(6):2468-74.

Ruan, E. A., et al. "Glutathione levels in chronic inflammatory disorders of the human colon." *Nutrition Research* (1997) 17(3):463-73.

Sjokin, K., Nilsson, E., Hallberg, A., et al. "Metaboism of N-acetyl-L-cysteine." *Biochem Pharm* (1989) 38:3981-5.

Yim, C. Y., Hibbs, J. B., Jr., McGregor, J. R., et al. "Use of N-acetylcysteine to increase intracellular glutathione during the induction of antitumor responses by IL-2." *J Immunol* (1994) 152:5796-805.

Zhang, H., Spapen, H., Nguyen, D. N., et al. "Protective effects of N-acetyl-L-cysteine in endotoxemia." *Am J Physiol* (1994) 266(5 pt 2):H1726-54.

Chapter 15. Tyrosine

Anderson, J. L. "The immune system and major depression." *Adv Neuroimmunol* (1996) 6(23):119-29.

Avraham, Y., Bonne, O., Berry, E. M. "Behavioral and neurochemical alterations caused by diet restriction—the effect of tyrosine administration in mice." *Brain Res* (1996) 732(1-2):133-44.

Cohen, S., Tyrrell, D. A., Smith, A. P. "Psychological stress and susceptibility to the common cold." *N Engl J Med* (1991) 325(9):606-12.

Deijen, J. B., Orlebeke, J. F. "Effect of tyrosine on cognitive function and blood pressure under stress." *Brain Res Bull* (1994) 33(3):319-23.

Deutsch, S. I., Rosse, R. B., Schwartz, B. L., et al. "L-tyrosine pharmacotherapy of schizophrenia: preliminary data." *Clin Neuropharmacol* (1994) 17(1):53-62.

Dollins, A. B., Krock, L. P., Storm, W. F., et al. "L-tyrosine ameliorates some effects of lower body negative pressure stress." *Physiol Behav* (1995) 57(2):223-30.

Elwes, R. D., Crewes, H., Chesterman, L. P., et al. "Treatment of narcolepsy with L-tyrosine: double-blind placebo-controlled trial." *Lancet* (1989) 2(8671):1067-9.

Gelenberg, A. J., Gibson, C. J. "Tyrosine for the treatment of depression." *Nutr Health* (1984) 3(3):163-73.

Gelenberg, A. J., Wojcik, J. D., Gibson, C. J., et al. "Tyrosine for depression." *J Psychiatr Res* (1982-3) 17(2):175-80.

Gelenberg, A. J., Wojcik, J. E., Growdon, J. H., et al. "Tyrosine for treatment of depression." *Am J Psychiatry* (1980) 137:622-32.

Kaneko, M., Watanabe, K., Kumashiro, H. "Plasma ratios of tryptophan and tyrosine to other large neutral amino acids in manic-depressive patients." *Jpn J Psychiatry Neurol* (1992) 46(3):711-20.

Licinio, J., Gold, P. W., Wong, M. L. "A molecular mechanism for stress-induced alterations in susceptibility to disease." *Lancet* (1995) 346(8967):104-6.

McCann, U. D., Penetar, D. M., Shaham, Y., et al. "Effects of catecholamine depletion on alertness and mood in rested and sleep deprived normal volunteers." *Neuropsychopharmacology* (1993) 8(4):345-56.

Mcgregor, N. R., Dunstan, R. H., Zerbes, M., et al. "Preliminary determination of a molecular basis of chronic fatigue syndrome." *Biochem Mol Med* (1996) 57(2): 73-80.

Moller, S. E. "Effect of oral contraceptives on tryptophan and tyrosine availability: evidence for a possible contribution to mental depression." *Neuropsychobiology* (1981) 7(4):192-200.

Mouret, J., Lemoine, P., Sanchez, P., et al. "Treatment of narcolepsy with L-tyrosine." *Lancet* (1988) 2(8626-8627):1458-9.

Neri, D. F., Wiegmann, D., Stanny, R. R., et al. "The effects of tyrosine on cognitive performance during extended wakefulness." *Aviat Space Environ Med* (1995) 66(4):313-9.

Owasoyo, J. O., Neri, D. F., Lamberth, J. G. "Tyrosine and its potential use as a countermeasure to performance decrement in military sustained operations." *Aviat Space Environ Med* (1992) 63(5):364-9.

Rauch, T. M., Lieberman, H. R. "Tyrosine pretreatment reverses hypothermia-induced behavioral depression." *Brain Res Bull* (1990) 24(1):147-50.

Reeves, P. G., O'Dell, B. L. "The effect of dietary tyrosine levels on food intake in zinc-deficient rats." *J Nutr* (1984) 114(4):761-7.

Reinstein, D. K., Lehnert, H., Scott, N. A., et al. "Tyrosine prevents behavioral and neurochemical correlates of an acute stress in rats." *Life Sci* (1984) 34(23):2225-31.

Risch, S. C. "Recent advances in depression research: from stress to molecular biology and brain imaging." *J Clin Psychiatry* (1997) 58 (suppl 5):3-6.

Sajo, E., Amodia, D., Stewart, P. "A historically controlled trial of tyrosine for cocaine dependence." *J Psychoactive Drugs* (1996) 28(3):305-9.

Salter, C. A. "Dietary tyrosine as an aid to stress resistance among troops." *Mil Med* (1989) 154(3):144-6.

Schweiger, U., Warnhoff, M., Pirke, K. M. "Brain tyrosine availability and the depression of central nervous norepinephrine turnover in acute and chronic starvation in adult male rats." *Brain Res* (1985) 335(2):207-12.

Shukitt-Hale, B., Stillman, M. J., Lieberman, H. R. "Tyrosine administration prevents hypoxia-induced decrements in learning and memory." *Physiol Behav* (1996) 59(4-5):867-71.

Shurtleff, D., Thomas, J. R., Schrot, J., et al. "Tyrosine reverses a cold-induced working memory deficit in humans." *Pharmacol Biochem Behav* (1994) 47(4):935-41.

Stone, A. A., Bovbjerg, D. H. "Stress and humoral immunity: a review of the human studies." *Adv Neuroimmunol* (1994) 4(1):49-56.

Chapter 16. Lutein

Bent S, Padula A, Moore D, Patterson M, Mehling W. Valerian for sleep: a systematic review and meta-analysis. Am J Med. 2006 Dec; 119(12):1005-12. Review.

Bone, R. A., Landrum, J. T., Friedes, L. M., et al. "Distribution of lutein and zeaxanthin stereoisomers in the human retina." *Exp Eye Res* (1997) 64(2):211-8.

Christen, W. G., Glynn, R. J., Hennekens, C. H. "Antioxidants and age-related eye disease." *AEP* (1996) 6(1):60-6.

Fuhrman, B., Elis, A., Aviram, M. "Hypocholesterolemic effect of lycopene and beta-carotene is related to suppression of cholesterol synthesis and augmentation of LDL receptor activity in macrophages." *Biochem Biophys Res Commun* (1997) 233(3):658-62.

Gartner, C., Stahl, W., Sies, H. "Lycopene is more bioavailable from tomato paste than from fresh tomatoes." *Am J Clin Nutr* (1997) 66(1):116-22.

Gerster, H. "Antioxidant vitamins in cataract prevention." *Z Ernahrungswiss* (1989) 28:56-75.

_________. "The potential role of lycopene for human health." *J Am Coll Nutr* (1997) 16(2):109-26.

Hall, I. H., Starnes, C. O., Jr., Lee, K. H., et al. "Mode of action of sesquiterpene lactones as anti-inflammatory agents." *J Pharm Sci* (1980) 69(5):537-43.

Hammond, B. R., Jr., Fuld, K., Snodderly, D. M. "Iris color and macular pigment optical density." *Exp Eye Res* (1996) 62(3):293-7.

Hammond, B. R., Jr., Wooten, B. R., Snodderly, D. M. "Cigarette smoking and retinal carotenoids: implications for age-related macular degeneration." *Vision Res* (1996) 36(18):3003-9.

_________. "Density of the human crystalline lens is related to the macular pigment carotenoids, lutein and zeaxanthin." *Optom Vis Sci* (1997) 74(7):499-504.

Heinamaki, A. A., Muhonen, A. S., Piha, R. S. "Taurine and other free amino acids in the retina, vitreous, lens, iris-ciliary body, and cornea of the rat eye." *Neurochem Res* (1986) 11(4):535-42.

Khachik, F., Beecher, G. R., Smith, J. C., Jr. "Lutein, lycopene, and their oxidative metabolites in chemoprevention of cancer." *J Cell Biochem Suppl* (1995) 22:236-46.

Khachik, F., Bernstein, P. S., Garland, D. L. "Identification of lutein and zeaxanthin oxidation products in human and monkey retinas." *Invest Ophthalmol Vis Sci* (1997) 38(9):1802-11.

Krinsky, N. I. "Antioxidant functions of carotenoids." *Free Radic Biol Med* (1989) 6:617-35.

Landrum, J. T., Bone, R. A., Joa, H., et al. "A one-year study of the macular pigment: the effect of 140 days of a lutein supplement." *Exp Eye Res* (1997) 65(1):57-62.

Malinow, M. R., Feeney-Burns, L., Peterson, L. H., et al. "Diet-related macular anomalies in monkeys." *Invest Ophthalmol Vis Sci* (1980) 19(8):857-63.

Mares-Perlman, J. A., Brady, W. E., Klein, R., et al. "Serum antioxidants and age-related macular degeneration in a population-based case-control study." *Arch Ophthalmol* (1995) 113(12):1518-23.

Martin, K. R., Failla, M. L., Smith, J. C., Jr. "Beta-carotene and lutein protect HepG2 human liver cells against oxidant-induced damage." *J Nutr* (1996) 126(9):2098-106.

Morin AK, Jarvis Cl, Lynch AM. Therapeutic options for sleep-maintenance and sleep-onset insomnia. Pharmacotherapy. 2007 Jan;27(1):89-110.

Sapp, R. J., Christianson, J. S., Maier, L., et al. "Carotenoid replacement therapy in Drosophila: recovery of membrane, opsin and visual pigment." *Exp Eye Res* (1991) 53(1):73-9.

Scott, K. J., Thurnham, D. I., Hart, D. J., et al. "The correlation between the intake of lutein, lycopene and beta-carotene from vegetables and fruits, and blood plasma concentrations in a group of women aged 50-65 years in the UK." *Br J Nutr* (1996) 75(3):409-18.

Seddon, J. M., Ajani, U. A., Sperduto, R. D., et al. "Dietary carotenoids, vitamin A, C, and E, and advanced age-related macular degeneration: Eye Disease Case-Control Study Group." *JAMA* (1994) 272(18):1413-20.

Snodderly, D. M. "Evidence for protection against age-related macular degeneration by carotenoids and antioxidant vitamins." *Am J Clin Nutr* (1995) 62(suppl 6):1448S-61S.

Taylor, A. "Role of nutrients in delaying cataracts." *Ann NY Acad Sci* (1992) 669:111-23.

Tokunaga S, Takeda Y, Niimoto T, Nishida N, Kubo T, Ohno T, Matsuura Y, Kawahara Y, Shinomiya K, Kamei C. Effect of Valerian Extract Preparation (BIM) on the Sleep-Wake Cycle in Rats. Biol Pharm Bull. 2007;30(2):363-6.

Yeurn, K. J., Taylor, A., Tang, G., et al. "Measurement of carotenoids, retinoids, and tocopherols in human lenses." *Invest Ophthalmol Vis Sci* (1995) 36(13):2756-61.

Yolton, D. P. "Nutritional effects of zinc on ocular and systemic physiology." *J Am Optom Assoc* (1981) 52(5):409-14.

Chapter 17. Quercetin

Alarcon de la Lastra, C., Martin, M. J., Motilva, V. "Antiulcer and gastroprotective effects of quercetin: a gross and histologic study." *Pharmacology (Switzerland)* (1994) 48:56-62.

Baumann, J., Bruchhausen, F., Wurm, G. "Flavonoids and related compounds and inhibitors of arachidonic acid peroxidation." *Prostaglandins* (1980) 20:627-39.

Bronner, C., Landry, Y. "Kinetics of the inhibitory effect of flavonoids on histamine secretion from mast cells." *Agents Actions* (1985) 16(3-4):147-51.

Clark, W., Mackay, E. "Effect of flavonoid substances on histamine toxicity, anaphylactic shock and histamine-enhanced capillary permeability to dye." *J Allergy* (1950) 21:133-47.

Ennis, M., Truneh, A., White, J. R., Pearce, F. L. "Inhibition of histamine secretion from mast cells." *Nature* (1981) 289(5794):186-7.

Ezeamuzie, I. C., Assem, E. S. "Modulation of the effect of histamine-releasing lymphokine on human basophils." *Agents Actions* (1984) 14(3-4):501-5.

Fewtrell, C. M., Gomperts, B. D. "Quercetin: a novel inhibitor of Ca2+ influx and exocytosis in rat peritoneal mast cells." *Biochim Biophys Acta* (1977) 469(1):52-60.

Jaber R. Respiratory and allergic diseases: from upper respiratory tract infections to asthma. Prim Care. 2002 Jun;29(2):231-61. Review.

Kaul, T., Middleton, E., Ogra, P. L. "Antiviral effects of flavonoids on human viruses." *J Med Virol* (1985) 15:71-79.

Leung, K. B., Barrett, K. E., Pearce, F. L. "Differential effects of anti-allergic compounds on peritoneal mast cells of the rat, mouse and hamster." *Agents Actions* (1984) 14(3-4):461-7.

Liebovitz, Brian. "Bioflavonoids part 2: medical applications." *Nutrition Update* (1990) 4(2).

Middleton, E., Jr., Drzewiecki, G. "Flavonoid inhibition of human basophil histamine release stimulated by various agents." *Biochem Pharmacol* (1984) 33(21):3333-8.

Middleton, E., Drzewiechi, G., Krishnarao, D. "Quercetin: an inhibitor of antigen-induced human basophil histamine release." *J Immunol* (1981) 127(2):546-50.

Middleton, E., Jr., Kandaswami, C. "Effects of flavonoids on immune and inflammatory cell functions." *Biochem Pharmacol* (1992) 43:1167-79.

Ogasawara, H., Fujitani, T., Drzewiecki, G., Middleton, E., Jr. "The role of hydrogen peroxide in basophil histamine release and the effect of selected flavonoids." *J Allergy Clin Immunol* (1986) 78(2):321-8.

Pearce, F. L., Befus, A. D., Bienenstock, J. "Mucosal mast cells. III. Effect of quercetin and other flavonoids on antigen-induced histamine secretion from rat intestinal mast cells." *J Allergy Clin Immunol* (1984) 73(6):819-23.

Theoharides TC. Treatment approaches for painful bladder syndrome/interstitial cystitis. Drugs. 2007;67(2):215-35.

Welton, A. F., Tobias, L. D., Fiedler-Nagy, C., et al. "Effect of flavonoids on arachidonic acid metabolism." *Prog Clin Biol Res* (1986) 213:231-242.

Chapter 18. Kava

Alschuler, L. "Kava root: herbal treatment for anxiety conditions." *Am J Nat Med* (1997) 4(10):22.

Backhaus, C., Krieglstein, J. "Extract of kava (Piper methysticum) and its methysticin constituents protect brain tissue against ischemic damage in rodents." *Eur J Pharmacol* (1992) 215(2-3):265-9.

Bahrami H, Melia M, Dagnelie G. Lutein supplementation in retinitis pigmentosa: PC-based vision assessment in a randomized double-masked placebo-controlled clinical trial [NCT00029289]. BMC Ophthalmol. 2006 Jun 7;6:23.

Balderer, G., Borbely, A. A. "Effect of valerian on human sleep." *Psychopharmacology (Berl)* (1985) 87(4):406-9.

Black PN, Morgan-Day A, McMillan TE, Poole PJ, Young RP. Randomised, controlled trial of N-acetylcysteine for treatment of acute exacerbations of chronic obstructive pulmonary disease [ISRCTN21676344] BMC Pulm Med. 2004 Dec 6;4:13.

Blumenthal, M. "Kava: The peaceful herb from the South Pacific." *Natural Pharmcacy* (1997) 12-15.

Bone, K. "Kava—a safe herbal treatment for anxiety." *British J of Phytotherapy.* (1993) 3(4):147-53.

Brown, D. "Valerian: A possible substitute for benzodiazepines?" *Quart Rev Nat Med* (1993) winter quarter, pp. 17-18.

Cawte, J. "Psychoactive substances of the South Seas: betel, kava and pituri." *Aust N Z J Psychiatry* (1985) 19(1):83-7.

Czekalla, J., Gastpar, M., Hubner, W. D., et al. "The effect of hypericum extract on cardiac conduction as seen in the electrocardiogram compared to that of imipramine." *Pharmacopsychiatry* (1997) 30 (suppl 2):86-8.

Dimpfel, W., Hofmann, R. "Pharmacodynamic effects of St. John's wort on rat intracerebral field potentials." *Eur J Med Res* (1995) 1(3):157-67.

Ernst, E. "St. John's wort, an anti-depressant? A systematic, criteria-based review." *Phytomed* (1995) 2:67-71.

Gleitz, J., Beile, A., Wilkens, P., et al. "Antithrombotic action of the kava pysone (+)-kavain prepared from Piper methysticum on human platelets." *Planta Med* (1997) 63(1):27-30.

Hansel, R. (Trans. Clay, A., Reichert, R.) "Kava-kava in modern drug research: portrait of a medicinal plant." *Quart Rev of Natural Medicine* (Winter 1996):259-74.

Harrer, G., Sommer, H. "Treatment of mild/moderate depressions with *Hypericum*." *Phytomed* (1994) 1:3-8.

Jamieson, D. D., Duffield, P. H. "The antinociceptive action of kava components in mice." *Clin Exp Pharmacol Physiol* (1990) 17:495-508.

Kasper, S. "Treatment of seasonal affective disorder (SAD) with hypericum extract." *Pharmacopsychiatry* (1997) 30(suppl 2):89-93.

Kinzler, E., Kromer, J., Lehmann, E. "Effect of a special kava extract in patients with anxiety-, tension-, and excitation states of non-psychotic genesis: double blind study with placebos over four weeks." *Arzneimittel-forschung* (1991) 41(6):584-8.

Kvansakul J, Rodriguez-Carmona M, Edgar DF, Barker FM, Kopcke W, Schalch W, Barbur JL. Supplementation with the carotenoids lutein or zeaxanthin improves human visual performance Ophthalmic Physiol Opt. 2006 Jul;26(4):362-71.

Leathwood, P. D., Chauffard, F., et al. "Aqueous extract of valerian reduces latency to fall asleep in man." *Planta Medica* (1985) 51:144-8.

Lehmann, E., Kinzler, E., Friedemann, J. "Efficacy of a special kava extract (*Piper methysticum*) in patients with states of anxiety, tension and excitedness of non-mental origin—a double-blind placebo-controlled study of four weeks treatment." *Phytomed* (1996) 3:113-9.

Leuschner, J., Muller, J., Rudmann, M. "Characterisation of the central nervous depressant activity of a commercially available valerian root extract." *Arzneimittelforschung* (1993) 43(6):638-41.

Lindahl, O., Lindwall, L. "Double blind study of a valerian preparation." *Pharmacol Biochem Behav* (1989) 32(4):1065-6.

Martinez, B., Kasper, S., Ruhrmann, S., et al. "*Hypericum* in the treatment of seasonal affective disorders." *J Ger Psychiatry Neurol* (1994) 7(suppl 1):S29-S33.

Norton, S. A., Ruze, P. "Kava dermopathy." *J Am Acad Dermatol* (1994) 31(1):89-97.

Rodriguez-Carmona M, Kvansakul J, Harlow JA, Kopcke W, Schalch W, Barbur JL. The effects of supplementation with lutein and/or zeaxanthin on human macular pigment density and colour vision. Ophthalmic Physiol Opt. 2006 Mar;26(2):137-47.

Rosenthal JM, Kim J, de Monasterio F, Thompson DJ, Bone RA, Landrum JT, de Moura FF, Khachik F, Chen H, Schleicher RL, Ferris FL 3rd, Chew EY. Dose-ranging study of lutein supplementation in persons aged 60 years or older. Invest Ophthalmol Vis Sci. 2006 Dec;47(12):5227-33. Erratum in: Invest Ophthalmol Vis Sci 20007 Jan;48(1):17, de Monastario, Francisco [corrected to de Monasterio, Francisco].

Saletu, B., Grünberger, J., Linzmayer, L., et al. "EEG-brain mapping, psychometric and psychophysiological studies on the central effects of kavain—a kava plant derivative." *Human Psychopharmacol* (1989) 4:169-90.

Schulz, H., Stolz, C., Muller, J. "The effect of valerian extract on sleep polygraphy in poor sleepers: a pilot study." *Pharmacopsychiatry* (1994) 27(4):147-51.

Singh, Y. N. "Kava: an overview." *J Ethnopharmacol* (1992) 37(1):13-45.

Thiede, H. M., Walper, A. "Inhibition of MAO and COMT by hypericum extracts and hypericin." *J Geriatr Psychiatry Neurol* (1994) 7 Suppl 1:S54-S56.

Volz, H. P. "The anxiolytic efficacy of the kava special extract WS 1490 using long-term therapy—a randomized, double-blind study." *Quart Rev Nat Med* (Fall 1996):185.

Volz, H. P., Kieser, M. "Kava-kava extract WS 1490 versus placebo in anxiety disorders—a randomized placebo-controlled 25-week outpatient trial." *Pharmacopsychiatry* (1997) 30(1):1-5.

Warnecke, G. "Psychosomatic dysfunctions in the female climacteric: clinical effectiveness and tolerance of kava extract WS 14901." *Fortschr Med* (1991) 109(4):119-22.

Woelk, H., Kapoula, S., Lehrl, S., et al. "Treatment of patients from anxiety—double-blind study: kava special extract versus benzodiazepines." *Z Allgemeinmed* (1993) 69:271-7.

Chapter 19. Phosphatydyl Serine and Acetyl-L-Carnitine

Allegro, L., Favaretto, V., Ziliotto, G. "Oral phosphatidylserine in elderly subjects with cognitive deterioration—an open study." *Clin Trials J* (1987) 24:104-8.

Amaducci, L., et al. "Phosphatidylserine in the treatment of Alzheimer's disease: results of a multicenter study." *Psychopharmacol Bull* (1988) 24:130-4.

Aporti, F., et al. "Age-dependent spontaneous EEG bursts in rats: effects of brain phosphatidylserine." *Neurobiology of Aging* (1986) 7:115-120.

Borghese, C. M., et al. "Phosphatidylserine increases hippocampal synaptic efficacy." *Brain Res Bull* (1993) 31:697-700.

Caffarra, P., Santamaria, V. "The effects of phosphatidylserine in subjects with mild cognitive decline: an open trial." *Clin Trials J* (1987) 24:109-14.

Calvani, M., Carta, A. "Clues to the mechanism of action of acetyl-L-carnitine in the central nervous system." *Dementia* (1991) 2:1-6.

Calvani, M., Carta, A., Caruso, G., et al. "Action of acetyl-L-carnitine in neurodegeneration and Alzheimer's disease." *Ann NY Acad Sci* (1992) 663:483-6.

Cenacchi, B., et al. "Cognitive decline in the elderly: a double-blind, placebo-controlled multicenter study on efficacy of phosphatidylserine administration." *Aging Clin Exp Res* (1993) 5:123-33.

________. "Human tolerability of oral phosphatidylserine assessed through laboratory examinations." *Clin Trials J* (1987) 24:125-30.

Cocito, L., Bianchetti, A., Bossi, L., et al. "GABA and phosphatidylserine in human photosensitivity: a pilot study." *Epilepsy Research* (1994) 17:49-53.

Crook, T. H., Tinklenberg, J., Yesavage, J., Petrie, W., Nunzi, M. G., Massari, D. C. "Effects of phosphatidylserine in age-associated memory impairment." *Neurology* (1991) 41(5):644-9.

Crook, T. H., et al., "Effects of phosphatidylserine in Alzheimer's disease." *Psychopharmacol Bull* (1992) 28:61-6.

Delwaide, P. J., et al. "Double-blind randomized controlled study of phosphatidylserine in demented subjects." *Acta Neurol Scand* (1986) 73:136-40.

DeSimone, C., Tzantzoglou, S., Famularo, G., et al. "High dose L-carnitine improves immunologic and metabolic parameters in AIDS patients." *Immunopharmacol Immunotoxicol* (1993) 15:1-12.

DeSimone, C., Tzantzglou, S., Jirillo, E., et al. "L-carnitine deficiency in AIDS patients." *AIDS* (1992) 6:203-5.

Gecele, M., Francesetti, G., Meluzzi, A. "Acetyl-L-carnitine in aged subjects with major depression: clinical efficacy and effects on the circadian rhythm of cortisol." *Dementia* (1991) 2:333-7.

Goa, K. L., Brogden, A. "L-carnitine, a preliminary review of its pharmacokinetics, and its therapeutic use in ischaemic cardiac disease and primary and secondary carnitine deficiencies in relationship to its role in fatty acid metabolism." *Drugs* (1987) 34:1-24.

Granata, Q., DiMichele, J. "Phosphatidylserine in elderly subjects." *Clin Trials J* (1987) 24:99-103.

Kidd, P. M. *Phosphatidylcholine (PC): Versatile Membrane Nutrient*. Lucas Meyer, Inc., Decatur, IL, (1996).

________. *Phosphatidylserine (PS): A Remarkable Brain Cell Nutrient* 2d ed. Lucas Meyer, Inc., Decatur, IL (1997).

Loeb, C., et al. "Preliminary evaluation of the effect of GABA and phosphatidylserine in epileptic patients." *Epilepsy Res* (1994) 1:209-12.

Lowitt, S., Malone, J. I., Salem, A. F., et al. "Acetyl-L-carnitine corrects the altered peripheral nerve function of experimental diabetes." *Metabolism* (1995) 44:677-80.

Monteleone, P., et al. "Effects of phosphatidylserine on the neuroendocrine response to physical stress in humans." *Neuroendocrinol* (1990) 52:243-8.

Onofrj, M., Fulgente, T., Melchionda, D., et al. "L-acetylcarnitine as a new therapeutic approach for peripheral neuropathies with pain." *Int J Clin Pharm Res* (1995) 15:9-15.

Palmieri, G., et al. "Double-blind controlled trial of phosphatidylserine in subjects with senile mental deterioration." *Clin Trials J* (1987) 24:73-83.

Quatraro, A., Roca, P., Donzella, C., et al. "Acetyl-L-carnitine for symptomatic diabetic neuropathy." *Diabetologia* (1995) 38(1):123.

Rai, G., Wright, G., Scott, L., et al. "Double-blind, placebo controlled study of acetyl-L-carnitine in patients with Alzheimer's dementia." *Curr Med Res Opin* (1990) 1:638-47.

Ransmayr, G., et al. "Double-blind controlled trial of phosphatidylserine in patients with senile mental deterioration." *Clin Trials J* (1987) 24:62-72.

Sano, M., Bell, K., Cote, L., et al. "Double-blind parallel design pilot study of acetyl levocarnitine in patients with Alzheimer's disease." *Arch Neurol* (1992) 49:1137-41.

Sima, A. A., Ristic, H., Merry, A., et al. "Primary preventive and secondary interventionary effects of acetyl-L-carnitine on diabetic neuropathy in the bio-breeding Worchester rat." *J Clin Invest* (1996) 97(8):1900-7.

Sinforiani, E., et al. "Cognitive decline in aging brain: therapeutic approach with phosphatidylserine." *Clin Trials J* (1987) 24:115-24.

Spagnoli, A., Lucca, U., Menasce, G., et al. "Long-term acetyl-L-carnitine treatment in Alzheimer's disease." *Neurology* (1991) 41:1726-32.

Tempesta, E., Casella, I., Pirrongelli, C., et al. "L-acetylcarnitine in depressed elderly subjects: a cross-over study vs. placebo." *Drugs Exp Clin Res* (1987) 13:417-23.

Tempesta, E., Troncon, R., Janiri, L., et al. "Role of acetyl-L-carnitine in the treatment of cognitive deficit in chronic alcoholism." *Int J Clin Pharm Res* (1990) 10(1-2):101-7.

Villardita, C., et al. "Multicentre clinical trial of brain phosphatidylserine in elderly patients with intellectual deterioration." *Clin Trials J* (1987) 24:84-93.

White, H. L., Scates, P. W. "Acetyl L-carnitine as a precursor of acetylcholine." *Neurochem Res* (1990) 14: 597-601.

Chapter 20. Branched Chain Amino Acids

Bigard, A. X., Lavier, P., Ullmann, L., et al. "Branched-chain amino acid supplementation during repeated prolonged skiing exercises at altitude." *Int J Sport Nutr* (1996) 6(3):295-306.

Blackburn, G. L., Moldawer, L. L., Usui, S., et al. "Branched chain amino acid administration and metabolism during starvation, injury, and infection." *Surgery* (1979) 86(2):307-15.

Blazer, S., Reinersman, G. T., Askanazi, J., et al. "Branched-chain amino acids and respiratory pattern and function in the neonate." *J Perinatol* (1994) 14(4):290-5.

Blomstrand, E., Ek, S., Newsholme, E. A. "Influence of ingesting a solution of branched-chain amino acids on plasma and muscle concentrations of amino acids during prolonged submaximal exercise." *Nutrition* (1996) 12:485-90.

Blomstrand, E., Hassmen, P., Ek, S., et al. "Influence of ingesting a solution of branched-chain amino acids on perceived exertion during exercise." *Acta Physiol Scand* (1997) 159:41-9.

Blomstrand, E., Newsholme, E. "Effect of branched-chain amino-acid supplementation on the exercise-induced change in aromatic aminoacid concentration in human muscle." *Acta Physiol Scand* (1992) 146:293-8.

Bugge, M., Bengtsson, F., Nobin, A., et al. "Amino acids and indoleamines in the brain after infusion of branched-chain amino acids to rats with liver ischemia." *J Parenter Enteral Nutr* (1986) 10(5):474-8.

Calders, P., Pannier, J. L., Matthys, D. M., et al. "Pre-exercise branched-chain amino acid administration increases endurance performance in rats." *Med Sci Sports Exerc* (1997) 29(9):1182-6.

Carli, G., Bonifazi, M., Lodi, L., et al. "Changes in the exercise-induced hormone response to branched chain amino acid administration." *Eur J Appl Physiol* (1992) 64(3):272-7.

Chua, B., Siehl, D. L., Morgan, H. E. "Effect of leucine and metabolites of branched chain amino acids on protein turnover in heart." *J Biol Chem* (1979) 254(17):8358-62.

Davis, J. M. "Carbohydrates, branched-chain amino acids, and endurance: the central fatigue hypothesis." *Int J Sport Nutr* (1995) 5 Suppl:S29-S38.

Frexes-Steed, M., Warner, M. L., Bulus, N., Flakoll, P., Abumrad, N. N. "Role of insulin and branched-chain amino acids in regulating protein metabolism during fasting." *Am J Physiol* (1990) 258 (6 pt 1):E907-17.

Garlick, P. J., Grant, I. "Amino acid infusion increases the sensitivity of muscle protein synthesis in vivo to insulin: effect of branched-chain amino acids." *Biochem J* (1988) 254(2):579-84.

Hassmen, P., Blomstrand, E., Ekblom, B., et al. "Branched-chain amino acid supplementation during 30-km competitive run: mood and cognitive performance." *Nutrition* (1994) 10(5):427-8.

Kawamura, I., Sato, H., Ogoshi, S., et al. "Use of an intravenous branched chain amino acid enriched diet in the tumor-bearing rat." *Jpn J Surg* (1985) 15(6):471-6.

Kirvela, O., Takala, J. "Postoperative parenteral nutrition with high supply of branched-chain amino acids: effects on nitrogen balance and liver protein synthesis." *J Parenter Enteral Nutr* (1986) 10(6):574-7.

Kirvela, O., Thorpy, M., Takala, J., Askanazi, J., et al. "Respiratory and sleep patterns during nocturnal infusions of branched chain amino acids." *Acta Anaesthesiol Scand* (1990) 34(8):645-8.

Lemon, P. W. "Do athletes need more dietary protein and amino acids?" *Int J Sport Nutr* (1995) suppl 5:S39-S61.

Louard, R. J., Barrett, E. F., Gelfand, R. A. "Effect of infused branched-chain amino acids on muscle and whole-body amino acid metabolism in man." *Clin Sci (Colch)* (1990) 79(5):457-66.

Manner, T., Wiese, S., Katz, D. P., Skeie, B., Askanazi, J. "Branched-chain amino acids and respiration." *Nutrition* (1992) 8(5):311-5.

Marchesini, G., Zoli, M., Dondi, C., et al. "Anticatabolic effect of branched-chain amino acid-enriched solutions in patients with liver cirrhosis." *Hepatology* (1982) 2(4):420-5.

Meeusen, R., De Meirleir, K. "Exercise and brain neurotransmission." *Sports Med* (1995) 20(3):160-88.

Sayegh, R., Schiff, I., Wurtman, J., Spiers, P., McDermott, J., Wurtman, R. "The effect of a carbohydrate-rich beverage on mood, appetite, and cognitive function in women with premenstrual syndrome." *Obstet Gynecol* (1995) 86(4 pt 1):520-8.

Schena, F., Guerrini, F., Tregnaghi, P., et al. "Branched-chain amino acid supplementation during trekking at high altitude: the effects on loss of body mass, body composition, and muscle power." *Eur J Appl Physiol* (1992) 65(5):394-8.

Skeie, B., Petersen, A. J., Manner, T., Askanazi, J., et al. "Branched-chain amino acids increase the seizure threshold to picrotoxin in rats." *Pharmacol Biochem Behav* (1992) 43(3):669-71.

Soreide, E., Skeie, B., Kirvela, O., Lynn, R., Ginsberg, N., Manner, T., Katz, D. P., Askanazi, J. "Branched-chain amino acid in chronic renal failure patients: respiratory and sleep effects." *Kidney Int* (1991) 40(3):539-43.

Stewart, J. K., Koerker, D. J., Goodner, C. J. "Effects of branched chain amino acids on spontaneous growth hormone secretion in the baboon." *Endocrinology* (1984) 115(5):1897-900.

Struder, H. K., Hollmann, W., Duperly, J., et al. "Amino acid metabolism in tennis and its possible influence on the neuroendocrine system." *Br J Sports Med* (1995) 29(1):28-30.

Takala, J., Askanazi, J., Weissman, C., et al. "Changes in respiratory control induced by amino acid infusions." *Crit Care Med* (1988) 16(5):465-9.

Tanaka, H., West, K. A., Duncan, G. E., et al. "Changes in plasma tryptophan/ branched chain amino acid ratio in responses to training volume variation." *Int J Sports Med* (1997) 18(4):270-5.

Uretzky, G., Vinograd, I., Freund, H. R., et al. "Protective effect of branched chain-enriched amino acid formulation in myocardial eschemia." *Isr J Med Sci* (1989) 25(1):3-6.

Wagenmakers, A. J. "Amino acid metabolism, muscular fatigue and muscle wasting: speculations on adaptations at high altitude." *Int J Sports Med* (1992) 13 (Suppl 1):S110-13.

Wurtman, J. J., Brzezinski, A., Wurtman, R. J., et al. "Effect of nutrient intake on premenstrual depression." *Am J Obstet Gynecol* (1989) 161(5):1228-34.

Chapter 21. Black Cohosh, Red Clover, Licorice

Dittmar, F., Böhnert, K. J., Peeters, M., et al. "Premenstrual syndrome: treatment with a phytopharmaceutical." *Therapiewoche Gynäkol* (1992) 5(1):60-8.

Dodge, J. A., Glasebrook, A., et al. "Environmental estrogens: receptor binding, cholesterol lowering and bone metabolic effects." *J Bone Mineral Res* (1994) 9 (suppl 1):134.

Duda, R. B., Kessel, B., Curtin, M., et al. "The use of herbal remedies and alternative therapies by breast cancer patients." (meeting abstract) *Proc Annu Meet Am Soc Clin Oncol* (1995) 14:A70.

Duker, E. M., Kopanski, L., Jarry, H. et al. "Effects of extracts from *Cimifuga racemosa* on gonadotropin release in menopausal women and ovariectomized rats." *Planta Medica* (1991) 57:420-4.

Eagon, C. L., Elm, M. S., Eagon, P. K. "Estrogenicity of traditional Chinese and Western herbal remedies." *Proc Annu Meet Am Assoc Cancer Res* (1996) 37:A1937.

Jarry, H., Harnischfeger, G. "Studies on the endocrine efficacy of the constituents of *Cimicifuga racemosa*. 1. Influence on the serum concentration of pituitary hormones in ovariectomied rats." *Planta Med* (1985) 1:46-9.

Jarry, H., Harnischfeger, G., Duker, E. "Studies on the endocrine efficacy of the constituents of *Cimicifuga racemosa*. II. *In vitro* binding of compounds to estrogen receptors." *Planta Med* (1985) 4:316-9.

Lemon, H. M. "Pathophysiologic considerations in the treatment of menopausal symptoms with estrogens: the role of estriol in the prevention of mammary carcinoma." *Acta Endocrinol* (1980) 233(suppl):17-27.

Liske, E. "Therapeutic efficacy and safety of Cimicifuga racemosa for gynecologic disorders." *Adv Ther* (1998) 15(1):45-53.

Miksicek, R. J. "Commonly occurring plant flavonoids have estrogenic activity." *Molecular Pharmacology* (1993) 44:37-43.

Peteres-Welter, C., Albrecht, M. "Menstrual abnormalities and PMS: *Vitex agnus-castus* in a study of application." *Therapiewoche Gynäkol* (1994) 7:49-52.

Propping, D., Katzorke, T., Belkien, L. "Diagnosis and therapy of corpus luteum deficiency in general practice." *Therapiewoche Gynäkol* (1988) 38:2992-3001.

Ruiz-Larrerea, M. B., Mohan, A. R., Paganga, G., et al. "Antioxidant activity of phytoestrogenic isoflavones." *Free Radic Res* (1997) 26(1):63-70.

Chapter 22. Saw Palmetto

Belaiche, P., Leivoux, O. "Clinical studies on the palliative treatment of prostatic adenoma with extract of Urtica root." *Phytother Res* (1991) 5:267-9.

Bensadoun, H. "Medical treatment of benign hypertrophy of the prostate." *Presse Med* (1995) 24(32):1485-9.

Berges, R. R., Windeler, J., Trampisch, H. J., et al. "Randomized, placebo-controlled, double-blind clinical trial of beta-sitosterol in patients with benign prostatic hyperplasia: Beta-sitosterol Study Group." *Lancet* (1995) 345:1529-32.

Berry, S. J., Coffey, D. S., Walsh, P. C., et al. "The development of human benign prostatic hyperplasia with age." *J Urol* (1984) 132:474-9.

Boccafoschi, C., Annoscia, S. "Comparison of Serenoa repens extract with placebo by controlled clinical trial in patients with prostatic adenomatosis." *Urologia* (1983) 50:1257-68.

Braeckman, J. "The extract of *Serenoa repens* in the treatment of benign prostatic hyperplasia: a multicenter open study." *Curr Ther Res* (1994) 55:776-85.

Briley, M., Carilla, E., Roger, A. "Inhibitory effect of Permixon on testosterone 5-alpha reductase activity of the rat ventral prostate." *Br J Pharmacol* (1984)83:401-10.

Byrnes, C. A., Morton, A. S., Liss, C. L., et al. "Efficacy, tolerability, and effect on health-related quality of life of finasteride versus placebo in men with symptomatic benign prostatic hyperplasia: a community based study. CUSP investigators. Community-based study of proscar." *Clin Ther* (1995) 17(5):956-69.

Carbin, B. E., Larsson, B., Linahl, O. "Treatment of benign prostatic hyperplasia with phytosterols." *Br J Urol* (1990) 66(6):639-41.

Carilla, E., Briley, M., Fauran, F., et al. "Binding of Permixon, a new treatment for prostatic benign hyperplasia, to the cytosolic androgen receptor in the rat prostate." *J Steroid Biochem* (1984) 20(1):521-3.

Carraro, J. C., Raynaud, J. P., Koch, G., et al. "Comparison of phytotherapy (Permixon) with finasteride in the treatment of benign prostate hyperplasia: a randomized international study of 1,098 patients." *Prostate* (1996) 29(4): 231-40; discussion 241-2.

Casarosa, C., Cosci di Coscio, M., Fratta, M. "Lack of effects of a lyposterolic extract of *Serenoa repens* on plasma levels of testosterone, follicle-stimulating hormone, and luteinizing hormone." *Clin Ther* (1988) 10(5):585-8.

Champhault, G., Patel, J. C., Bonnard, A. M. "A Double-blind trial of an extract of the plant *Serenoa repens* in benign prostatic hyperplasia." *Br J Clin Pharm* (1984) 18:461-2.

Cirillo-Marucco, E., Pagliarulo, A., Tritto, G., et al. "Extract of Serenoa repens (PermixonR) in the early treatment of prostatic hypertrophy." *Urologia* (1983) 5:1269-77.

Emili, E., Lo Cigno, M., and Petrone, U. "Clinical trial of a new drug for treating hypertrophy of the prostate (Permixon)." *Urologia* (1983) 50:1042-8.

Eri, L., Tveter, K. "Alpha-blockade in the treatment of symptomatic benign prostatic hyperplasia." *J Urol* (1995) 154:923-34.

Gerber, G. S., Zagaja, G. P., Bales, G. T., et al. "Saw palmetto (Serenoa repens) in men with lower urinary tract symptoms: effects on urodynamic parameters and voiding symptoms." *Urology* (1998) 51(6):1003-7.

Habib, F. K., Ross, M., Lewenstein, A., et al. "Identification of a prostate inhibitory substance in a pollen extract." *Prostate* (1995) 26(3):133-9.

Hyrb, D. J., Khan, M. S., Romas, N. A., et al. "The effect of extracts of the roots of the stinging nettle (Urtica Dioica) on the interaction of SHBG with its receptor on human prostatic membranes." *Planta Med* (1995) 61(1):31-2.

Koch, E., Biber, A. "Pharmacological effects of *Sabal* and *Urtica* extracts as basis for a rational medication of benign prostatic hyperplasia." *Urologe* (1994) 34:90-5.

Kondas, J., Philipp, V., Dioszeghy, G. "Sabal serrulata extract (Strogen forte) in the treatment of symptomatic benign prostatic hyperplasia." *Int Urol Nephrol* (1996) 28(6):767-72.

Krzeski, T., Kazon, M., Borkowski, A., et al. "Combined extracts of Urtica dioica and Pygeum africanum in the treatment of benign prostatic hyperplasia: double-blind comparison of two doses." *Clin Ther* (1993) 15(6):1011-20.

Kupeli, B., Soygur, T., Aydos, K., et al. "The role of cigarette smoking in prostatic enlargement." *British J Urol* (1997) 80:201-4.

Lowe, F. C., Ku, J. C. "Phytotherapy in treatment of benign prostatic hyperplasia: a critical review." *Urology* (1996) 48(1):12-20.

Lucchetta, G., Weill, A., Becker, N., et al. "Reactivation of the secretion from the prostatic gland in cases of reduced fertility: biological study of seminal fluid modifications." *Urol Int* (1984) 39(4):222-4.

Mattei, F. M., Capone, M., Acconcia, A. "*Serenoa repens* extract in the medical treatment of benign prostatic hypertrophy." *Urologia* (1988) 55:547.

Plosker, G., Brogden, R. "Serenoa repens (Permixon): a review of its pharmacology and therapeutic efficacy in benign prostatic hyperplasia." *Drugs and Aging* (1996) 9(5):379-95.

Reece Smith, H., Memon, A., Smart, C. J., et al. "The value of permixon in benign prostatic hypertrophy." *Br J Urol* (1986) 58(1):36-40.

Shimada, H., Tyler, V. E., McLaughlin, J. L. "Biologically active acylglycerides from the berries of saw-palmetto (Serenoa repens)." *J Nat Prod* (1997) 60(4):417-8.

Chapter 23. Nutrients of the Future

Alkylglyerols

Alexander, P., Connell, D. I., Brohult, A., et al. "Reduction of radiation induced shortening of lifespan by a diet augmented with alkoxyglycerol esters and essential fatty acids." *Gerontologia* (1959) 3:147.

Brohult, A., Brohult, J., Brohult, S. "Regression of tumor growth after administration of alkoxyglycerols." *Acta Obstet Gynecol Scand* (1978):57:79.

Brohult, A., Brohult, J., Brohult, S., et al. "Effects of alkoxyglycerols on the frequency of injuries following radiation therapy for carcinoma of the uterine cervix." *Obstet Gynecol Scand* (1977) 56:441.

________. "Reduced mortality in cancer patients after administration of alkoxyglycerols." *Acta Obstet Gynecol Scand* (1986) 65:779-85.

Burns, C. P., Spector, A. A. "Effects of lipids on cancer therapy." *Nutr Rev* (1990) 48:233-40.

Palmblad, J., Samuelsson, J., Brohult, J., "Interactions between alkylglycerols and human neutrophil granulocytes." *Scand J Lab Invest* (1990) 50:363-70.

Theoharides TC. Treatment approaches for painful bladder syndrome/interstitial cystitis. Drugs. 2007;67(2):215-35.

Modified Citrus Pectin

Linehan, W. M. "Inhibition of prostate cancer metastasis: a critical challenge ahead." *J Natl Cancer Inst* (1995) 87(5):331-2.

Naik, H., Pilat, M. J., Donat, T., et al. "Inhibition of in vitro tumor cell-endothelial adhesion by modified citrus pectin: a pH modified natural complex carbohydrate." (Meeting abstract) *Proc Annu Meet Am Assoc Cancer Res* (1995) 36:A377.

Pienta, K. J., Naik, H., Akhtar, A., et al. "Inhibition of spontaneous metastasis in a rat prostate cancer model by oral administration of modified citrus pectin." *J Natl Cancer Inst* (1995) 87(5):348-53.

Platt, D., Raz, A. "Modulation of the lung colonization of B15-F1 melanoma cells by citrus pectin." *J Natl Cancer Inst* (1992) 84(6):438-42.

CALCIUM D-GLUCARATE

Abou-Issa, H., Moeschberger, M., el-Masry, W., et al. "Relative efficacy of glucarate on the initiation and promotion phases of rat mammary carcinogenesis." *Anticancer Res* (1995) 15(3):805-10.

Dwivedi, C., Oredipe, O. A., Barth, R. F., et al. "Effects of the experimental chemopreventative agent, glucarate, on intestinal carcinogenesis in rats." *Carcinogenesis* (1989) 10(8):1539-41.

Lin, S., Young, C. W., Tong, W. P. "High performance liquid chromatographic analysis of D-glucarate in support of the Phase I chemopreventive trial of calcium glucarate." (meeting abstract) *Proc Annu Meet Am Assoc Cancer Res* (1993) 34:A1749.

Walaszek, Z., Hanausek, M., Adams, A. K., et al. "Antiproliferative effects of calcium d-glucarate (CG) and d-glucaro-1, 4-lactone (GL) on the rat mammary gland and colon and mouse skin." (meeting abstract) *Proc Annu Meet Am Assoc Cancer Res* (1990) 31:A735.

________. "Effect of Calcium D-glucarate on development of the rat mammary gland and its sensitivity to chemical carcinogenesis." (meeting abstract) *Proc Annu Meet Am Assoc Cancer Res* (1992) 33:A981.

Walaszek, Z., Szemraj, J., Adams, A. K., et al. "Reduced levels of D-glucaric acid in mammary tumor-bearing hosts and the effect of its supplementation during estrogen replacement and tamoxifen therapy." (meeting abstract) *Proc Annu Meet Am Assoc Cancer Res* (1996) 37:A1254.

Pycnogenol

Bagchi, D., Garg, A., Krohn, R. L., et al. "Oxygen free radical scavenging abilities of vitamins C and E, and a grape seed proanthocyanidin extract in vitro." *Res Commun Mol Pathol Pharmacol* (1997) 95(2):179-89.

Maffei Facino, R., Carini, M., Aldini, G., et al. "Sparing effect of procyanidins from Vitis vinifera on vitamin E: in vitro studies." *Planta Med* (1998) 64(4):343-7.

Rong, Y., Li, L., Shah, V., et al. "Pycnogenol protects vascular endothelial cells from t-butyl hydroperoxide induced oxidant injury." *Biotechnol Ther* (1994-5) 5(3-4):117-26.

Whitehead, T. P., Robinson, D., Allaway, S., et al. "Effect of red wine ingestion on the antioxidant capacity of serum." *Clin Chem* (1995) 41(1):32-5.

Resveratrol

Bertelli, A. A., Giovannini, L., Giannessi, D., et al. "Antiplatelet activity of synthetic and natural resveratrol in red wine." *Int J Tissue React* (1995) 17(1):1-3.

Chen, C. K., Pace-Asciak, C. R. "Vasorelaxing activity of resveratrol and quercetin in isolated rat aorta." *Gen Pharmacol* (1996) 27(2):363-6.

Constant, J. "Alcohol, ischemic heart disease, and the French paradox." *Coron Artery Dis* (1997) 8(10):645-9.

Gehm, B. D., McAndrews, J. M., et al. "Resveratrol, a polyphenolic compound found in grapes and wine, is an agonist for the estrogen receptor." *Proc Natl Acad Sci USA* (1997) 94(25):14138-43.

Jang, M., Cai, L., Udeani, G. O., et al. "Cancer chemopreventive activity of resveratrol, a natural product derived from grapes." *Science* (1997) 275(5297):218-20.Jang, M. S., Lee, S. K., You, M., et al. "Resveratrol, a novel dietary cancer chemoprotective agent." (meeting abstract) *Proc Annu Meet Am Assoc Cancer Res* (1996) 37:1897.

Kawada, N., Seki, S., Inoue, M., et al. "Effect of antioxidants, resveratrol, quercetin, and N-acetylcysteine, on the functions of cultured rat hepatic stellate cells and Kupffer cells." *Hepatology* (1998) 27(5):1265-74.

Mgbonyebi, O. P., Russo, J., Russo, I. H. "Antiproliferative effect of synthetic resveratrol on human breast epithelial cells." *Int J Oncol* (1998) 12(4):865-9.

Pace-Asciak, C. R., Hahn, S., Diamandis, E. P., et al. "The red wine phenolics trans-resveratrol and quercetin block human platelet aggregation and eicosanoid synthesis: implications for protection against coronary heart disease." *Clin Chim Acta* (1995) 235(2):207-19.

Green Tea

Blot, W. J., Li, J. Y., Taylor, P. R. "Nutrition intervention trials in Linxian, China: supplementation with specific vitamin/mineral combination, cancer incidence and disease specific mortality in the general population." *J Natl Cancer Inst* (1993) 85:1483-93.

Carlin, B. I., Pretlow, T. G., Pretlow, T. P., et al. "Green tea polyphenols inhibit growth of prostate cancer xenograft CWR 22: implications for prostate cancer chemoprevention." (meeting abstract) *Proc Annu Meet Am Assoc Cancer Res* (1996) 37:A1915.

Hibasami, H., Komiya, T., Achiwa, Y., et al. "Induction of apoptosis in human stomach cancer cells by green tea catechins." *Oncol Rep* (1998) 5(2):527-9.

Imai, K., Nakachi, K. "Cross sectional study of effects of drinking green tea on cardiovascular and liver diseases." *BMJ* (1995) 310(6981):693-6.

Imai, K., Suga, K., Nakachi, K. "Cancer-preventive effects of drinking green tea among a Japanese population." *Prev Med* (1997) 26(6):769-75.

Ji, B. T., Chow, W. H., Hsing, A. W., et al. "Green tea consumption and the risk of pancreatic and colorectal cancers." *Int J Cancer* (1997) 70(3):255-8.

Mukhtar, H., Katiyar, S. K., Agarwal, R. "Green tea and skin-anticarcinogenic effects." *J Invest Dermatol* (1994) 102(1):3-7.

Ruch, R. J., Cheng, S. J., Klaunig, J. E. "Prevention of cytotoxicity and inhibition of intercellular communication by antioxidant catechins isolated from Chinese green tea." *Carcinogenesis* (1989) 10(6):1003-8.

Licorice

Baschetti, R. "Chronic fatigue syndrome and liquorice." (letter) *NZ Med J* (1995) 108(998):156-7.

Demitrack, M. A., Dale, J. K., Straus, S. E., et al. "Evidence for impaired activation of the hypothalamic-pituitary-adrenal axis in patients with chronic fatigue syndrome." *J Clin Endocrinol Metab* (1991) 73:1224-34.

Fuhrman, B., Buch, S., Vaya, J., et al. "Licorice extract and its major polyphenol glabridin protect low-density lipoprotein against lipid peroxidation: in vitro and ex vivo studies in humans and in atherosclerotic apolipoprotein E-deficient mice." *Am J Clin Nutr* (1997) 66(2):267-75.

Suzuki, F., Kobayashi, M., Pollard, R. B. "Inhibitory effect of glycyrrhizin (GR), an active component of licorice roots, on an experimental pulmonary metastasis in mice inoculated with B16 melanoma." (meeting abstract) *Proc Annu Meet Am Assoc Cancer Res* (1997) 38:A802.

Suzuki, F., Schmitt, D. A., Utsunomiya, T., et al. "Stimulation of host resistance against tumors by glycyrrhizin, an active component of licorice roots." *In vivo* (1992) 6(6):589-96.

Utsunomiya, T., Kobayashi, M., Pollard, R.B., et al. "Glycyrrhizin, an active component of licorice roots, reduces morbidity and mortality of mice infected with lethal doses of influenza virus." *Antimicrob Agents Chemother* (1997) 41(3):551-6.

Van Marle, J., Aarsen, P. N., Lind, A., et al. "Deglycyrrhizinised liquorice (DGL) and the renewal of rat stomach epithelium." *Eur J Pharmacol* (1981) 72(2-3):219-25.

Vaya, J., Belinky, P. A. Aviram, M. "Antioxidant constituents from licorice roots: isolation structure elucidation and antioxidative capacity toward LDL oxidation." *Free Radic Biol Med* (1997) 23(2):302-13.

Aloe Vera

Chithra, P., Sajithlal, G. B., Chandrakasan, G. "Influence of Aloe vera on the glycosaminoglycans in the matrix of healing dermal wounds in rats." *J Ethnopharmacol* (1998) 59(3):179-86.

________. "Influence of Aloe vera on the healing of dermal wounds in diabetic rats." *J Ethnopharmacol* (1998) 59(3):195-201.

Lipoic Acid

Barbiroli, B., Medori, R., Tritschler, H. J., et al. "Lipoic (thioctic) acid increases brain energy availability and skeletal muscle performance as shown by *in vivo* 31P-MRS in a patient with mitochondrial cytopathy." *J Neurol* (1995) 242(7):472-7.

Estrada, D. E., Ewart, H. S., Tsakiridis, T., et al. "Stimulation of glucose uptake by the natural coenzyme alpha-lipoic acid/thioctic acid: participation of elements of the insulin signaling pathway." *Diabetes* (1996) 45:1798-1804.

Jacob, S., Henriksen, E. J., Tritschler, H. J., et al. "Improvement of insulin-stimulated glucose-disposal in type 2 diabetes after repeated parenteral administration of thioctic acid." *Exp Clin Endocrinol Diabetes* (1996) 104:284-8.

Nagamatsu, M., Nickander, K. K., Schmelzer, J. D. "Lipoic acid improves nerve blood flow, reduces oxidative stress, and improves distal nerve conduction in experimental diabetic neuropathy." *Diabetic Care* (1995) 18:1160-6.

Streeper, R. S., Henriksen, E. J., Jacob, S., et al. "Differential effects of lipoic acid stereoisomers on glucose metabolism in insulin-resistant skeletal muscle." Am J Physiol (1997) 273 (1 pt 1):E185-91.

Strodter, D., Lehmann, E., Lehmann, U., et al. "The influence of thioctic acid on metabolism and function of the diabetic heart." *Diabetes Res Clin Pract* (1995) 29:19-26.

Ziegler, D., Hanefield, M., Ruhnau, K. J., et al. "Treatment of symptomatic diabetic peripheral neuropathy with the anti-oxidant alpha-lipoic acid:

a 3-week multicenter randomized controlled trial. (ALADIN Study)." *Diabetologia* (1995) 38:1425-33.

CONJUGATED LINOLEIC ACID

Belury, M. A. "Conjugated dienoic linoleate: a polyunsaturated fatty acid with unique chemoprotective properties." *Nutr Rev* (1995) 53(4 pt 1):83-9.

Ip, C., Chin, S. F., Scimeca, J. A., et al. "Mammary cancer prevention by conjugated dienoic derivative of linoleic acid." *Cancer Res* (1991) 51(22):6118-24.

Ip, C., Scimeca, J. A., Thompson, H. J. "Conjugated linoleic acid: a powerful anticarcinogen from animal fat sources." *Cancer* (1994) 74(suppl 3):1050-4.

Kohlmeier, L., Simonsen, N., Mottus, K. "Dietary modifiers of carcinogenesis." *Environ Health Perspect* (1995) 103 (suppl 8):177-84.

Liu, K. L., Belury, M. A. "Conjugated linoleic acid reduces arachidonic acid content and PGE2 synthesis in murine keratinocytes." *Cancer Lett* (1998) 127(1-2):15-22.

Nicolosi, R. J., Rogers, E. J., Kritchevsky, D., et al. "Dietary conjugated linoleic acid reduces plasma lipoproteins and early aortic atherosclerosis in hypercholesterolemic hamsters." *Artery* (1997) 22(5):266-77.

Park, Y., Albright, K. J., Liu, W., et al. "Effect of conjugated linoleic acid on body composition in mice." *Lipids* (1997) 32(87):853-8.

Parodi, P. W. "Cows' milk fat components as potential anticarcinogenic agents." *J Nutr* (1997) 127(6):1055-60.

HYDROXYCITRIC ACID (HCA)

Sullivan, A. C., Dairman, W., Triscari, J. "(—)-Threo-Chlorocitric acid: a novel anorectic agent." *Pharmacol Biochem Behav* (1981) 15(2):303-10.

PYRUVATE

Ivy, J. L., Cortez, M. Y., Chandler, R. M., et al. "Effects of pyruvate on the metabolism and insulin resistance of obese Zucker rats." *Am J Clin Nutr* (1994) 59(2):331-7.

Kashiwagi, A., Nishio, Y., Asahina, T., et al. "Pyruvate improves deleterious effects of high glucose on activation of pentose phosphate pathway and glutathione redox cycle in endothelial cells." *Diabetes* (1997) 46(12):2088-95.

Seymour, A. M., Chatham, J. C. "The effects of hypertrophy and diabetes on cardiac pyruvate dehydrogenase activity." *J Mol Cell Cardiol* (1997) 29(10):2771-8.

Stanko, R. T., Mullick, P., Clarke, M. R., et al. "Pyruvate inhibits growth of mammary adenocarcinoma 13762 in rats." *Cancer Res* (1994) 54(4):1004-7.

Stanko, R. T., Robertson, R. J., Galbreath, R. W., et al. "Enhanced leg exercise endurance with a high-carbohydrate diet and dihydroxyacetone and pyruvate." *J Appl Physiol* (1990) 69(5):1651-6.

Stanko, R. T., Tietze, D. L., Arch, J. E. "Body composition, energy utilization, and nitrogen metabolism with a 4.25-MJ/d low-energy diet supplemented with pyruvate." *Am J Clin Nutr* (1992) 56(4):630-5.

ARGININE

Adams, M. R., McCredie, R., Jessup, W., et al. "Oral L-arginine improves endothelium-dependent dilatation and reduces monocyte adhesion to endothelial cells in young men with coronary artery disease." *Atherosclerosis* (1997) 129(2):261-9.

Ceremuzynski, L., Chamlec, T., Herbaczynska-Cedro, K. "Effect of supplemental oral L-arginineon exercise capacity in patients with stable angina pectoris." *Am J Cardiol* (1997) 80(3):331-3.

Giugliano, D., Marfella, R., Coppola, L., et al. "Vascular effects of acute hyperglycemia in humans are reversed by L-arginine: evidence for reduced availability of nitric oxide during hyperglycemia." *Circulation* (1997) 95(7):1783-90.

Heys, S. D., Segar, A., Payne, S., et al. "Dietary supplementation with L-arginine: modulation of tumour-infiltrating lymphocytes in patients with colorectal cancer." *Br J Surg* (1997) 84(2):238-41.

Kubota, T., Imaizumi, T., Oyama, J., et al. "L-arginine increases exercise-induced vasodilation of the forearm in patients with heart failure." *Jpn Circ J* (1997) 61(6):471-80.

Moody, J. A., Vernet, D., Laidlaw, S., et al. "Effects of long-term oral administration of L-arginine on the rat erectile response." *J Urol* (1997) 158(3 pt 1):942-7.

Smith, S. D., Wheeler, M. A., Foster, H. E., Jr., et al. "Improvement in interstitial cystitis symptom scores during treatment with oral L-arginine." *J Urol* (1997) 158 (3 pt 1):703-8.

Wascher, T. C., Graier, W. F., Dittrich, P., et al. "Effects of low-dose L-arginine on insulin-mediated vasodilatation and insulin sensitivity." *Eur J Clin Invest* (1997) 27(80):690-5.

SAMe

Bressa, G. M. "s-adenosyl-L-methionine (SAMe) as antidepressant: meta-analysis of clinical studies." *Acta Neurol Scand Suppl* (1994) 154:7-14.

Buchwald, D., Garrity, D. "Comparison of patients with chronic fatigue syndrome, fibromyalgia, and multiple chemical sensitivities." *Arch Intern Med* (1994) 154:2049-53.

Caruso, I., Fumagalli, M., Boccassini, L., et al. "Antidepressant activity of s-adenosyl-L-methionine." (letter) *Lancet* (1984) 1 (8382):904.

Di Benedetto, P., Iona, L. G., Zidarich, V. "Clinical evaluation of s-adenosyl-L-methionine versus transcutaneous electrical nerve stimulation in primary fibromyalgia." *Curr Ther Res* (1993) 53(2):222-9.

Grassetto, M., Varotto, A. "Primary fibromyalgia is responsive to s-adenosyl-L-methionine." *Curr Ther Res* (1994) 55(7) 797-806.

Jacobsen, S., Danneskiold-Samsøe, B., Andersen, R. B. "Oral s-adenosyl-L-methionine in primary fibromyalgia: double-blind clinical evaluation." *Scand J Rheumatol* (1991) 20(4):294-302.

Salmaggi, P., et al. "Double-blind, placebo-controlled study of s-adenosyl-L-methionine in depressed postmenopausal women." *Psychother Psychosom* (1993) 59(1):34-40.

Index

B

D

E

H

I

J

K

L

M

N

O

P

Q

R

S

T

U

V

W

Y

Z

Dr. Richard N. Firshein

Richard N. Firshein D.O., is board certified in Family Medicine, and a UCLA trained and certified medical acupuncturist. He is the author of three groundbreaking books: *Reversing Asthma*, which details his comprehensive program for the treatment and prevention of asthma; *The Nutraceutical Revolution: 20 cutting edge nutrients to design your own whole-life program*; and Dr. Firshein's "*7 Steps towards an Asthma Free Child*". His books have been translated into numerous languages such as Italian, Spanish,Mandarin and Japanese.

Dr. Firshein is considered a leading authority and pioneer in the field of Integrative Medicine and is the medical director of The Firshein Center for Comprehensive Medicine, in New York City. Dr. Firshein treats a wide range of conditions including asthma and allergies, cardiovascular disease, arthritis, diabetes, osteoporosis, hormone imbalances, thyroid conditions, and chronic pain. His comprehensive programs combine nutraceutical supplementation, personal diets, acupuncture, and traditional medicine.

He has served as an Assistant Professor of Family Medicine at the New York College of Osteopathic Medicine, and is a well known lecturer and writer. He is the author of over 50 articles on natural approaches to health, was a contributing editor for Psychology Today and was a contributor for several magazines including Complete Wellness and Natural Health. He was host of the radio show *House Calls* in New York City for over 10 years. His work has been featured in numerous news shows and popular magazines such as the CBS news, NBC, and FOX, as well as Good Housekeeping, Self, and Vogue. He is also the founder of DrCity.com, and Healeos.com, dynamic health 2.0 information and medical resource websites. He currently holds a patent for his research into the benefits of alkylglycerols and cancer therapy.

For information about specific nutraceutical /vitamins or supplements that Dr Firshein recommends, or for more information about Dr Richard Firshein or the Firshein Center go to www.DrFirshein.com, or www.Firsheincenter.com. For more information about this book, go to www.vitaminprescriptionforlife.com

LaVergne, TN USA
11 January 2011
211960LV00004B/26/P